BASIC GUIDE TO DENTAL PROCEDURES

Second Edition

Carole Hollins

General Dental Practitioner
Member of the British Dental Association
Former Chairman and presiding examiner for the National Examining Board
for Dental Nurses

WILEY Blackwell

Library of Congress Cataloging-in-Publication Data

Hollins, Carole, author.
  Basic guide to dental procedures / Carole Hollins. – Second edition.
    p. ; cm.
  Includes index.
  ISBN 978-1-118-92455-6 (cloth)
  I. Title.
  [DNLM: 1. Dentistry–methods–Handbooks. 2. Dental Assistants–Handbooks. WU 49]
  RK56
  617.6–dc23
                                                                2015007740

A catalogue record for this book is available from the British Library.

Wiley also publishes its books in a variety of electronic formats. Some content that appears in print may not be available in electronic books.

Typeset in 9/11pt SabonLTStd by SPi Global, Chennai, India
Printed and bound in Malaysia by Vivar Printing Sdn Bhd

1 2015

Contents

How to use this book

As the title suggests, the book has been written as an introductory guide to the more usual dental procedures carried out in a modern dental practice. It does not attempt to explain the full theoretical and clinical technique behind these procedures, rather it aims to give a sufficient overview of them, with the use of 'before and after' colour photographs to hopefully make the book useful for helping to explain certain dental procedures to patients. In this second edition, each chapter has been updated as necessary in line with the latest dental techniques and materials available to the profession.

However, the main readership is envisaged to be dental care professionals, especially those unqualified or inexperienced dental nurses who may not have access to viewing many of the procedures described, as many practices continue to specialise in providing dental care only in certain areas of dentistry. It should be used, then, in conjunction with the excellent textbooks already available for dental nurse training, where more detail of instruments used and other underpinning knowledge is provided. By popular request, photographic examples of the instruments and materials, which may be required for various procedures, have been included in this edition, and while the images used provide guidance for those undertaking OSCE-style training and assessment, they are not intended to be exhaustive in their content.

The text in each section is laid out to explain the reasons behind the treatment described, the relevant dental background, the basics of how each procedure is carried out and any aftercare information necessary. It is beyond the remit of the book to cover every current technique in every dental discipline discussed, so it is hoped that the text provides at least the basic information required for the reader to gain an understanding of the procedure, before seeking a greater depth of knowledge elsewhere.

The inclusion of information on extended duties for dental nurses in this edition is of particular relevance to the United Kingdom-based readership. Examples have been given throughout the chapter of the type and extent of 'in-house' training that may be provided in a broad selection of these duties, as well as examples of suggested recording sheets that may be used to provide evidence of monitoring and competency in various of the necessary skills discussed. It is hoped that the information provided will help UK dental practices to train and extend the useful skills of its workforce, in an effort to develop their dental team and widen their provision of dental services for the ultimate benefit of their patients.

Wherever possible the correct dental terminology has been adhered to, but as the dental knowledge of the expected readership will vary widely, a glossary of terms has been updated and included to clarify certain definitions in the context to which they have been referred to in the text.

Chapter 1

Preventive techniques

REASON FOR PROCEDURE

Preventive techniques are aimed at preventing the onset of dental caries in teeth, to maintain the dental health of a patient.

The two procedures discussed are:

- Application of fissure sealants
- Application of topical fluorides – full mouth or specific teeth

BACKGROUND INFORMATION OF PROCEDURE – FISSURE SEALANTS

Any surface area of a tooth that cannot be cleaned easily by the patient can allow food debris, and ultimately plaque, to accumulate there and allow caries to develop by acting as a stagnation area. Patients usually clean their teeth by tooth brushing, flossing, the use of other interdental cleaning aids, mouthwashing, or any combination of these techniques.

The usual sites that can act as stagnation areas are the occlusal pits and fissures of posterior teeth (Figure 1.1), and especially the first permanent molars which erupt at around 6 years of age.

These teeth are particularly prone to caries because:

- They are the least accesible teeth for cleaning, being at the back of the young patient's mouth
- They erupt at an age when a good oral hygiene regime is unlikely to have been developed, so may be cleaned poorly by the patient
- Younger patients often have a diet containing more sugars than an adult, as the concept of dietary control will not be appreciated

Basic Guide to Dental Procedures, Second Edition. Carole Hollins.
© 2015 John Wiley & Sons, Ltd. Published 2015 by John Wiley & Sons, Ltd.

PREVENTIVE TECHNIQUES

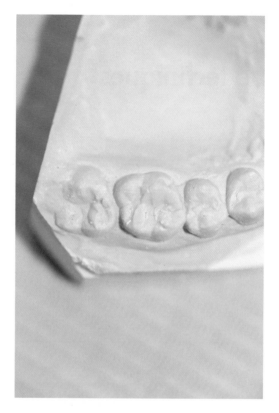

Figure 1.1 Molar tooth model showing occlusal fissure system

DETAILS OF PROCEDURE – FISSURE SEALANTS

The occlusal pit or fissure needs to be eliminated to prevent it acting as a stagnation area, and this is achieved by closing the inaccesible depth with a sealant material.

The materials used are either unfilled resins, composites, or glass ionomer cements, or a combination of these two materials (known as a compomer).

The usual instruments and materials that may be laid out for a fissure sealant procedure are shown in Figure 1.2.

TECHNIQUE:

- The tooth is kept isolated from saliva contamination, as materials will not adhere to the tooth when it is wet
- Isolation techniques include the use of cotton wool rolls and low speed suction techniques using a saliva ejector (Figure 1.3)

- The occlusal fissures and pits are chemically roughened with acid etch to allow the microscopic bonding of the sealant material to the enamel
- The etch is washed off and the tooth is dried; the etched surface will appear chalky white
- Unfilled resin is run into the etched areas to seal the fissures or pits, and then locked into the enamel structure by setting with a curing lamp
- If any demineralisation of the fissure is present, one of the alternative materials listed above is used to replace the enamel surface

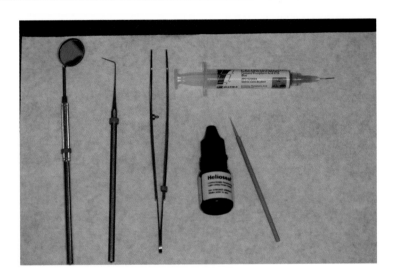

Figure 1.2 Fissure sealant instruments and materials

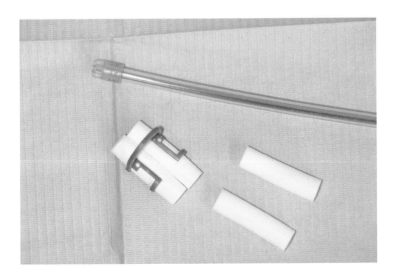

Figure 1.3 Tooth isolation techniques

BACKGROUND INFORMATION OF PROCEDURE – TOPICAL FLUORIDE

Other very difficult to clean areas of the teeth are the points where they have contact with each other in the dental arch – the interproximal (interdental) areas.

There are certain oral health products available specifically for cleaning these areas, such as dental floss and interdental brushes, but they require a certain amount of dexterity and determination by the patient to be used effectively.

All fluoridated toothpastes provide some protection of these areas from caries, but some patients require additional full mouth fluoride protection by the professional application of a topical fluoride varnish or gel.

They are:

- Children and vulnerable adults with high caries rates
- Physically disabled patients who are unable to achieve a good level of oral hygiene
- Medically compromised patients for whom tooth extractions are too dangerous to be carried out (haemophiliacs, patients with some heart defects)

DETAILS OF PROCEDURE – FULL MOUTH TOPICAL FLUORIDE APPLICATION

A high concentration of fluoride is required to be applied to the interproximal areas that is viscous enough not to be washed away quickly by saliva, so that it can be taken into the enamel structure of the tooth and make it more resistant to caries. The usual material used is a sticky fluoride varnish or gel, such as that shown in Figure 1.4.

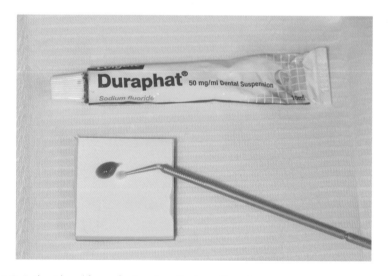

Figure 1.4 Fluoride gel for professional application – Duraphat

TECHNIQUE:

- The operator and the patient wear suitable personal protective equipment
- The teeth are polished with a pumice slurry to remove any plaque present and allow the maximum tooth contact with the fluoride
- The polish is thoroughly washed off and the teeth are dried
- Adequate soft tissue retraction and moisture control are provided by the dental nurse, so that the dry tooth surfaces are accessible and the gel will not be displaced by accident during the procedure
- The viscous fluoride gel is manually applied to all available surfaces of each tooth, using one or more applicator buds and one arch at a time

DETAILS OF PROCEDURE – SPECIFIC TOOTH TOPICAL FLUORIDE APPLICATION

In some patients, individual teeth may show signs of previous acid attack from certain foods and drinks as a 'brown spot' lesion on the enamel surface (Figure 1.5). Other patients may have gingival recession present, which exposes the root surface of a tooth to dietary acids and sugars, therefore making it vulnerable to attack by dental caries (see Figure 5.8). These specific areas can be protected by the direct application of a localised fluoride varnish such as that shown in Figure 1.4, using a similar technique to that of a full mouth application as described earlier.

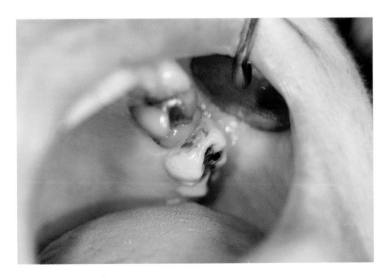

Figure 1.5 Brown spot lesion indicating previous enamel damage

Chapter 2

Oral hygiene instruction

Oral hygiene instruction is given to patients to ensure that they are maximising their efforts to remove plaque from their teeth, to minimise the damage caused by periodontal disease and caries.

Dietary advice is also given to help patients avoid foods and drinks that are particularly damaging to their teeth – those high in refined sugars or those that are acidic.

When the advice is correctly followed on a regular basis, the patients can enjoy a well cared for and pain-free mouth, as well as avoiding the expense of reparative dental treatment.

The procedures discussed are:

- Use of disclosing agents
- Toothbrushing
- Interdental cleaning

BACKGROUND INFORMATION OF PROCEDURE – DISCLOSING AGENTS

Disclosing agents are harmless vegetable dyes supplied in liquid or tablet form and in various colours, usually red or blue (Figure 2.1).

They act by staining any plaque on the tooth surface to their own colour (Figure 2.2), thus making it far easier to show the presence and location of the plaque to the patient, as plaque is normally a creamy white colour and may be difficult to see otherwise (Figure 2.3).

Once stained, suitable oral hygiene instruction can be given to remove the plaque effectively. The dyes do not stain the teeth themselves, nor any restorations.

Basic Guide to Dental Procedures, Second Edition. Carole Hollins.
© 2015 John Wiley & Sons, Ltd. Published 2015 by John Wiley & Sons, Ltd.

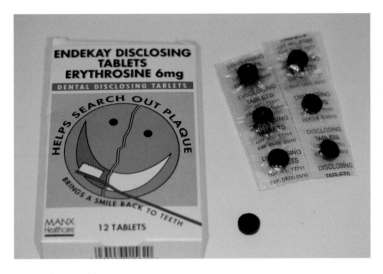

Figure 2.1 Disclosing tablets

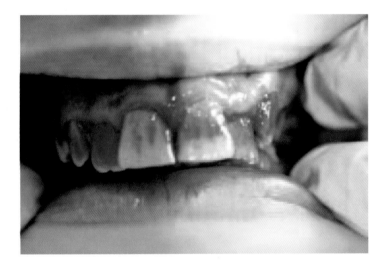

Figure 2.2 Disclosed teeth showing the presence of plaque

DETAILS OF PROCEDURE – DISCLOSING AGENTS

The agents can initially be used at the practice by the oral health team so that the correct problem areas can be identified and suitable cleaning advice given. The patient can then use the agents at home to check their progress on a regular basis. The commonest agents used are disclosing tablets.

ORAL HYGIENE INSTRUCTION

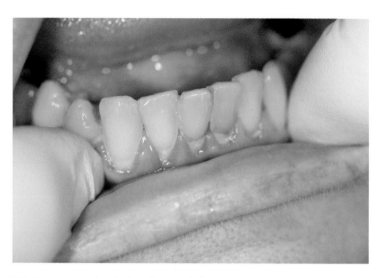

Figure 2.3 Appearance of undisclosed gingival plaque

TECHNIQUE:

- A protective bib is placed over the patients so that their clothing is not inadvertently marked
- The patients are given one disclosing tablet and asked to chew it for about 1 min
- After this time, they are asked to spit out the chewed tablet and saliva, but are instructed not to rinse their mouth out
- Using a patient-mirror, any stained plaque is pointed out by the oral health team and the worst areas noted (very often the gingival margins)
- Detailed advice is then given on how to improve their tooth brushing and cleaning techniques to eliminate the plaque from these areas
- The patients can follow these instructions immediately so that all the stained plaque is removed while under the supervision of the oral health team
- With the plaque easily visible due to the disclosing agent, the patients are able to see their own progress and develop the skill to maintain good oral hygiene

BACKGROUND INFORMATION OF PROCEDURE – TOOTHBRUSHING

Toothbrushing is the commonest method used by patients to remove plaque from the easily accessible flat surfaces of the teeth, but not from the interdental areas.

Many toothbrushing techniques have been suggested over the years – especially side to side brushing and rotary brushing – but the technique used is immaterial as long as the plaque is removed successfully without causing damage to the tooth surface. Disclosing agents can be used to determine the most successful method for a patient.

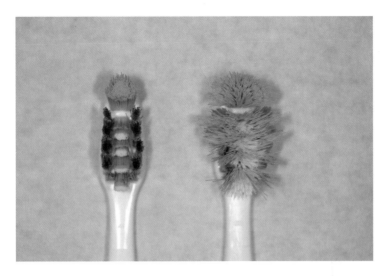

Figure 2.6 Comparison of new and worn toothbrush

BACKGROUND INFORMATION OF PROCEDURE – INTERDENTAL CLEANING

The surfaces of the teeth that remain untouched by toothbrushing are the contact points, or interdental areas (Figure 2.7). Plaque accumulates here just as easily as the flat surfaces of the teeth, and even more so when restorations extend into the interdental areas as microscopically they provide more potential for stagnation areas to occur.

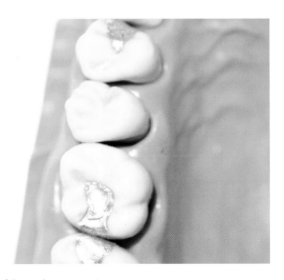

Figure 2.7 Contact points of the teeth

ORAL HYGIENE INSTRUCTION

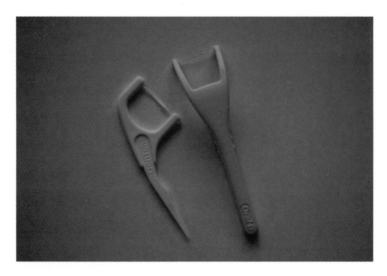

Figure 2.8 Interdental 'flossettes'

Although toothbrushes are too large to clean interdentally, other oral health products have been designed to do so:

- Tape or floss
- Manual interdental brushes
- Dental woodsticks
- Some specialised electric toothbrush heads
- Some mouthwashes

The first four are used to physically clean plaque from the interdental areas, while some mouthwashes can be vigorously rinsed and swished through the interdental areas by the patient to dislodge larger particles of debris.

A certain amount of manual dexterity is required by the patient to use dental tape or floss effectively, and a lack of dexterity is often the cause of patients abandoning the technique. Some products have been developed to help, whereby a fork design holds a small piece of tape or floss firmly while it is used with one hand to enter and clean the interdental areas (Figure 2.8). This removes the need by the patient for wrapping the tape around the fingers and holding it firmly while trying to access the interdental areas.

DETAILS OF PROCEDURE – FLOSSING

This is the technique used by the majority of patients who routinely clean interdentally, despite it being the most difficult to achieve.

Some tapes and flosses are waxed to assist easier entry into tight interdental areas, and others are impregnated with fluoride so that the interdental surfaces of the teeth are protected once accessed (Figure 2.9).

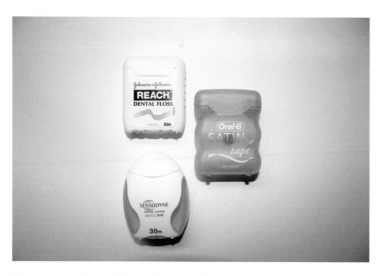

Figure 2.9 Examples of dental floss and tape products

TECHNIQUE:

- Ideally the patient should carry out flossing with the aid of a mirror, in a well-lit room
- A piece of tape or floss (approximately 20 cm) is removed from the holder and wrapped around both index fingers, leaving a central portion between the hands (Figure 2.10)
- This is held over both thumb pads and guided into each interdental area, one at a time
- Once in the area, the thumbs are used to adapt the tape to first the surface of one tooth then the other forming the contact point (Figure 2.11)
- While in contact with the tooth surface, the tape is drawn from side to side to wipe any plaque from each surface
- As the tape is dirtied, it is loaded off one finger and onto the other so that a clean portion is available for the next interdental area
- Tape is more gentle on the gingivae than floss if the patient is heavy-handed or if force is required to access some tight interdental areas, but some patients may find tape too thick to use effectively

DETAILS OF PROCEDURE – INTERDENTAL BRUSHING

This is an alternative and useful technique of cleaning the interdental areas for patients who have contact points wide enough to admit a specially designed interdental brush into the area. Several 'bottle-brush' style designs of interdental brush are available and a widely-used example is shown in Figure 2.12. These brushes are provided in a variety of colour-coded width sizes so that patients with spaced teeth can successfully use larger brushes to clean their interdental areas, while patients with tight contact points are also able to insert the smallest design of brush to clean their interdental areas (Figure 2.13).

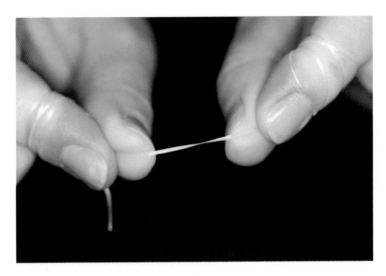

Figure 2.10 Correct positioning of floss around fingers

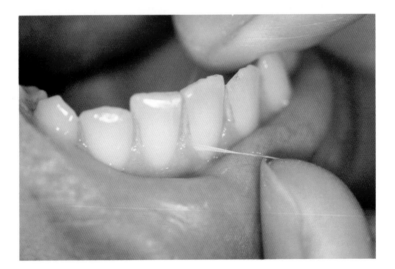

Figure 2.11 Flossing technique

TECHNIQUE:

- Ideally the patient should carry out interdental brushing with the aid of a mirror, in a well-lit room
- The patient should be advised by the oral health team on the correct size of interdental brush to use

- Some patients may require to use more than one size of brush for different areas of their mouth, while other patients may need to use only one size of interdental brush for cleaning one specific area of their mouth
- Depending on the area of the mouth to be cleaned, the brush head can be angled to make its insertion into the interdental area easier to achieve – this is particularly useful when cleaning between posterior teeth (Figure 2.14)
- The head is pushed into the interdental area, then used in a backwards and forwards motion to clean plaque from each side of the adjacent teeth and to dislodge any food debris present
- The brush can also be rotated while inserted in the interdental area to give better tooth contact and debris removal
- Any visible debris on the brush bristles must be removed by rinsing before the next contact point is accessed, otherwise plaque and food will be transferred from one area to another
- Dislodged food particles in the mouth can be spat into the sink or swallowed
- The interdental brush can be rinsed clean and re-used until it becomes ineffective at cleaning or the bristles become bent, and should then be replaced

Some good quality electric tooth brushes have specifically designed interdental cleaning attachments that can be used by the patient in a similar way to the manual ones, to ensure that plaque and food debris are removed from the contact points (Figure 2.15).

Again, the interdental area must be wide enough to allow their safe use, and the patient should follow the manufacturer's instructions or ideally be instructed by the oral health team on their correct use.

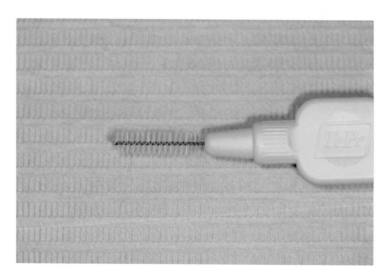

Figure 2.12 Interdental brush design

ORAL HYGIENE INSTRUCTION

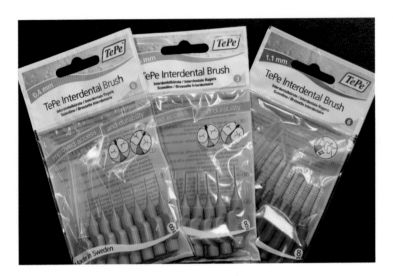

Figure 2.13 Size range of interdental brushes

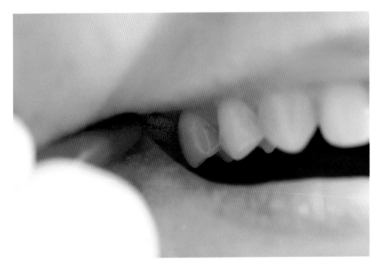

Figure 2.14 Use of interdental brush for posterior cleaning

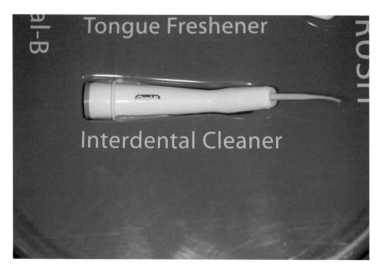

Figure 2.15 Electric brush attachment for interdental cleaning

Chapter 3

Scaling and polishing

REASON FOR PROCEDURE

Everyone's mouth contains a variety of bacteria, some of which react with saliva and the food that is eaten to produce a sticky film called plaque. Plaque forms wherever the food debris becomes lodged in the mouth, the usual areas being along the gum margin (see Figure 2.3) and in difficult to clean areas called stagnation areas.

Plaque lying along the gum margin will irritate the soft tissue and eventually cause inflammation of the gum, or gingivitis. Regular toothbrushing and interdental cleaning by the patient will remove the plaque and prevent this from happening.

However, if the plaque is not removed, it gradually hardens by absorbing minerals from the patient's saliva and becomes calculus (tartar). Calculus cannot be removed by toothbrushing alone, and the dentist, therapist or hygienist will need to remove it by scaling the teeth. When the plaque or calculus lies attached to the tooth surface above the gum line it is called 'supragingival' (Figure 3.1).

If the calculus is left untouched, it gradually forms further and further down the side of the tooth root as the gum tissue is destroyed, and eventually the supporting structures of the tooth (the jaw bone and periodontal ligaments) are also destroyed and the tooth becomes loose in its socket. This is called periodontal disease, or periodontitis, and the plaque and calculus are referred to as 'subgingival'.

The more advanced the damage to the periodontal tissues, the more difficult it is for the oral health team to treat, and the more likely that long term problems including tooth loss will occur.

The procedures discussed are:

- Simple scaling of supragingival debris
- Deep scaling and debridement of subgingival debris
- Polishing

Basic Guide to Dental Procedures, Second Edition. Carole Hollins.
© 2015 John Wiley & Sons, Ltd. Published 2015 by John Wiley & Sons, Ltd.

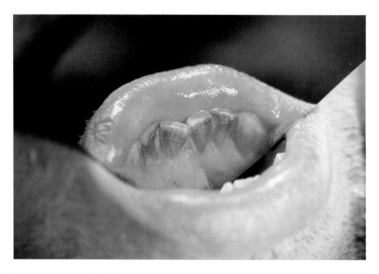

Figure 3.1 Supragingival calculus

BACKGROUND INFORMATION OF PROCEDURE – SCALING

The dentist, therapist or hygienist can scale a patient's teeth using hand instruments or electrical scalers, or a combination of both. The aim of the procedure is to remove all the calculus and plaque from around each tooth so that the supporting structures are no longer irritated and inflamed, and repair themselves.

If the calculus has extended down the side of the root and under the gum (subgingival), its removal is more difficult to achieve. Electric scalers vibrate ultrasonically and have a spray of water at their tip to help remove the calculus both from the tooth root and out from under the gum (Figure 3.2).

Some patients find the vibration and cold water uncomfortable and may choose to have a scaling procedure carried out under local anaesthetic.

DETAILS OF PROCEDURE – SIMPLE SCALING

The presence of supragingival plaque and calculus will have been noticed by the dentist during routine examination of the patient's mouth. The amount present and whether local anaesthesia is required will help to determine if a second appointment will be needed, or if the scaling can be completed during the examination appointment. The dentist, therapist or hygienist will act as the operator to carry out the procedure while assisted by the dental nurse.

Supragingival scaling removes plaque and calculus deposits from the enamel surface of the teeth down to the gingival margins of the teeth. The hand instruments used are shaped accordingly, to fit around the shape of the teeth (sickle and Jaquette scalers), or

SCALING AND POLISHING

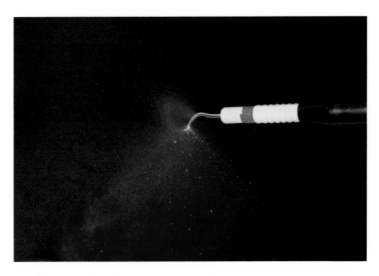

Figure 3.2 Ultrasonic scaler showing water spray effect

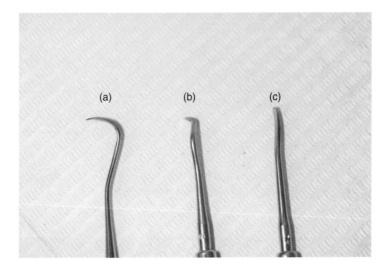

Figure 3.3 Supragingival scalers. (a) Sickle scaler. (b) Jaquette scaler. (c) Push scaler

are shaped like a fine chisel (push scaler) to be pushed between the anterior teeth to remove interdental calculus (Figure 3.3).

In addition, a high speed suction tip and tissues or gauze sheets to wipe the debris from the instruments are required.

The instruments and materials that may be required to carry out a simple scale and polish procedure are shown in Figure 3.4.

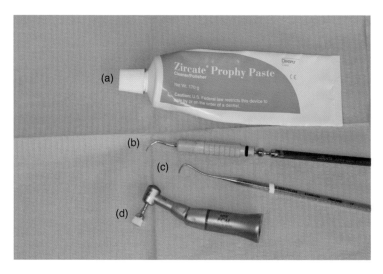

Figure 3.4 Instruments and materials for simple scale and polish procedure. (a) Prophylaxis paste. (b) Ultrasonic scaler. (c) Hand scalers. (d) Polishing brush with handpiece

TECHNIQUE:

- The oral health team and the patient wear personal protective equipment (Figure 3.5)
- Local anaesthetic is given if required
- Hand and/or electric scalers are made ready
- If an electric scaler is used, the dental nurse uses high speed suction to remove water and debris from the patient's mouth as the scaling is carried out
- The operator will systematically scale each tooth that has calculus present, using vision and tactile sensation to determine when it has been fully removed
- The scaler is worked from the bottom edge of the calculus upwards in a scraping motion, so that it is dislodged 'en masse'
- The instrument is then reapplied to remove any remaining specks of calculus until a smooth tooth surface is achieved (Figure 3.6)
- The process causes some amount of bleeding of the gums as they are in an inflamed state, but scaling does not cut into the gums themselves
- The gums will return to their healthy pink appearance within days of the calculus being removed

DETAILS OF PROCEDURE – DEEP SCALING AND DEBRIDEMENT

The presence of subgingival plaque and calculus is determined by the dentist while carrying out a basic periodontal examination of the teeth, and the presence and depth of any periodontal pockets recorded. Plaque retention factors such as overhanging fillings are also noted.

SCALING AND POLISHING

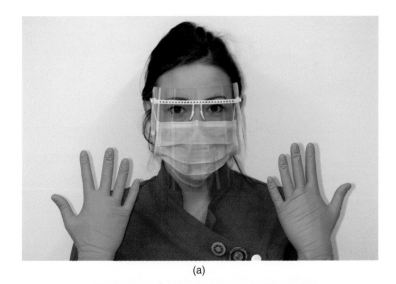

(a)

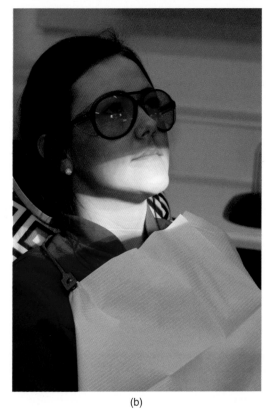

(b)

Figure 3.5 Personal protective equipment. (a) Oral health team members – gloves, mask and eye protection. (b) Patient – bib and safety glasses

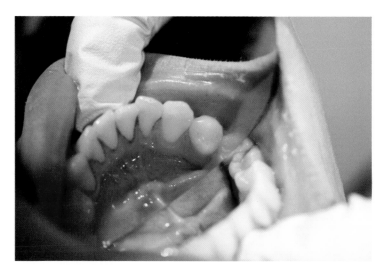

Figure 3.6 Appearance after completion of supragingival scaling

SCALING AND POLISHING

Deep scaling and debridement is usually carried out under local anaesthetic and in a few sections of the mouth at a time, and the number of areas to be treated determines the number of appointments required. Subgingival scaling removes plaque and calculus deposits from the root surfaces of teeth within the periodontal pockets. In addition, the instruments are also used to remove a layer of contaminated cementum from the root surfaces during debridement, and the debris created is then irrigated from the pockets and aspirated from the mouth.

The instruments used to achieve subgingival scaling and debridement have to be long enough to reach the base of each periodontal pocket, and be thin enough to do so without tearing the soft tissues, and are called curettes (Figure 3.7). The ultrasonic scaler unit has interchangeable heads so that it can be used for both supragingival and subgingival scaling and debridement procedures.

TECHNIQUE:

- The oral health team and the patient wear personal protective equipment
- Local anaesthetic is administered as required, the particular equipment and materials that may be required to do so are shown in Figure 3.8
- Currettes and the ultrasonic unit are made ready
- The dental nurse uses high speed suction to remove water and debris from the patient's mouth as the scaling and debridement are carried out
- The operator will systematically deep-scale each root in the anaesthetised mouth section that has calculus present, using vision and tactile sensation to determine when it has been fully removed
- The currette is worked from the bottom edge of the calculus upwards in a scraping motion, so that it is dislodged 'en masse'
- The instrument will then be reapplied to remove a layer of contaminated cementum from the root surface during debridement, the process being repeated until a smooth root surface is achieved
- Deep pockets may be irrigated with antiseptic mouthwash solutions by some operators, to assist in the destruction and removal of the periodontal bacteria

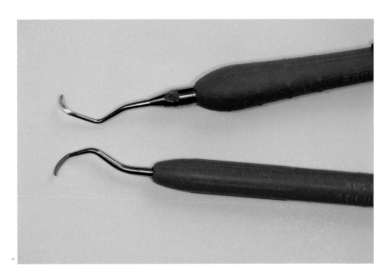

Figure 3.7 Currettes for subgingival scaling and debridement

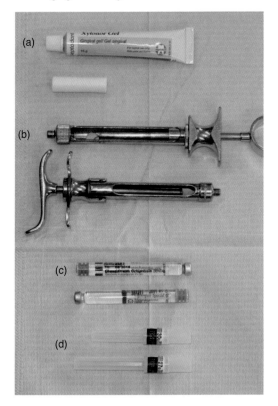

Figure 3.8 Local anaesthetic equipment. (a) Topical anaesthetic and cotton wool roll. (b) Syringe – aspirating or non-aspirating. (c) Cartridge – content specific to patient need. (d) Needle – long or short

BACKGROUND INFORMATION OF PROCEDURE – POLISHING

Whether calculus is present or not, everyones' teeth can stain from time to time by exposure to normal dietary substances such as tea, coffee, red wine and highly coloured foods. Smokers can also develop unsightly dark staining from tobacco tar products.

The process of professional polishing of the anterior teeth using special abrasive pastes can easily remove all but the most tenacious of these surface stains, giving the teeth a cleaner and brighter appearance.

Obviously, continued exposure to the staining agents will cause the discolouration to develop again with time, but it can usually be kept under control if the patient has a good and regular oral hygiene routine.

Polishing causes no surface damage to the teeth.

DETAILS OF PROCEDURE – POLISHING

Polishing is usually carried out at the end of a course of treatment, and especially once scaling has been completed. The use of bristle brushes or rubber cups in the dental handpiece (Figure 3.9) to apply the abrasive polishing paste gives a greater cleaning effect than if it were applied using a toothbrush.

The pastes are often flavoured for the benefit of the patient, and feel quite gritty in the mouth.

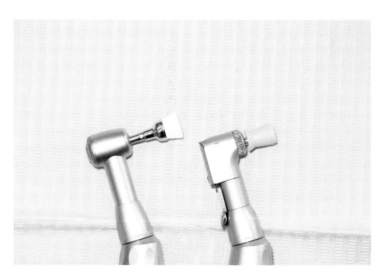

Figure 3.9 Polishing brush and cup in dental hand pieces

SCALING AND POLISHING

SCALING AND POLISHING

TECHNIQUE:

- If not already in place, the operator, nurse and patient wear personal protective equipment
- Either a bristle brush or rubber cup will be locked into the dental handpiece, and then dabbed into the polishing paste so that a small amount is picked up
- With the lips held out of the way, the rotating brush/cup will be moved across the front surface of each anterior tooth, from one contact point to the next until the stains are removed
- The patient may feel a not unpleasant tickling sensation in each tooth
- The brush will be worked over the whole tooth surface, and especially into the contact points of the teeth where stains usually accumulate
- Fresh paste is picked up on the brush for each tooth
- Once the procedure is complete, the patient can rinse the gritty paste out of the mouth

Chapter 4

Diagnostic techniques

REASON FOR PROCEDURE

When a patient attends a dental appointment for a dental examination, the dentist has to check the oral health and determine the presence and location of any caries, periodontal disease or oral soft tissue problems. While the visual skills of the dentist are of paramount importance in identifying problems of the oral tissues, it is often necessary for diagnostic techniques to be implemented so that a definitive diagnosis can be made.

The three techniques discussed are:

- Use of dental hand instruments
- Dental radiographs
- Study models

BACKGROUND INFORMATION OF PROCEDURE – INSTRUMENTS

A variety of dental hand instruments called probes have been designed to aid the dentist in detecting the presence of both caries and periodontal disease.

Those used to detect caries have sharp points that can be run over the tooth surface to find any softened areas of the enamel, which indicates that demineralisation has occurred and the area has undergone carious attack.

Those used to detect periodontal disease are blunt-ended and have graded depth markings on them, so that the gums are not pierced during use and any gum pockets discovered can be depth recorded.

DETAILS OF PROCEDURE – INSTRUMENTS

Frank carious cavities in teeth are easily visible to the dentist when they occur on uncovered and easily accesible surfaces of those teeth (Figure 4.1), but more difficult areas

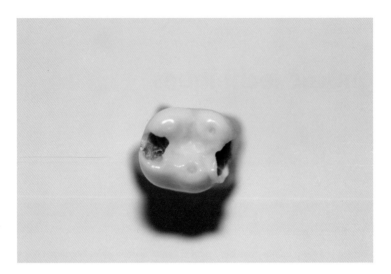

Figure 4.1 Cavity in tooth

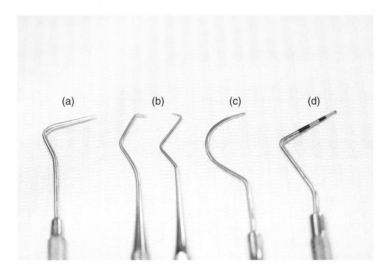

Figure 4.2 Diagnostic probes. (a) Right angle probe. (b) Briault probe. (c) Sickle probe. (d) Periodontal BPE probe

to examine require the use of dental probes. All have been designed so that their pointed ends are bent at various angles so that all surfaces of each tooth can be easily probed by the dentist (Figure 4.2).

TECHNIQUE:

- The patient is placed in the dental chair at a suitable angle for the dentist, with the dental inspection light providing good illumination when the mouth is open

- Visual examination is carried out first so that any suspicious tooth surfaces are detected
- Each suspect area is then revisited and the probe end is run over the tooth surface
- A hard, scratchy surface indicates sound enamel
- A soft, non-scratchy surface indicates the presence of dental caries
- The dentist will be able to determine the presence of either by tactile sensation through the probe to the hand
- The dental nurse will record the findings of the dental examination on a manual chart or its computer alternative, and either can be referred to at a later date to monitor the improvement or deterioration of the patient's dental condition and any treatment that has been provided by the oral health team to treat any caries found

Periodontal disease is often more difficult to detect by vision alone as the gums of some patients appear to be quite healthy and exhibit no bleeding when touched. The presence of periodontal pockets alongside the tooth roots indicates that some destruction of the supporting tissues of the tooth has occurred – and the deeper the pocket, the more severe the destruction.

The pockets are not visible to the naked eye, but can be easily detected using a periodontal probe (see Figure 4.2).

TECHNIQUE:

- The patient is placed in the dental chair at a suitable angle for the dentist, with the dental inspection light providing good illumination when the mouth is open
- Visual examination is carried out first, including the presence of any plaque or calculus and the identification of any tooth mobility
- Each suspect tooth/gum junction is then inspected for periodontal pocketing by 'walking' the blunt-ended probe around the gingival crevice
- A healthy gingival crevice is no deeper than 2 mm and does not bleed when probed
- Where a periodontal problem exists, the probe sinks easily below the tooth-gum junction and the area bleeds on probing
- The probe may sink for several millimetres and greater depths indicate more severe periodontal disease (Figure 4.3)
- Sometimes the probe may also detect specks of subgingival calculus on the tooth root
- The dental nurse records the findings of the periodontal examination on a manual chart or its computer alternative, and either can be referred to at a later date to monitor the improvement or deterioration of the patient's periodontal condition

BACKGROUND INFORMATION OF PROCEDURE – DENTAL RADIOGRAPHS

Radiographs provide the dentist with a method of seeing within the dental tissues themselves, without having to drill or cut into those tissues beforehand.

DIAGNOSTIC TECHNIQUES

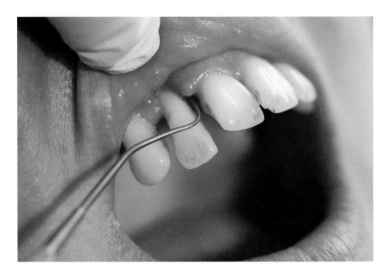

Figure 4.3 BPE probe inserted in periodontal pocket

They are an invaluable diagnostic technique for determining the presence or absence of dental disease, as well as such widely varied features as unerupted teeth, jaw or tooth fractures, extra teeth, foreign bodies and so on.

A wide variety of images can be produced depending on the type of radiographic view required, ranging from a single tooth to the whole oral cavity. Where a single tooth or just a few teeth are to be viewed, an intra-oral radiograph is taken, which can then either be chemically processed to produce an image or transmitted with specialist digital equipment to a computer screen for immediate viewing.

Examples of the types of radiograph discussed are shown in Figure 4.4 and are:

- Bitewings
- Periapicals
- Occlusals

When a more extensive area is to be radiographed, an extra-oral dental pantomograph (DPT) view is taken, using a cassette containing intensifying screens to reduce the X-ray exposure of the patient. The image produced will show all the teeth in both the upper and lower jaws, as well as the surrounding bony anatomy (Figure 4.5).

A specialist cephalometric view can also be taken in certain orthodontic cases, so that measurements can be made of the angulation of the teeth, jaws and skull to each other to determine the severity of the malocclusion, and the likelihood of the need for orthognathic surgery to correct the jaws. The view produced is referred to as a lateral skull image (Figure 4.6).

DETAILS OF PROCEDURE – DENTAL RADIOGRAPHS

When an intra-oral view is taken, it is important that there is no distortion of the film or the image produced, as can happen if the film is bent in the mouth or if the angulation of

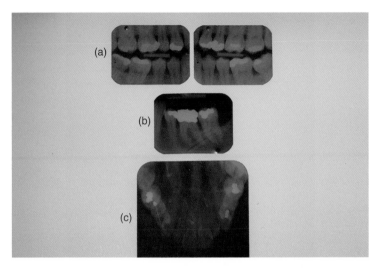

Figure 4.4 Examples of intra-oral radiographic views. (a) Bitewings. (b) Periapical. (c) Upper occlusal

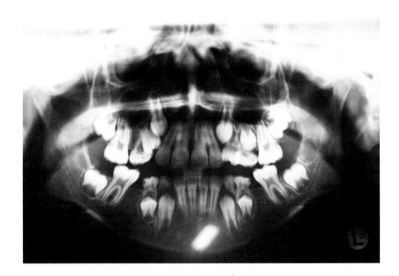

Figure 4.5 Dental pantomograph

the X-ray machine cone is incorrect. Therefore the film is placed into one of a variety of holders before being positioned in the patient's mouth, so that the film is held in parallel to the tooth being exposed and prevents distortion, as well as allowing the cone angulation to be set correctly.

If a digital radiograph is to be produced, the sensor unit is treated in the same manner.

DIAGNOSTIC TECHNIQUES

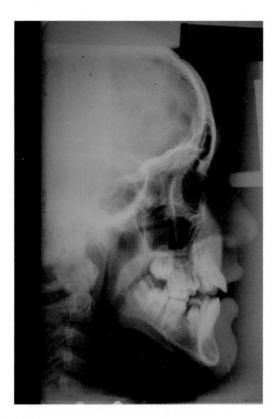

Figure 4.6 Lateral skull view

TECHNIQUE:

- The patient is seated comfortably in the dental chair, usually in an upright position or nearly so
- All removable prostheses are taken out of the mouth, as they superimpose their image over the teeth and make diagnosis difficult
- The X-ray machine exposure and time settings are chosen by the operator, depending on which tooth and view is being taken
- A suitable holder is chosen, depending on whether a bitewing, anterior or posterior periapical view is required (Figure 4.7)
- Occlusal views do not require the use of a holder, as the patient is able to bite onto the film packet itself and hold it correctly in place during exposure
- The intra-oral film is correctly inserted into the holder so that the front of the film faces the X-ray cone
- The holder and film are then gently but accurately positioned in the patient's mouth, so that the tooth to be viewed lies between the film holder and the X-ray cone, and in parallel with both (Figure 4.8)

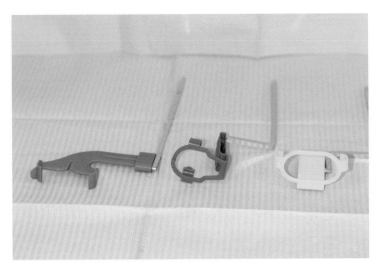

Figure 4.7 Examples of film holders. (a) Bitewing holder. (b) Anterior periapical holder. (c) Posterior periapical holder

- The final position of the X-ray cone is checked before all personnel except the patient move outside the 2 metre safety zone
- The patient is told to remain completely still during the exposure, which is identified by a ringing or buzzing sound
- The operator presses the X-ray machine button to expose the film, releasing it only when the audio alarm ends
- A digital X-ray view is produced immediately on the computer screen
- An ordinary film is removed from the patient's mouth and holder, and taken to be chemically processed either manually or in an automatic processor
- The processed radiograph can be viewed on a viewer within 5 min, and a diagnosis made

When a DPT is to be taken, the patient has to be correctly positioned within the headset of the X-ray machine, so that the film produced is in focus throughout and so that no positional distortions are produced (Figure 4.9). The exposure time is usually in the region of 15 s, but a reduced X-ray dose to the patient is achieved by the use of intensifying screens within the cassette.

The film is chemically processed to produce the image, either manually or automatically. These views are often taken for orthodontic diagnosis of missing or unerupted teeth, as well as to identify jaw fractures and pathology.

BACKGROUND INFORMATION OF PROCEDURE – STUDY MODELS

When a patient has a complicated occlusion, it is easier for the dentist to visualise this by copying the dental arches and the way they bite together by producing a set of study

DIAGNOSTIC TECHNIQUES

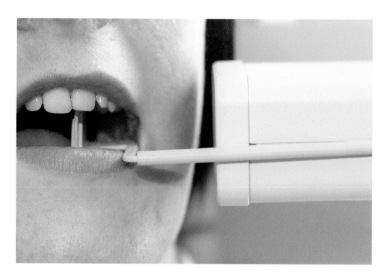

Figure 4.8 Film packet and holder in place ready for exposure

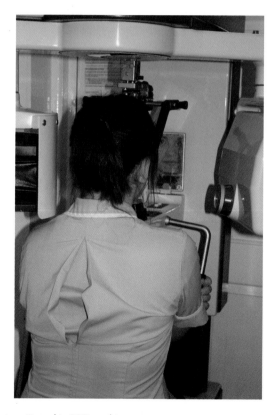

Figure 4.9 Patient positioned in DPT machine

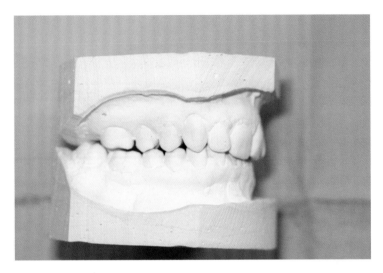

Figure 4.10 Set of simple study models

models (Figure 4.10). These can then be viewed from all angles by the dentist, without the hinderance of the patient's lips, cheeks and tongue.

Often, unexpected details are discovered that were not evident just by viewing the patient in the dental chair, such as abnormal wear patterns on the teeth.

Diagnostic study models are invaluable aids to the dentist for the following situations:

- Orthodontics
- Multiple crown restorations
- Bridges
- Implants
- Bruxism (tooth grinding)
- Denture design

DETAILS OF PROCEDURE – STUDY MODELS

When producing diagnostic study models, an impression has to be taken of each arch of the patient's dentition that is accurate without being prohibitively expensive. The impression material of choice is alginate, which is sufficiently elastomeric to be accurate as well as being relatively inexpensive. Correctly sized stock trays are adequate to hold the impression material, and a wax wafer bite allows the accurate positioning of the two models produced.

The materials and equipment that may be required for a set of simple study models are shown in Figure 4.11.

In more complicated cases, the models are often mounted on an articulator by the laboratory technician so that jaw movements can be reproduced and a more in-depth occlusal analysis carried out.

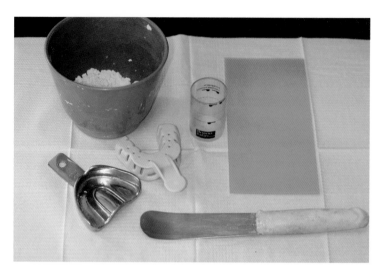

Figure 4.11 Equipment and materials for taking a set of simple study models

TECHNIQUE:

- The patient is usually seated upright in the dental chair, so that excess material does not cause gagging during the procedure
- A protective bib is placed over the patient
- All removable prostheses are taken out of the mouth, unless their presence is required for the occlusal analysis
- A wax wafer bite is taken if necessary, using warmed pink wax
- Upper and lower stock trays are sized to the patient's dental arches, so that each arch is fully covered by the tray without being uncomfortable or actually choking the patient
- A stiff, bubble-free mix of alginate is prepared and loaded into one of the trays and then inserted into the patient's mouth to fully cover one of the dental arches
- The patient is advised to breathe through the nose while the impression is being taken, not to swallow, and to keep the lips and cheeks in a relaxed state
- Once set, the impression is carefully removed from the mouth in the tray and disinfected as necessary
- The process is repeated for the opposing arch
- Study models are cast in dental stone from the impressions, ideally within 24 h of the impressions being taken

The technique of taking alginate impressions for study models is one that can be carried out by suitably trained dental nurses as an extended duty, and the full procedure is discussed further in Chapter 13.

Chapter 5

Tooth restoration with fillings

REASON FOR PROCEDURE

When a tooth is attacked by caries, a process of demineralisation occurs in the hard tissues of the tooth, starting in the enamel outer layer. This opens the inner dentine layer to infection by the bacteria involved in caries, and as this layer contains nerve endings, the patient feels hot and cold sensitivity and eventually pain. Once painful, there is a loss of function as the patient avoids chewing with the affected tooth.

The caries attack progresses further into the tooth until it reaches the pulp chamber, eventually causing an abscess and the death of the tooth, unless the tooth is dentally treated by filling before the pulp chamber is breached.

A tooth may also require a filling if it fractures, whether caries is involved or not, as a fractured tooth may also become sensitive to hot and cold food, or cause soft tissue trauma to areas within the oral cavity.

The purpose of the filling procedure is to ultimately restore the tooth to its normal function, and this involves the elimination of any caries first, as well as the elimination of any discomfort or pain experienced by the patient.

The procedures discussed are:

- Amalgam fillings
- Composite fillings
- Glass ionomer fillings

BACKGROUND INFORMATION OF PROCEDURE – AMALGAM FILLINGS

Amalgam is a metallic material used for fillings, produced by the mixing of an alloy powder (containing mainly silver) with a small amount of liquid mercury. This produces a malleable material that can be inserted fully into the tooth cavity and then carved to the shape of the tooth surface. Once set, it forms a solid plug in the cavity that is hard enough

Basic Guide to Dental Procedures, Second Edition. Carole Hollins.
© 2015 John Wiley & Sons, Ltd. Published 2015 by John Wiley & Sons, Ltd.

to chew on, as well as sealing the tooth's sensitive inner layers from further exposure to hot and cold stimulants.

As the material is metallic in appearance, it tends not to be used for anterior fillings as far more acceptable aesthetic substances are produced for use here, using tooth-coloured filling materials.

DETAILS OF PROCEDURE – AMALGAM FILLINGS

The procedure is normally carried out under local anaesthetic so that the patient feels neither pain nor thermal stimulation in the tooth. The effects of the local anaesthetic wear off after several hours, by which time the dental treatment has been completed painlessly.

The instruments and materials required to administer a local anaesthetic are shown in Figure 3.8.

During the procedure, the dental nurse provides good moisture control in the oral cavity using high speed suction equipment, so that the dentist has a clear field of vision at all times. The suction equipment is used to remove saliva, debris from the tooth and water from the dental handpiece that cools the drill while in use.

The instruments and materials required to carry out an amalgam filling procedure are shown in Figure 5.1.

TECHNIQUE:

- The dentist, nurse and patient wear personal protective equipment for safety reasons and this usually consists of goggles and mask for the dental team, and a protective bib and safety glasses for the patient (see Figure 3.5)
- Local anaesthetic is administered and allowed to take full effect
- All caries is removed from the tooth cavity using a combination of high and low speed dental handpieces with drills and occasionally with the additional use of cutting hand instruments
- This produces a firm tooth cavity surface into which the filling can be placed, which is then undercut to prevent loss of the completed filling
- Depending on the depth of the finished cavity, a protective lining may be placed over its base so that the pulp beneath is not exposed to thermal irritation through the metallic filling
- The walls of the cavity can also be sealed using a light-cured resin-type material, which improves the tooth resistance to thermal stimulation and assists in reducing marginal leakage of the set filling
- If more than one tooth surface has been destroyed by the caries, a metal matrix band is placed around the tooth and tightened, to allow the amalgam to be pushed into the cavity from one surface without it squeezing out of the other
- The mixed amalgam is inserted into the cavity in increments by the dental team, starting at its deepest point and gradually filling the cavity to the surface of the tooth
- After each increment, the dentist uses hand instruments to push the plastic amalgam material into all the cavity depths so that no voids remain – these air spaces weaken the filling and allow future fracture, if present
- The dental nurse uses the high speed suction to remove all excess amalgam from the area, as the dentist carves and shapes the surface of the filling
- Once completed, the shaping of the filling should allow the patient to bite together without prematurely contacting it, but so that the tooth can still be used for chewing
- The patient is advised not to attempt chewing until the local anaesthetic has worn off, otherwise there is the risk of biting oneself
- By this time, the amalgam is hardened and fully set (Figure 5.2)

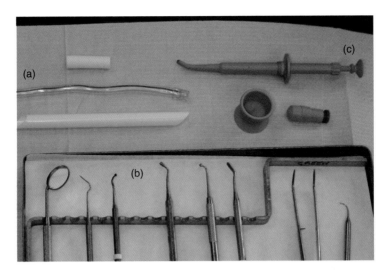

Figure 5.1 Instruments and materials for amalgam filling procedure. (a) Moisture control items. (b) Hand instruments. (c) Amalgam capsule, well and carrier

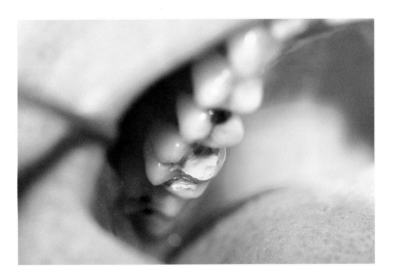

Figure 5.2 Completed amalgam filling

BACKGROUND INFORMATION OF PROCEDURE – COMPOSITE FILLINGS

Composite is a tooth-coloured filling material that is available in many shades to match a very wide range of tooth colours. It can be polished, once set, to produce a shiny surface that matches tooth enamel superbly and is therefore an excellent material to be used for anterior fillings. Some modern types of composite are also strong and wear-resistant enough to be used as a posterior filling material instead of amalgam.

TOOTH RESTORATION WITH FILLINGS

Unlike amalgam, composite is not freshly mixed and then allowed to set with time, but rather it is used in its ready-mixed plastic state to fill a cavity, and then set (or cured) by exposure to a blue curing lamp. This gives the dentist more time to fully adapt the plastic material to the tooth as required, before using the curing lamp to harden it in a controlled manner.

Although composite is far superior to amalgam aesthetically, it can take longer to use and the procedure is technique-sensitive. In addition, only certain types of composite are strong enough to be used in larger cavities in posterior teeth as the chewing forces generated here are considerable.

DETAILS OF PROCEDURE – COMPOSITE FILLINGS

Again, local anaesthesia is usually administered before dental treatment begins, and a dental nurse provides moisture control throughout the procedure, as composite is particularly sensitive to moisture contamination from saliva, blood or irrigation water.

Indeed, some dentists choose to isolate the tooth completely from the rest of the oral cavity while placing composite fillings, by using a rubber dam. This allows the tooth to be restored to project through the rubber dam sheet while keeping all other oral structures away from it, thus preventing saliva contamination of the tooth while the filling is placed.

The instruments required to apply rubber dam to a tooth are shown in Figure 5.3

The equipment and materials required to carry out a composite filling procedure are shown in Figure 5.4.

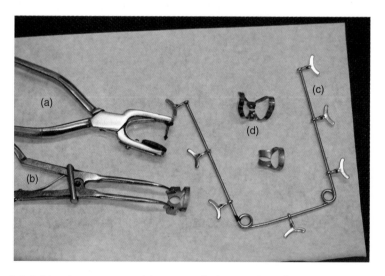

Figure 5.3 Rubber dam instruments. (a) Dam punch. (b) Dam clamp forceps, with clamp. (c) Dam frame. (d) Selection of other clamps

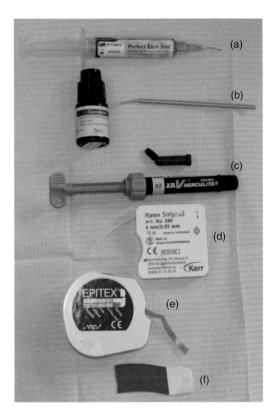

Figure 5.4 Equipment and materials for composite filling procedure. (a) Acid etchant. (b) Resin and applicator. (c) Composite material example. (d) Transparent matrix strip. (e) Finishing strip. (f) Articulating paper

TECHNIQUE:

- The dentist, nurse and patient wear personal protective eqiupment, and ideally the patient's safety glasses are orange-tinted to counteract the blue curing lamp
- Local anaesthetic is administered and allowed to take full effect
- A rubber dam is placed if required (Figure 5.5)
- All caries is removed from the tooth cavity as before, but then the preparation can be minimal as the composite material bonds to enamel and no undercuts are required to hold the filling in place
- A lining may be placed in deeper cavities to prevent chemical irritation of the pulp by the filling material
- The required shade is chosen using a shade guide in natural light (this may be taken beforehand if a rubber dam is placed)
- The exposed enamel edges of the cavity are covered in acid etch to chemically roughen their surfaces

(continued)

TOOTH RESTORATION WITH FILLINGS

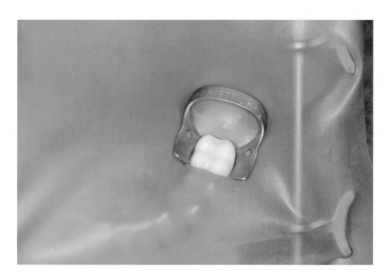

Figure 5.5 Rubber dam in place on lower molar tooth

TECHNIQUE: (*Continued*)

- The etch is washed off, the edges dried, and then unfilled resin is wiped over them and cured with the blue lamp for a short time to produce a sticky layer of material
- The resin forms a bond between the enamel and the filling material, locking the latter into place
- A transparent matrix strip is used to avoid overspill as the composite is placed into the cavity, in 2 mm increments that are individually cured to ensure full setting of the overall filling
- The matrix is transparent to allow the curing light beam to pass through it
- Coloured articulating paper is used to identify any premature contacts on any biting surfaces of the filling, and these are removed to allow the patients to achieve their correct bite
- Polishing strips, discs, and burs are used to produce the final shiny surface of the completed filling (Figure 5.6 shows an old composite filling, as a new one is very difficult to see because of their superb aesthetics)
- Although the filling is fully set once cured, the patient is advised not to attempt chewing until the local anaesthetic has worn off, to avoid soft tissue injury

BACKGROUND INFORMATION OF PROCEDURE – GLASS IONOMER FILLINGS

Glass ionomer is another tooth-coloured filling material available for tooth restoration, although the shade range is more limited than for composite. It is also less translucent and cannot be polished to give a shiny surface, so the final aesthetics produced are inferior to those achieved with composite materials.

The advantage that glass ionomer has over other filling materials is that it is adhesive to all tooth surfaces – enamel, dentine, and cementum – and is therefore invaluable in filling

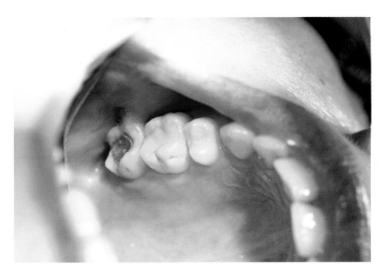

Figure 5.6 Completed composite filling – old filling shown as new one is not easily visible

cavities where only minimal, if any, tooth preparation is possible. This is a particular advantage when filling abrasion cavities produced at the necks of the teeth, often by over-zealous toothbrushing by the patient.

It is also useful in filling the deciduous teeth of young patients who often do not tolerate the administration of local anaesthetic. It is of special value here as it releases fluoride into the cavity and helps to slow or stop the progression of the caries.

It is usually provided as a powder of glass-like material to be mixed by hand with an acidic liquid, or as a capsule containing both to be mixed mechanically; some set chemically with time while others set after exposure to the blue curing lamp. Attempts to adjust the surface of the filling once set produce a chalky appearance, so accurate placement of a light-cure type requiring no adjustment produces the best aesthetic result.

The equipment and materials required to carry out a glass ionomer filling procedure are shown in Figure 5.7.

DETAILS OF PROCEDURE – GLASS IONOMER FILLINGS

As little or no tooth preparation is required with this material unless caries is present, local anaesthesia may not always be required. However, good moisture control is imperative to the filling setting properly, so a rubber dam may well be placed in adult patients.

TECHNIQUE:

- The dentist, nurse and patient wear personal protective equipment
- Local anaesthetic is administered if caries removal is necessary

(continued)

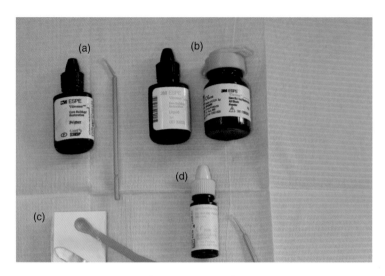

Figure 5.7 Equipment and materials for glass ionomer filling procedure. (a) Conditioning liquid and applicator. (b) Powder and liquid filling material example. (c) Waxed pad, spatula, and measuring scoop. (d) Varnish and applicator

TECHNIQUE: (*Continued*)

- A rubber dam is placed if required
- Any caries is fully removed if present, otherwise no tooth preparation is required
- The cavity is conditioned by wiping it over fully with polyacrylic liquid, to remove dirt and any preparation debris and allow chemical bonding of the filling to the tooth
- The conditioner is washed off and the cavity dried
- Deeper cavities are lined to prevent chemical irritation of the pulp
- The mixed filling material is applied and fully adapted to the cavity so that no adjustment is required once set
- Light-cured types of glass ionomer are cured as necessary, while chemically cured types are kept dry while setting occurs with time
- The set surface is coated with a waterproof varnish to prevent the filling drying out once set (Figure 5.8)

AFTERCARE OF FILLINGS

No matter how well placed, microscopically the edges of a filling provide a new surface area for plaque and oral bacteria to adhere to, giving the potential for further carious attack if not removed regularly.

Consistently high standards of oral hygiene must be maintained by the patient to prevent this happening, especially interdentally if the filling extends between the teeth. This involves the use of a good toothbrushing technique with a good quality fluoridated

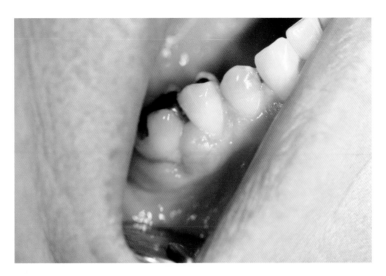

Figure 5.8 Completed glass ionomer filling on lower molar

toothpaste, as well as the use of floss, tape or interdental brushes. Ideally, a plaque suppressing mouthwash should also be used routinely.

The standard of oral hygiene achieved should be monitored and reinforced as necessary at regular dental examinations. Where techniques are poor and calculus has developed, this should be fully removed by scaling and polishing the teeth.

Patients should also be advised to alter their diet when they have experienced caries previously. Their intake of foods and drinks high in refined sugars or acids should be reduced as far as possible, and confined to mealtimes to allow the natural buffering action of saliva to minimise any carious attack.

Failure to comply with these oral health instructions is likely to result in further caries and the need for further fillings in the future.

Chapter 6

Tooth restoration with crowns, bridges, veneers or inlays

REASON FOR PROCEDURE – CROWNS

Each time a tooth is restored with a filling, some of the tooth tissue is removed. Eventually, this compromises the strength of the remaining tooth and it may begin to fracture under normal occlusal forces. This especially occurs when teeth have been root treated, so it is usual for heavily filled and root filled teeth to be crowned before fracture occurs.

In other cases, a tooth may be poorly shaped and require elective crowning to be more aesthetically pleasing. Similarly, a tooth may be too poorly shaped to assist in the retention of, say, a denture, but can be made so by elective crowning.

BACKGROUND INFORMATION OF PROCEDURE – CROWNS

Posterior crowns are sometimes constructed from non-precious or precious metals such as yellow gold. These metallic materials provide maximum strength to withstand occlusal forces and have no risk of fracture. More modern posterior crowns and anterior crowns are made of either tooth-coloured ceramic throughout, or have porcelain bonded to a substructure of metal, and these give an aesthetically pleasing result when shaded and matched accurately with the adjacent teeth. Although modern techniques of crown construction are superb, it is possible for ceramic crowns to fracture or to break away from their metallic substructure, so that repairs or even replacements are required. This can occur in patients with especially heavy bites or in those who grind their teeth.

DETAILS OF PROCEDURE – CROWNS

Unless the tooth to be crowned has been root treated and is therefore non-vital, crown preparation is usually carried out under local anaesthetic so that the patient feels neither

Basic Guide to Dental Procedures, Second Edition. Carole Hollins.
© 2015 John Wiley & Sons, Ltd. Published 2015 by John Wiley & Sons, Ltd.

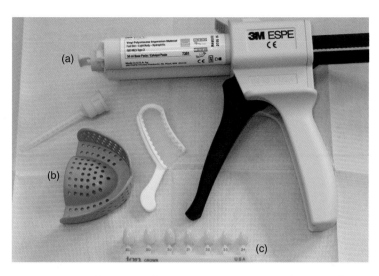

Figure 6.1 Equipment and materials for crown preparation procedure. (a) Elastomer based impression material example. (b) Selection of impression trays. (c) Temporary crown form example

pain nor thermal stimulation in the tooth throughout the procedure. The equipment and materials required to administer local anaesthetic are shown in Figure 3.8.

The prepared tooth requires thermal protection by being covered with a temporary crown material such as acrylic, as the crown has to be individually constructed by a technician before it can be fitted.

During the preparation procedure, a dental nurse provides good moisture control in the oral cavity using high speed suction equipment. This provides a clear field of vision for the dentist, as well as making the patient more comfortable by removing water, saliva and tooth debris from the mouth.

The instruments required to carry out a crown preparation procedure are shown in Figure 5.1b.

The equipment and materials required to carry out a crown preparation procedure are shown in Figure 6.1.

TECHNIQUE:

- The dentist, nurse and patient wear personal protective equipment, as usual
- Local anaesthetic is administered and allowed to take full effect
- The shade and shape of crown are chosen by the dentist and patient, using a shade guide
- A rubber dam is placed if required
- All sides and the occlusal surface of the tooth are reduced by a uniform amount using a bur in the high speed handpiece, so that space is created for the crown to be constructed and fitted over the remaining tooth without altering the patient's occlusion
- The side reduction is completed to produce a near parallel tooth core, to give maximum retention of the crown on cementation (Figure 6.2)
- Once the tooth preparation is complete, impressions are taken of both arches and the patient's normal biting position is recorded

(continued)

TECHNIQUE: (*Continued*)

- Impression of the opposing arch can be taken in alginate, but that of the working arch has to be in a very accurate, non-tearing elastomeric material such as a silicone or polyether
- When satisfactory impressions have been produced, the tooth core is coated with a temporary acrylic material or fitted with a temporary crown form, to prevent sensitivity and to restore some degree of aesthetics while the permanent crown is constructed (Figure 6.3)
- Once the crown has been constructed, the patient reattends for its cementation

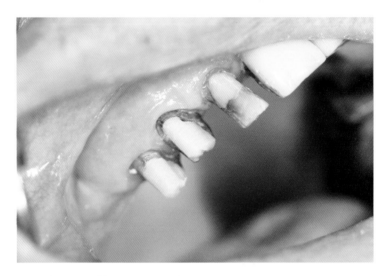

Figure 6.2 Teeth prepared for crown procedure

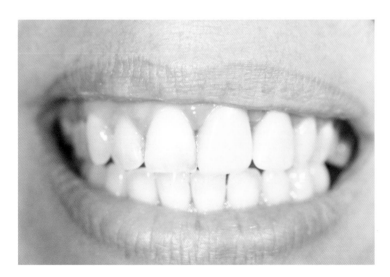

Figure 6.3 Temporary crowns in place on the upper left incisors

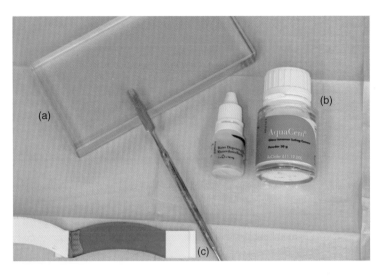

Figure 6.4 Equipment and materials for crown cementation procedure. (a) Mixing pad and spatula. (b) Luting cement example. (c) Articulating paper

The equipment and materials required to cement a permanent crown are shown in Figure 6.4.

- Again, local anaesthetic is administered and a rubber dam placed if required
- On removal of the temporary material, the crown is tried onto the tooth core and checked for accuracy of fit, shade and occlusion
- If satisfactory, the crown is cemented permanently onto the tooth core using one of a variety of luting cements (Figure 6.5)

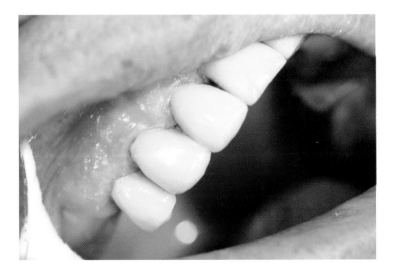

Figure 6.5 Cemented crowns

AFTERCARE OF CROWNS

As with fillings, microscopically all fixed prosthetic restorations provide a surface area for the attachment of plaque and oral bacteria. As crown margins are deliberately placed at the gingival margin to give superior aesthetics, any plaque accumulation can potentially cause either caries of the underlying tooth core or periodontal disease down the root of the tooth.

A consistently high standard of oral hygiene around crown margins is therefore imperative. This involves good toothbrushing using a good quality fluoride toothpaste, and successful interdental cleaning using floss or tape. As many crowns are placed specifically to close existing interdental spaces, it is unlikely that the use of interdental brushes is possible.

Regular use of a plaque-suppressing mouthwash should also be encouraged, and the oral hygiene standard achieved by the patient can be monitored and reinforced at regular dental examinations. Any calculus found to be present should be fully removed by scaling and polishing the teeth.

As always, a diet high in sugars and acids should be reduced to an absolute minimum, and confined to mealtimes only.

BACKGROUND INFORMATION OF PROCEDURE – BRIDGES

A bridge is a fixed restoration used to replace one or a few missing teeth in a dental arch, although in advanced cases multiple bridges can be fitted to provide full mouth rehabilitation.

Various designs of bridges are available, and that used in each case has to be determined by the dentist on its merits.

For patients with only a few missing teeth and a low biting force in the area of the bridge, a minimal amount of tooth preparation can be carried out and an acid etch retained bridge placed. Where occlusal forces are likely to dislodge this type of restoration, a more conventional design is used, where the adjacent teeth are prepared as for crowns and the missing teeth incorporated into the whole structure.

Bridges are usually constructed of porcelain bonded to a metallic substructure, although some modern, all ceramic materials are also available.

DETAILS OF PROCEDURE – BRIDGES

As minimal tooth preparation is carried out for an acid etch bridge preparation, it is often not necessary for local anaesthetic to be administered. With more conventional designs involving whole tooth preparation, it is usual for local anaesthetic to be administered for any vital teeth involved.

As always, a dental nurse provides good moisture control in the oral cavity throughout the bridge preparation procedure.

The instruments, equipment and materials required for a bridge preparation are as for those detailed previously for a crown preparation (see Figures 5.1b and 6.1).

TECHNIQUE:

- The dentist, nurse and patient wear personal protective equipment
- Local anaesthetic is administered if necessary, and allowed to take full effect
- The design of the bridge will have been discussed and determined previously, and the shade is now chosen
- A rubber dam is placed if required
- If an acid etch bridge is being provided, a small area of enamel at the back of the retaining adjacent teeth is removed to provide room for the technician to construct the retaining metal wings to hold the bridge in place
- These have to be constructed so as not to interfere with the patient's normal occlusion
- When a more conventional bridge is being provided, each retaining tooth is reduced to a core as for a crown preparation, using the same technique and design principles (see Figure 6.2)
- Once prepared, an impression of the working arch is taken in a highly accurate material such as silicone or polyether, and one of the opposing arch is taken in alginate
- The bite and jaw movements can be recorded simply, or with the help of articulated study models, depending on the complexity of the case
- The prepared teeth are temporarily covered to prevent sensitivity, as with crown preparations
- In complex cases, the metallic substructure of the bridge (if used) is tried in for accuracy of fit before the porcelain is bonded to it, as this avoids costly full remakes if problems do occur
- Once the bridge is fully constructed, the patient reattends for its cementation

The equipment and materials required to cement a bridge are shown in Figure 6.4.

- Local anaesthetic is administered and a rubber dam placed as necessary
- On removal of the temporary coverings, the bridge is tried onto the retaining teeth and checked for accuracy of fit, shade and occlusion
- The replaced missing tooth (or teeth) is checked for its fit against the bony ridge of the dental arch, to ensure that the area can be easily cleaned by the patient
- Once satisfactory, an acid etch retained bridge is cemented using one of a variety of light cured bonding materials
- A conventional bridge is cemented using one of a variety of luting cements

AFTERCARE OF BRIDGES

All of the aftercare advice for crowns is similarly applicable to bridges, but additional oral hygiene techniques also need to be employed when maintaining the pontic areas of a bridge. The pontic is the section of the bridge that replaces the missing tooth or teeth, and rests on the ridge of the dental arch itself, once the bridge is cemented in place.

The point where the pontic rests on the gingiva is a difficult area to clean and may accumulate plaque and oral bacteria quite easily. This causes gingival inflammation unless the plaque is removed, either by vigorous mouthwashing or by physically cleaning the underside of the pontic, using floss or tape.

Where the pontic has retainers on both sides so that the bridge is a solid structure, superfloss can be threaded beneath the pontic and used to clean its underside. Superfloss

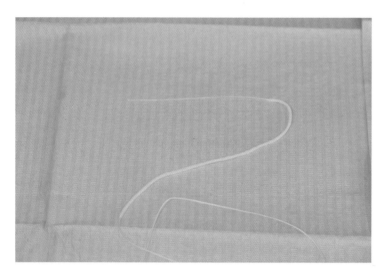

Figure 6.6 Superfloss for cleaning beneath a bridge pontic

has a stiff end for threading as described, which is attached to an expanded spongy section that then runs into normal floss (Figure 6.6). It has been designed specifically to clean bridges in this way.

BACKGROUND INFORMATION OF PROCEDURE – VENEERS

A less invasive technique than conventional crown preparation for improving the aesthetics of a tooth is to place veneers. These are thin layers of porcelain that are acid etch cemented to the front surface of any number of anterior teeth, to improve a patient's appearance by correcting dark or malaligned teeth, or both.

They have no other functional purpose than a cosmetic one, and their fragility and ease of fracture or loss dictates their case suitability. Patients with aberrant occlusal habits or heavy bites are usually unsuitable for veneers.

Although usually constructed of porcelain, it is possible to place either composite or acrylic veneers on a temporary basis.

Nowadays, a patient with well-aligned but discoloured anterior teeth may also undergo professional tooth whitening to improve their appearance, rather than undergo the relatively invasive procedure of having porcelain veneers fitted (see Chapter 12).

DETAILS OF PROCEDURE – VENEERS

As minimal tooth preparation is carried out for a veneer, it is often not necessary for local anaesthetic to be administered. Indeed it is frequently root filled, discoloured teeth that have veneers placed to improve aesthetics, as full crown preparations on these teeth can sometimes compromise them enough to cause fracture with time.

A dental nurse provides good moisture control in the oral cavity throughout the veneer preparation procedure.

The instruments, equipment, and materials required for a veneer preparation are those shown in Figures 5.1b and 6.1, although a temporary crown form is unnecessary in veneer cases.

TECHNIQUE:

- The dentist, nurse and patient wear personal protective equipment
- Local anaesthetic is administered as necessary, and allowed to take full effect
- The shade and shape of the veneer are chosen by the dentist and patient, and the need for any opaquing technique if a particularly dark tooth is involved is decided upon
- This may be necessary to prevent the tooth discolouration from being visible through the thin porcelain veneer, once fitted
- A rubber dam is placed if required (see Figure 5.3)
- The labial (front) surface of each tooth to be veneered is reduced uniformly using a bur in the high speed handpiece (Figure 6.7)
- This is to provide the technician with sufficient space to construct the veneer so that the restoration remains in line with the adjacent teeth, rather than projecting further forwards than required
- Once the veneer preparation is complete, a highly accurate working impression is taken in a material such as silicone or polyether
- If the occlusion of the prepared tooth has been altered, then an opposing alginate impression and bite record is also taken
- The prepared tooth surface can be temporarily covered with glass ionomer or composite to avoid sensitivity and improve aesthetics, but this is sometimes not carried out with non-vital teeth
- Once the veneer has been constructed, the patient reattends for its cementation

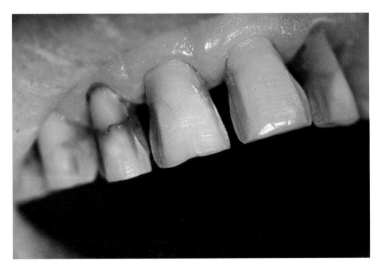

Figure 6.7 Tooth preparation for veneers

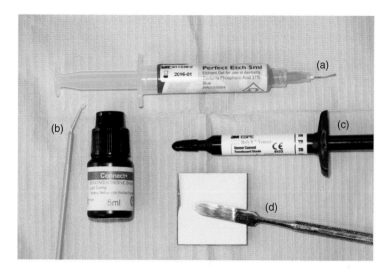

Figure 6.8 Equipment and materials for veneer cementation procedure. (a) Acid etchant. (b) Resin and applicator. (c) Veneer luting cement example. (d) Mixing pad and spatula

The equipment and materials required to cement a veneer are shown in Figure 6.8.

- Local anaesthetic is administered and a rubber dam placed if required
- On removal of any temporary covering placed, the veneer is placed onto the tooth and checked for accuracy of fit, shade and shape
- The final shade can be accurately achieved by the use of various tooth-coloured cements if necessary
- The veneer is secured to the tooth using one of a variety of light-cured bonding materials (Figure 6.9)

AFTERCARE OF VENEERS

As with other restorations, veneers can be subject to plaque and oral bacteria accumulations at their margins. Their aftercare advice is similar as for crowns, whereby a consistently good standard of plaque removal is required to prevent caries developing at the veneer margins and periodontal problems developing at the ginival margins.

This is achieved using a thorough toothbrushing technique with fluoride toothpaste, careful interdental cleaning using floss or tape, and the regular use of a plaque-suppressing mouthwash.

Regular dental examinations should be carried out, where oral hygiene techniques can be reinforced as necessary, as well as any scaling and polishing carried out to remove any accumulated calculus deposits.

Diet advice includes the reduction in intake of sugars and acids to a minimum, as well as for them to be confined to mealtimes only.

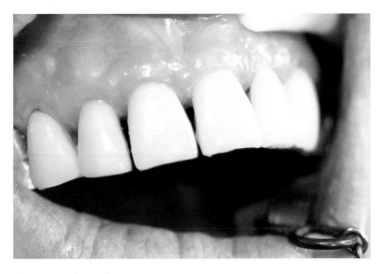

Figure 6.9 Cemented porcelain veneers

Patients should also be advised of the potential fragility of veneers in certain circumstances. Actions such as biting finger nails and habits such as holding pens in the mouth may be sufficient to crack a porcelain veneer and require its removal and remake. Patients should always be discouraged in these types of habits and activities anyway, as they are often sufficient to splinter fillings and slivers of enamel from the teeth.

REASON FOR PROCEDURE – INLAYS

An inlay is a device used to fill a prepared cavity in a tooth with a solid, pre-formed material rather than with a more conventional malleable filling material that can be manipulated into shape before setting, such as amalgam. The advantage of using an inlay in this situation is the greater strength of the material used versus that of conventional filling materials. This is of particular importance in patients with a very strong bite or in patients who habitually grind their teeth, as they tend to suffer from an increased incidence of filling fracture.

The inclusion of inlays in this chapter rather than with fillings is due to the similarity in the method of tooth preparation required as well as the materials available for inlay construction, both features being similar to those for crown and bridge work.

BACKGROUND INFORMATION OF PROCEDURE – INLAYS

As with crowns and bridges, inlays are constructed indirectly in a laboratory rather than at the chair side, using materials such as precious and non-precious metal alloys and ceramics.

Inlays are usually placed in posterior teeth which undergo heavy occlusal forces during normal chewing actions. These forces may be strong enough to fracture large conventional fillings, and allow caries to recur in the affected tooth through the fracture. Small uncomplicated cavities do not usually warrant the extra time and expense of restoring them with an inlay, and their use in anterior teeth has also declined with the development of better aesthetic anterior filling materials.

DETAILS OF PROCEDURE – INLAYS

Unless the tooth receiving the inlay has been root treated and is therefore non-vital, inlay preparation is usually carried out under local anaesthetic so that the patient feels neither pain nor thermal stimulation in the tooth throughout the procedure.

While the inlay is being constructed in the laboratory by the technician, a temporary filling material is placed to seal the cavity and prevent any food packing from occurring in it, as well as to protect the tooth from any uncomfortable thermal stimulation.

During the preparation procedure, a dental nurse provides good moisture control in the oral cavity, using high speed suction equipment. This provides a clear field of vision for the dentist, as well as making the patient more comfortable by removing water, saliva and tooth debris from the mouth.

The instruments required to carry out an inlay preparation procedure are shown in Figure 5.1b.

The same impression and bite recording techniques are used as for crown or bridge preparation procedures. The only additional equipment and material required is that for mixing and placing a temporary filling material to seal the cavity while the inlay is constructed.

TECHNIQUE:

- The dentist, nurse and patient wear personal protective equipment
- Local anaesthetic is administered as necessary, and allowed to take full effect
- The material used to construct the inlay is decided previously by the dentist and the patient, and if a ceramic is to be used the shade is chosen
- A rubber dam is placed if required (see Figure 5.3)
- Any existing filling is removed using ordinary cavity preparation burs in the high speed handpiece
- Similarly, any carious tooth tissue is removed down to sound dentine to leave a hollowed out cavity within the tooth, of varying shape and size dependent on the amount of caries removed
- The inner walls of the cavity must now be prepared to produce a near-parallel shape, by the infilling of any undercuts with an adhesive restorative material such as composite or glass ionomer (Figure 6.10)
- The walls must be near-parallel to allow the inlay to be seated accurately, while providing the maximum retention to prevent its inadvertent dislodgement during use

TOOTH RESTORATION WITH CROWNS, BRIDGES, VENEERS OR INLAYS

- Once the inlay preparation is complete, a highly accurate working impression is taken in a material such as silicone or polyether
- An opposing alginate impression and bite record are also taken so that the technician can construct the inlay surface to fit neatly into the occlusion
- The inlay cavity is then temporarily filled while the inlay is being constructed by the technician
- Once the inlay is available, the patient reattends for its cementation

The equipment and materials required to cement an inlay are the same as for a crown cementation, and are shown in Figure 6.4.

- Local anaesthetic is administered and a rubber dam placed if required
- The temporary filling material is carefully drilled out of the cavity, without altering the shape at all
- The inlay is placed in the cavity to ensure it seats fully, fills the cavity to the margins fully and sits accurately in the occlusion (Figure 6.11)
- Once satisfactory, the inlay is cemented into the cavity using a conventional luting cement or a dual-cure cement
- A final check is made of the seated restoration, using articulating paper to highlight any premature contacts

AFTERCARE OF INLAYS

As with other restorations, inlays can be subject to plaque and oral bacteria accumulations at their margins. Many inlays also involve extensions into the interdental areas of the dental arch to replace contact points between teeth, and these are particularly difficult regions to clean in the oral cavity. Consequently, in addition to the usual oral hygiene

TOOTH RESTORATION WITH CROWNS, BRIDGES, VENEERS OR INLAYS

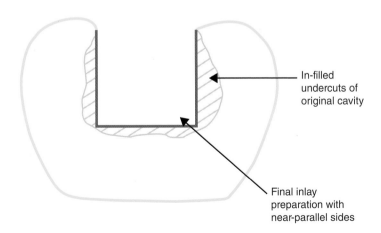

In-filled undercuts of original cavity

Final inlay preparation with near-parallel sides

Figure 6.10 Inlay preparation with in-filled undercuts

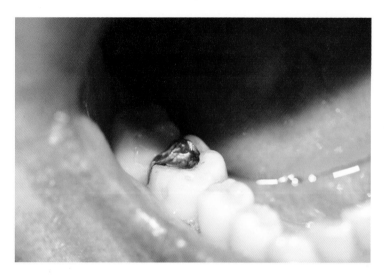

Figure 6.11 Inlay cemented in tooth

advice of effective and regular brushing using a fluoride toothpaste, these patients should also be advised to carry out regular interdental cleaning, using floss or tape, or a recommended size and design of interdental brush (see Figure 2.13).

The restoration is routinely checked for any signs of marginal leakage at each recall appointment.

Diet advice includes the reduction in intake of sugars and acids to a minimum, as well as for them to be confined to mealtimes only.

Chapter 7

Tooth restoration with endodontic techniques

Any event that results in the pulp tissue within the root canal of a tooth being at risk of inflammation or infection may eventually lead to the death of that tooth. Once a tooth has died, it is a source of either painless chronic infection or of acute and very painful infection – neither of which is amenable to the oral health of a patient.

Events that can occur resulting in the inflammation of the pulp (pulpitis) include the following:

- Deep caries lying close to, or exposing, the pulp
- Thermal injury, from the use of hand pieces without cooling irrigation, for example
- Chemical irritation from some restorative materials
- Trauma, which may have been severe enough to cause tooth fracture in some cases
- Prolonged irritation of the pulp tissue from very deep fillings within the tooth, which may transmit thermal and pressure shocks easily

The method available to the dentist for removing the symptoms and treating the tooth to save it from extraction is one of the following endodontic techniques:

- Pulp capping
- Pulpotomy
- Pulpectomy (conventional root canal treatment)

Occasionally a successful root-filled tooth may develop problems at a later date (sometimes years later) and result in a recurrent infection at the end of the root. This may be treated and the tooth saved from extraction by a surgical procedure called an apicectomy.

This is a technique carried out as a temporary measure to stabilise the tooth before proceeding to either pulpotomy or pulpectomy, to save it from extraction. It is necessary

---

when a small pulp exposure occurs unexpectedly during restorative dental treatment, or when a patient attends as an unscheduled emergency following trauma to the tooth, which has resulted in a very small pulp exposure.

The aim of pulp capping is to seal the exposed pulp from the oral cavity and the myriad of microorganisms within it, until time allows for a full endodontic procedure to be carried out to save the tooth.

DETAILS OF PROCEDURE – PULP CAPPING

If the pulp exposure occurred during restorative treatment, it is likely that a local anaesthetic has already been administered previously. If a recent trauma has caused the exposure, the tooth is likely to be concussed and unresponsive to stimulation, therefore not requiring a local anaesthetic procedure to be carried out anyway.

In any event, the tooth must be kept as clean as possible to prevent the introduction of microorganisms into the pulp chamber. Once completed, pulp capping prevents pain and infection developing before further treatment can be carried out.

TECHNIQUE:

- The dentist, nurse and patient wear personal protective equipment
- The tooth is isolated from any saliva contamination using appropriate moisture control techniques
- Any bleeding at the exposure site is arrested using sterile cotton wool pledgets, possibly soaked in a local anaesthetic solution containing a vasoconstrictor such as adrenaline
- Once bleeding has been arrested and the area is dry, a paste of calcium hydroxide material is carefully placed over the exposure site to fully cover and form a 'cap' over it
- The exposure site may be further protected by placing a second, more sturdy, cap over the calcium hydroxide material using an item such as a section of a glass ionomer matrix
- The remaining cavity or fracture site is then sealed with a sedative temporary dressing material to protect the calcium hydroxide cap and assist in reducing any inflammatory response by the pulp to the initial injury (Figure 7.1)

BACKGROUND INFORMATION OF PROCEDURE – PULPOTOMY

When trauma occurs to a permanent tooth in a young patient, it is often the case that the root canal is still wide open at the apex as the root is still growing – this can be determined by taking a radiograph.

When this is the case, the tooth often does not die as a result of the trauma, as the wide apex ensures that a good blood supply to the pulp is maintained during the inflammatory process and pulpal death is avoided. In these cases, only the potentially infected part of the pulp at the exposure site needs to be removed, while the apical blood supply ensures that the remainder of the pulp tissue heals itself.

The partial removal of pulp tissue from the pulp chamber only, and not the root canal, is called pulpotomy.

TOOTH RESTORATION WITH
ENDODONTIC TECHNIQUES

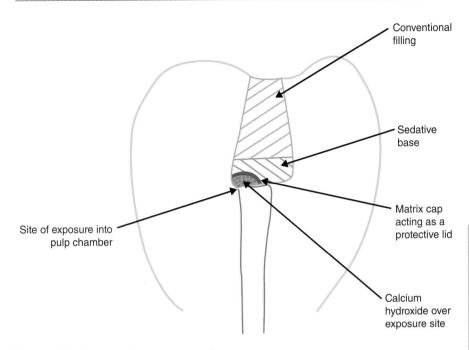

Conventional filling

Sedative base

Matrix cap acting as a protective lid

Site of exposure into pulp chamber

Calcium hydroxide over exposure site

Figure 7.1 Illustration of pulp capping technique

DETAILS OF PROCEDURE – PULPOTOMY

As the pulp tissue is still vital, local anaesthetic is required for the procedure. It is important to the success of the technique that any risk of contamination of the remaining pulp tissue is kept to an absolute minimum, so the dental nurse provides good moisture control throughout.

Similar additional equipment and materials as those used for a pulp capping procedure are required

TECHNIQUE:

- The dentist, nurse and patient wear personal protective equipment
- Local anaesthetic is administered and allowed to take full effect
- The tooth is isolated from saliva contamination, ideally using a rubber dam but this may not be possible on a young patient
- The pulp chamber is opened through the fracture site using a bur in the high speed hand piece
- The pulp tissue, within the pulp chamber only, is separated from that in the root canal using sharp sterile hand instruments or a sterile bur in the low speed hand piece

(continued)

TECHNIQUE: (Continued)

- Any bleeding of the amputated pulp stump is arrested using sterile cotton wool pledgets, possibly soaked in a vasoconstrictive local anaesthetic solution such as adrenaline
- Once dry, the pulp stump is covered with a calcium hydroxide lid of material that encourages the formation of a protective layer of secondary dentine to grow with time, and seal off the pulp tissue in the root canal from the injury site
- A stiff base material is placed over the calcium hydroxide lid to further protect the remaining pulp tissue from the oral environment
- The fracture site and tooth are then restored to full function and aesthetics, using one of the permanent restorative filling materials
- Depending on the degree of success of the technique, it may eventually be necessary to carry out a full root filling procedure on the tooth, but in the meantime the pulpotomy allows the root apex to close to a more normal size so that conventional root filling in future is more likely to be successful

BACKGROUND INFORMATION OF PROCEDURE – PULPECTOMY

When a permanent tooth undergoes an event causing pulpal inflammation in an adult patient, the end result is usually the death of the tooth. The closed root apex of an adult tooth prevents an adequate blood flow from helping to fight the inflammation and remove the excess fluids that build up during the inflammatory process. The ensuing swelling compresses the pulpal tissues within the root canal and tooth death occurs. An infection develops at the root apex that is referred to as a periapical abscess. If the infection develops quickly, it tends to be associated with swelling and pain and is an acute abscess, whereas a slowly developing chronic infection is often painless with no swelling, but often exhibits a discharging sinus tract which is referred to as a 'gum boil' by patients (Figure 7.2).

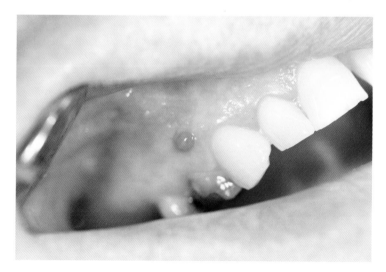

Figure 7.2 'Gum boil' appearance of a chronic infection

The patient therefore experiences varying degrees of pain and swelling throughout the tooth death process, and only a succesful pulpectomy procedure helps to avoid the extraction of the affected tooth.

The aim of pulpectomy, or root canal treatment, is to remove all of the pulpal tissue from the tooth and replace it with a sterile root filling material. This material must fully seal the root canal and prevent any contamination from causing further infection at the root apex.

DETAILS OF PROCEDURE – PULPECTOMY

Although a dead tooth should be unable to feel pain, many patients are more psychologically comfortable and relaxed during the procedure if a local anaesthetic is administered. The success of the pulpectomy technique depends very much on maintaining a sterile field to prevent contamination of the root canal system with saliva and oral microorganisms, and good moisture control is of paramount importance.

Often the full root canal treatment is carried out in one appointment, but if heavy infection is present or other difficulties occur, then it may be completed in more visits.

As well as a full conservation tray of instruments, the additional equipment and materials that may be required to carry out a pulpectomy procedure are shown in Figure 7.3.

TECHNIQUE:

- The dentist, nurse and patient wear personal protective equipment
- Local anaesthetic is administered as required and allowed to take full effect
- The tooth is isolated from the oral cavity, ideally by a rubber dam (see Figure 5.3)
- Access is gained to the pulp chamber and root canal system using a bur in the high speed hand piece
- All pulpal tissue is removed (extirpated) from the tooth using specialised endodontic barbed broach instruments
- The root canal system is enlarged laterally and to the root apex, using endodontic reamers or files, either by hand, with a slow speed hand piece and special files (or reamers), or more usually with specially designed endodontic hand pieces and their own specific files
- The walls of the root canal are also smoothed by the action of the endodontic files, to remove any infected tissue and surface irregularities that could harbour microorganisms in the future
- The root canal is irrigated throughout the preparation procedure to remove loose debris, lubricate the area, and avoid instrument fracture due to their snatching into the otherwise dry tooth structure and becoming stuck
- Once the root canal system is satisfactorily cleaned to the root apex and widened sufficiently to allow root filling, the decision is made whether to continue in a one-stage technique or to dress the root canal for a time with disinfecting medicaments
- Full length access to the root canal can be confirmed using an apex locator or by taking a periapical radiograph with a file inserted to a known length
- To root fill the canal, it is dried with paper points and then a gutta percha point smeared with a sealant material is inserted to the previously determined full working length of the root canal

(continued)

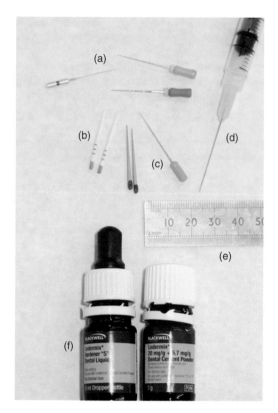

Figure 7.3 Equipment and materials for pulpectomy procedure. (a) Barbed broach and hand files. (b) Paper points. (c) Gutta percha points and finger spreader. (d) Irrigation syringe and needle. (e) Measuring ruler. (f) Sealing material example

TECHNIQUE: (*Continued*)

- Similar points are inserted laterally to fully obliterate both the full length and width of the root canal (obturation)
- This ensures that no spaces remain for microorganisms to linger and recontaminate the root canal in future
- The tooth is restored to full function and aesthetics, using one of the permanent restorative filling materials

AFTERCARE OF ROOT-TREATED TEETH

Although teeth that have undergone pulpectomy are now non-vital (dead), they can still be subject to carious attack if a consistently good standard of oral hygiene is not maintained, or if they are exposed to a diet high in sugars or acids. The patient feels no symptoms of thermal sensitivity or pain in these teeth, and only regular dental examinations will detect the presence of any caries.

If left undiagnosed, the root-treated tooth can become so undermined by caries that it fractures, usually catastrophically at the gingival margin of the tooth. It then requires extensive rebuilding, often involving the insertion of metal or carbon fibre posts into the root canal to anchor and support the rebuilt tooth.

Additionally, root-filled teeth can become brittle over time once their vitality is lost, and may then fracture more easily if their structure is not protected soon after the procedure has been completed. Many root filled teeth are therefore crowned as part of their restoration to full function (see Chapter 6). Similarly, when the endodontic procedure involves the removal of a considerable amount of tooth tissue to gain access to the root canal, a crown is likely to be placed to protect the remaining tooth and help restore it to full function.

However, if the tooth fractures catastrophically and is unrestorable, it requires extraction.

BACKGROUND INFORMATION OF PROCEDURE – APICECTOMY

Sometimes, a successfully root-filled tooth can develop an infection around the root apex many years after the initial procedure is carried out, and the associated infected tissues require removal if the tooth is to be saved from extraction. The tooth will often have already been restored using a crown (with or without a post cemented into the root canal) and access to the area of infection is best achieved by a direct surgical technique called an apicectomy.

The apicectomy procedure is therefore a second line treatment in conjunction with conventional root canal therapy, or after the failure of that conventional root canal therapy.

DETAILS OF PROCEDURE – APICECTOMY

The procedure is classed as a minor oral surgery technique and therefore performed under surgical conditions. Although the tooth involved is usually non-vital, local anaesthetic is still required as the oral soft tissues have to be cut open to provide access to the affected tooth root. Once the area of infection and the root apex have been removed from the surgical site, the cut end of the root stump has to be resealed to prevent further bacterial access and re-infection and this is often achieved by placing a conventional filling there.

Throughout the procedure the dental nurse provides adequate moisture control and careful soft tissue retraction, so that good visibility is provided and the patient's oral tissues are protected from possible trauma.

The instruments required for placing a conventional filling are shown in Figure 5.1b, and the available materials are discussed in Chapter 5.

The surgical instruments required to carry out a minor oral surgery procedure such as an apicectomy are shown in Figure 7.4.

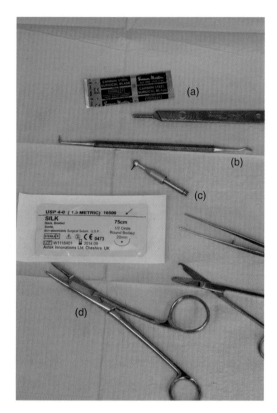

Figure 7.4 Examples of surgical instruments to carry out an apicectomy procedure. (a) Scalpel blade and handle. (b) Instruments to raise the tissue flap off the bone and remove infected soft tissue. (c) Micro-head with bur to prepare root cavity. (d) Suturing equipment

TECHNIQUE:

- The dentist, nurse and patient wear personal protective equipment
- Local anaesthetic is administered and allowed to take full effect
- The surgical site is disinfected using cotton wool rolls soaked in an appropriate solution, such as chlorhexidene
- A soft tissue flap is cut over the affected tooth and adjacent teeth to either side of it using the scalpel instrument, and is peeled off the underlying bone to expose the root apex area
- The flap is carefully retracted from the surgical site to allow good visibility and prevent trauma while the rotary instruments are in use
- A small window is cut into the bone so that the affected root apex and its associated infection are visible
- The infected soft tissue is removed and the root apex is cut off from the remaining root structure and removed from the surgical site
- The open end of the root canal that is then visible is prepared and filled using the micro-head and bur, and a conventional filling material

- Alternatively, specialised endodontic materials can be used to seal the root canal
- The bony cavity that remains is irrigated with sterile saline solution to remove any remaining debris
- The soft tissue flap is repositioned over the bone and carefully sutured back into place
- The sutures require removal in 7 to 10 days after the surgery

PATIENT AFTERCARE FOLLOWING MINOR ORAL SURGERY

Bruising, swelling and post-operative pain may all occur after any minor oral surgery procedure has been carried out, as the oral cavity has an extensive nerve and blood supply. Patients are told to expect any combination of these events over the first few post-operative days, and are given appropriate advice on the use of pain killers (analgesics) during this period.

A soft diet is usually recommended initially, and a good standard of oral hygiene must be maintained throughout the healing period, but without disturbing the sutures.

Hot salt water mouthwashes on a regular basis also assists greatly in the healing process, and these can be started the day after surgery and continued until the oral tissues have fully healed.

The patient should be advised to return to the surgery if any of the following events occur:

- Worsening pain, several days after the procedure
- Bleeding from the wound site
- Any discharge from the wound site
- Loss of the sutures so that the wound re-opens
- Extensive swelling, especially within the mouth rather than on the face

TOOTH RESTORATION WITH
ENDODONTIC TECHNIQUES

Chapter 8

Tooth extraction

Despite the best efforts of the dentist, there are times when a tooth is beyond restoration and it has to be extracted.Often in these circumstances, the patient could suffer from dental infection and pain if the tooth is allowed to remain. The cause of the infection or pain may be gross caries, severe trauma, periodontal disease, or failure of an endodontic technique.

There are also several reasons why a tooth may be electively extracted (that is, by choice rather than necessity) and these include the following:

- Prosthetic reasons, where the tooth is malaligned and preventing the placement of a denture or bridge
- Severe malalignment that cannot be corrected orthodontically
- To create space in a crowded dental arch so that other teeth can be aligned orthodontically
- Partially erupted and impacted teeth that cannot be adequately cleaned by the patient and suffer from repeated localised infection
- Retained deciduous teeth that prevent their adult successor from erupting correctly
- Patient choice, where the alternative is complicated and possibly expensive dental treatment

In most cases a tooth can be simply extracted by loosening it in the bony socket and removing it whole, but in more difficult cases a surgical procedure may be required, where either the bony socket or the tooth itself has to be cut away or into pieces, so that the tooth can be removed from the oral cavity.

The procedures discussed are:

- Simple extraction
- Surgical extraction

BACKGROUND INFORMATION OF PROCEDURE – SIMPLE EXTRACTIONS

A tooth is extracted by loosening it in its socket and then pushing it out of the socket, using a variety of dental extraction forceps, elevators, or luxators. To loosen the tooth

Basic Guide to Dental Procedures, Second Edition. Carole Hollins.
© 2015 John Wiley & Sons, Ltd. Published 2015 by John Wiley & Sons, Ltd.

there has to be access to the top of the root or roots for the dentist to hold onto with the extraction forceps – the tooth is never held by its crown as this would simply fracture during the procedure.

Alternatively, luxators can be used to sever the periodontal ligament attachment to the tooth and also widen the bony socket so that the tooth is loosened. It is then pushed out of the socket as the instrument is pushed apically.

Physical strength is less of an issue in successful tooth extraction than the skill of the dentist in loosening the tooth.

DETAILS OF PROCEDURE – SIMPLE EXTRACTIONS

No matter how loose a tooth, local anaesthetic should always be administered before an extraction procedure. This must be sufficient to numb not just the tooth but all of the surrounding gingiva if the procedure is to be painless for the patient.

The dental nurse provides good moisture control in the oral cavity using high speed suction, as well as providing head support to stabilise the patient and assist the dentist during the procedure.

Extraction forceps are designed to be used on certain teeth only, rather than universally, and there are therefore many patterns of design available, depending on the tooth to be extracted. Those required to extract a tooth are shown in Figure 8.1.

Examples of a luxator and various elevators are shown in Figure 8.2.

TECHNIQUE:

- A current radiograph of the tooth is displayed so that the dentist is aware of any root curvatures
- The dentist, nurse and patient wear personal protective equipment
- Local anaesthetic is administered and allowed to take full effect
- The dental chair is angled so that the dentist can apply suitable pressure to the tooth without straining, as tooth extraction requires some physical exertion
- The dental nurse supports the patient's head firmly but comfortably to prevent rocking movements, as these waste the physical effort of the dentist during the extraction
- The dentist uses extraction forceps, luxators and/or elevators to gradually loosen the periodontal attachment of the tooth root to the bony socket walls
- High speed suction is used by the dental nurse to remove any blood and keep the operative field visually clear for the dentist
- The tooth is firmly held by the forceps and removed from the oral cavity as the extraction is completed
- A bite pack is placed over the socket and the patient is instructed to bite down hard onto it to achieve haemostasis
- The tooth is inspected to ensure that it has been extracted whole, and that no fractured root fragments remain in the socket
- The socket is inspected once bleeding has stopped, to ensure no bony fractures to the socket wall have occurred – any loose sequestrae are removed
- Full verbal and written post-operative instructions (Figure 8.3) are given to the patient, to ensure the socket heals uneventfully

TOOTH EXTRACTION

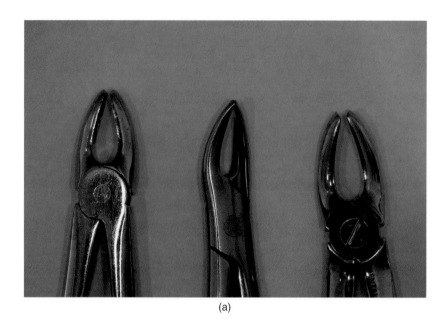

(a)

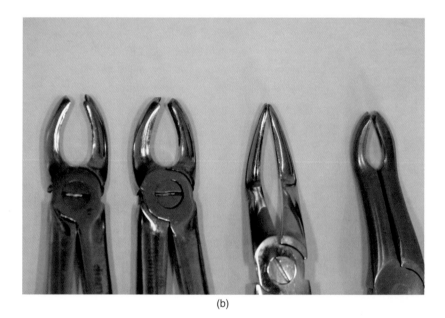

(b)

Figure 8.1 Examples of extraction forceps. (a) Upper anterior and premolar teeth/roots. (b) Upper molar teeth/roots. (c) Lower teeth and roots

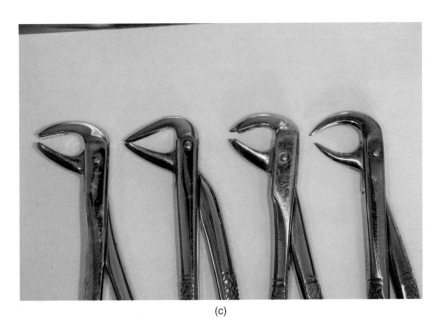

(c)

Figure 8.1 *(continued)*

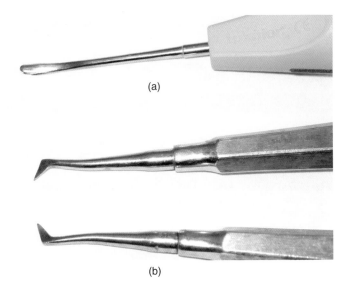

(a)

(b)

Figure 8.2 Examples of other extraction instruments. (a) Luxator. (b) Elevators

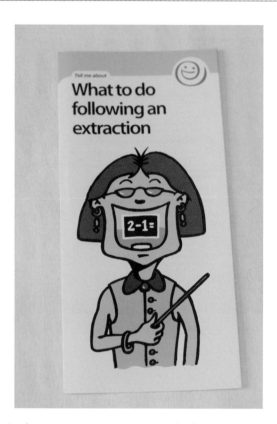

Figure 8.3 Example of written post-operative instruction leaflet

PATIENT AFTERCARE FOLLOWING A SIMPLE EXTRACTION

It is particularly important after an extraction for the patient to follow the post-operative advice that is given by the oral health team – that is why they are given both verbally at the surgery (so the patient can ask any questions) and also in a written format (so that they can be read again at home, and referred to by the patient as required).

Failure to follow the post-operative instructions is likely to result in a problem developing for the patient, usually a painful one. The instructions given are detailed below, with an explanation of their relevance and importance.

- Bite on the bite pack for a minimum of 15 min – this applies pressure to the torn blood vessels in the extraction site and assists in their constriction and in the control of haemorrhage from the wound
- Do nothing to encourage the wound to start bleeding again – therefore the patient should refrain from exercise, alcohol, hot drinks, mouth rinsing and touching the wound for the next 24 h
- Hot salt water mouth washes – these start the day after the extraction and should be carried out at least 3 times daily for 3 days, to help clean the wound and encourage healing

- Refrain from smoking – there is an increased risk of developing a post-operative infection in the wound if the patient smokes while it is still raw
- Eating – the patient can eat once the local anaesthetic has worn off, but avoid the extraction site and take warm, bland foods only, so that the tissues are not irritated during healing
- Analgesics – the patient can take pain killers if necessary, but must not exceed the correct dose and must avoid aspirin-based products as these act as anticoagulants and allow bleeding to recur
- Problems – if there is severe pain, swelling or recurrent bleeding, contact the surgery for emergency advice, and treatment where necessary

BACKGROUND INFORMATION OF PROCEDURE – SURGICAL EXTRACTIONS

When a tooth has decayed such that caries extends into the roots, it is likely to fracture during a simple extraction attempt. Similarly, a heavily filled tooth is weak to the forces applied during extraction and may also fracture and disintegrate during the procedure.

Some teeth, especially multi-rooted posterior ones, have curved roots that make simple extraction difficult, as attempts to elevate it from the socket in one direction often locks the curved root in place.

Partially erupted teeth (and obviously unerupted ones) are, by definition, not fully through the gingivae, so access to their roots for extraction purposes is impossible.

In all these cases, the dentist resorts to some form of surgical technique to extract the tooth involved, ideally without leaving any pieces in situ.

DETAILS OF PROCEDURE – SURGICAL EXTRACTIONS

When a simple extraction cannot be performed because of curved roots, the dentist can often simply section the tooth into two or three separate roots (hemisection or trisection, respectively) and elevate each one as a single root, without the need for peeling the gingiva from the underlying bone as a full surgical procedure.

In all other cases of surgical extraction, some degree of gingival and possibly bone removal is necessary, so again local anaesthetic is required. Specialised surgical instruments are employed, and the dental nurse uses high speed suction and fine surgical tips to maintain moisture control and provide a clear operative field for the dentist.

Examples of the surgical instruments required during a surgical extraction are shown in Figure 7.4, although the micro-head and bur are not required for an extraction procedure.

TOOTH EXTRACTION

TECHNIQUE:

- A current radiograph of the tooth is placed on display for the dentist's reference
- The dentist, nurse and patient wear personal protective equipment

(continued)

TECHNIQUE: (*Continued*)

- Local anaesthetic is administered and allowed to take full effect
- The dental chair is angled so that the dentist and nurse have clear visibility of the tooth without straining, as surgical extractions can take considerable time
- The dentist cuts the surrounding gingiva with a scalpel blade and peels it back from the underlying bone using surgical instruments
- The dental nurse retracts the soft tissues and uses high speed suction to maintain a clear operative field
- The tooth roots are assessed and bone may be removed to improve access to them, usually using a surgical bur and handpiece with copious irrigation
- Once sufficient bone has been removed, the dentist uses a variety of elevators, luxators and forceps to remove the roots
- Ideally all the tooth and root pieces are removed, but just occasionally, small but very deeply placed root fragments may remain inaccesible without some considerable bone removal
- A decision may be made to leave these *in situ* and keep them under observation radiographically, rather than proceed with excessive bone removal that could weaken the jaw itself
- The patient is informed of this decision at the time
- Once the tooth and root removal is completed, the socket is checked for any loose bony sequestrae, which are removed
- The gingival tissue flap is sutured back into place to cover the underlying bone and allow healing to occur
- The patient is instructed to clamp onto a bite pack placed over the socket until haemostasis has been achieved
- Full verbal and written post-operative instructions are given to the patient

PATIENT AFTERCARE FOLLOWING A SURGICAL EXTRACTION

All the instructions relevant to a simple extraction procedure are given for surgical cases too, and the following information is additionally provided to patients undergoing surgical extractions:

- Post-operative pain and swelling – these are likely to occur, as with any surgical procedure, and should be managed with routine pain killers and anti-inflammatories as necessary
- Sutures – the majority of surgical extractions involve the use of sutures to assist the soft tissues to fully heal, and they must not be interfered with by the patient, but require removal by the oral health team after 7 to 10 days (although some types are available which 'dissolve' over time and therefore do not require removal)
- Post-operative infection – the deeper oral tissues are vulnerable to post-operative infection until the surgical site has healed fully, and the need for the patient to follow the instructions correctly cannot be over-emphasised

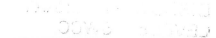

Chapter 9

Tooth replacement with dentures

REASON FOR PROCEDURE

Tooth replacement is necessary for several reasons, the main ones being to provide adequate masticatory function and to improve aesthetics. The absence of one or several teeth may also allow overloading of those remaining, so that excessive tooth wear or even tooth fractures occur. When a tooth is missing, those on either side of it can collapse into the space remaining so that the occlusion is altered, or those in the opposite dental arch can over-erupt into the space and cause unnatural wear of the remaining teeth.

Dentures are removable appliances made in several stages in a laboratory, designed to replace just one or several teeth, or a full dental arch in an edentulous patient. Unlike bridges, no tooth preparation is usually required for their construction as long as denture retention is available, and they can be removed from the patient's oral cavity for cleaning as necessary.

They are retained in the mouth by a film of saliva between the oral soft tissues and the denture surface providing suction, as well as by the muscular support of the cheeks, lips and tongue. When the patient has some natural teeth present, additional retention can also be provided by using metal clasps incorporated in the denture design to grip these standing teeth.

The base of the denture can be constructed using a pink or transparent acrylic material, or a very thin skeleton design of chrome-cobalt metal. The latter tends to be more comfortable to wear and more hygienic as less soft tissue is covered, but usually requires the additional retention provided by clasps on suitably positioned standing teeth.

The dentures discussed are:

- Full or partial acrylic dentures
- Full or partial chrome dentures
- Immediate replacement dentures

BACKGROUND INFORMATION OF PROCEDURE – ACRYLIC DENTURES

Acrylic dentures (Figure 9.1) are the more common type of dentures provided, as they are cheaper and more easily constructed than chrome dentures. They are also more easily

Basic Guide to Dental Procedures, Second Edition. Carole Hollins.
© 2015 John Wiley & Sons, Ltd. Published 2015 by John Wiley & Sons, Ltd.

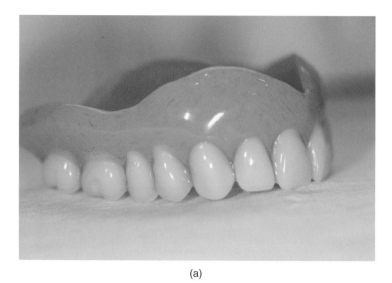

(a)

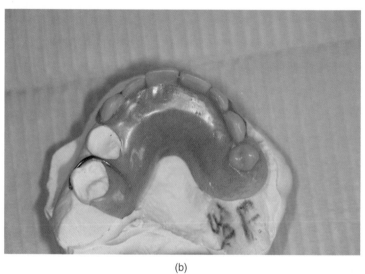

(b)

Figure 9.1 Examples of acrylic dentures. (a) Full upper denture. (b) Partial upper denture with clasp, on model

adjusted to fit as necessary, as well as being more amenable to relining and tooth addition as the patient's oral cavity alters with time. However, they can fracture during normal usage in patients with heavy bites, as well as if they are inadvertently dropped while out of the mouth.

None the less, acrylic dentures fulfil their necessary functions of restoring the patient's occlusion so that adequate mastication is possible, as well as improving their appearance, especially when anterior teeth are missing.

Whether one tooth, several teeth or all of the dental arch is to be replaced, the construction procedure for an acrylic denture is basically the same.

DETAILS OF PROCEDURE – ACRYLIC DENTURES

The denture construction normally takes up to five appointments, as each stage has to be sent to a laboratory for the next stage to be constructed. Where a partial denture is being made, the tooth shade is chosen to match that of the remaining standing teeth, but when full dentures are being provided, any shade can be chosen although the dentist tends to advise a natural creamy shade rather than a more unnatural stark white one.

TECHNIQUE:

- The dentist, nurse and patient wear personal protective equipment at each appointment
- The dental chair is kept upright for patient comfort, as well as being the ideal position for the dentist to access the oral cavity for this procedure
- Initial impressions are taken in alginate material and sent to the laboratory for study model casting and the provision of personalised impression trays to be constructed, as well as wax bite recording rims (Figure 9.2)
- The equipment and materials required for the impression-taking stage are shown in Figure 4.11
- At the next appointment, accurate impressions are taken in one of the elastomeric impression materials available, using the specially constructed impression trays, and the final decision on tooth shade and shape is made by the dentist and the patient
- Occlusal bite recording is carried out using the wax bite rims, so that a partially dentate patient has the same bite with the denture as without, and an edentulous patient can have the bite set at a comfortable position to allow speech and mastication, without the jaws being closed up or opened too much
- The equipment and materials required for the bite recording stage are shown in Figure 9.3
- Wax bite rims are warmed and stuck together during the bite recording process, and once placed onto the study models, the technician can reproduce the patient's bite accurately
- In complicated cases, the study models may be mounted onto an articulator at the laboratory
- At the next appointment, a waxed-up try-in of the denture is provided, with the teeth set at the previously recorded occlusion and in the shade and shape chosen (Figure 9.4)
- The fit of the denture is assessed for accuracy, although it feels slack to the patient as the wax base warms in the mouth
- The occlusion and aesthetics of the denture are assessed, and any minor adjustments carried out at the chairside by simply selectively warming the wax bases and adjusting the teeth as necessary
- If any major adjustments are required, the try-in is returned to the laboratory with details of the adjustments required, and a re-try appointment is arranged
- Once the dentist and patient are happy with the try-in, it is returned to the laboratory where a flasking process is carried out to replace the wax base with the permanent acrylic material, as the final construction stage of the denture

(continued)

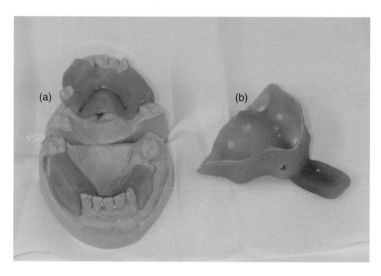

Figure 9.2 Second stage of denture construction. (a) Wax bite rims on models. (b) Special trays

TECHNIQUE: (*Continued*)

- If metal clasps are being used for additional retention with a partial denture, they are usually added at this final stage, although some laboratories add them at the try-in stage
- At the final appointment, the completed denture is checked for any sharp edges or specks on the fitting surface before being tried in the patient's mouth, as these would cause soft tissue trauma with time, if left
- The equipment and materials required for the fitting of the denture are shown in Figure 9.5
- The denture is then tried in the patient's mouth and assessed for accuracy of fit, function and aesthetics
- Minor occlusal adjustments can be carried out using an acrylic trimming bur and the slow speed handpiece, so that the patient has an even occlusion around the full dental arch
- Post-operative verbal and written care and cleaning instructions are given to the patient

BACKGROUND INFORMATION OF PROCEDURE – CHROME DENTURES

Chrome dentures (Figure 9.6) provide a strong alternative to acrylic in those patients with such a heavy bite that they continually fracture their denture base. As chrome can also be constructed as a relatively thin base compared to acrylic, it is also the material of choice in patients who gag easily while wearing dentures.

As the chrome is so strong, the denture can be designed to have minimal soft tissue coverage and be specifically designed not to cover the gingival margins of the teeth, where

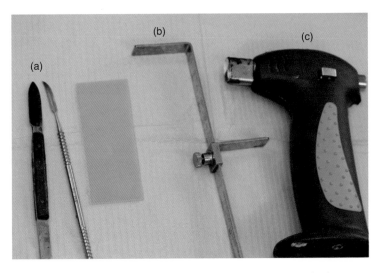

Figure 9.3 Equipment and materials for the bite recording stage. (a) Wax knife, carver and pink wax. (b) Bite gauge. (c) Heat source

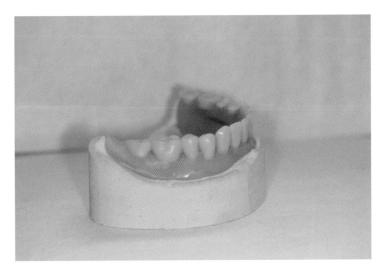

Figure 9.4 Try-in stage of lower full denture

TOOTH REPLACEMENT WITH DENTURES

plaque accumulates very easily. Consequently, chrome dentures are far more hygienic for the patient, and more tissue-friendly to the gingivae.

The construction of a chrome partial denture is similar to that of an acrylic one, but is less amenable to any inaccuracies of design and fit, as once the chrome-cobalt base has been cast, it cannot be added to or adjusted.

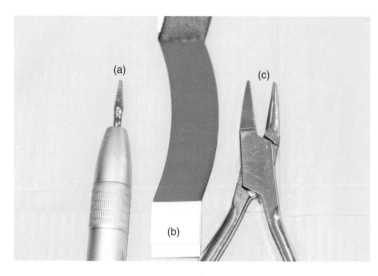

Figure 9.5 Equipment and materials for the fitting stage. (a) Straight hand piece and acrylic bur. (b) Articulating paper. (c) Pliers to adjust clasps

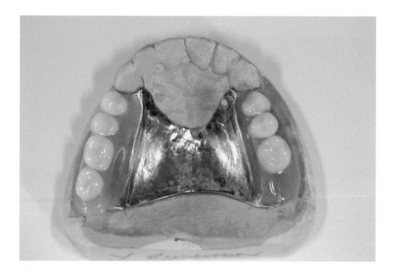

Figure 9.6 Example of chrome-cobalt partial denture on model

DETAILS OF PROCEDURE – CHROME DENTURES

The denture construction normally takes up to five appointments, with each stage being sent to a laboratory, as with acrylic dentures. Second impressions must be taken using the special trays made from the study models, as these must be accurate for the chrome base to be constructed well and to fit correctly.

TECHNIQUE:

- The dentist, nurse and patient wear personal protective equipment for each appointment
- The dental chair is kept upright for patient comfort and ease of access for the dentist
- Initial impressions are taken in alginate material and sent to the laboratory for casting of study models, construction of special impression trays and wax bite recording rims
- In partially dentate patients, the denture design is developed to make use of all naturally retentive features by placing clasps on suitable, undercut teeth
- At the next appointment, accurate impressions are taken in the special trays, using one of the many elastomeric impression materials available, such as silicone or polyether
- Occlusal bite recording is carried out using the wax rims, either to maintain the same occlusion or to adjust it accordingly for an edentulous patient
- Again, these can be mounted on an articulator in the laboratory by the technician, if necessary
- The final decision on shade and tooth shape is made by the dentist and the patient
- At the next appointment, the chrome-cobalt base design, including all clasps, is available to try in the patient's mouth for accuracy of fit and design
- Any discrepancies in the metal base requires a re-casting to be carried out by the laboratory
- The teeth may also have been added at this stage for a wax try-in, or may be added as an additional stage once the metal work has been approved
- The occlusion and aesthetics of the denture are assessed once the tooth try-in is received, and any minor adjustments made at the chairside (Figure 9.7)
- Once the dentist and patient are happy with both the metal and tooth try-in, it is returned to the laboratory for the flasking process to join the metal base to the acrylic gingivae and teeth
- At the final appointment, the completed denture is checked once again for accuracy of fit, function and aesthetics
- Minor occlusal adjustments can be carried out using an acrylic trimming bur and the slow speed handpiece, but the metal base should need no adjustments
- Post-operative verbal and written care and cleaning instructions are given to the patient

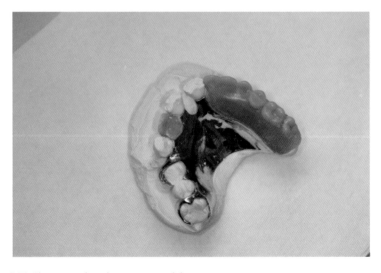

Figure 9.7 Chrome and tooth try-in on model

BACKGROUND INFORMATION OF PROCEDURE – IMMEDIATE REPLACEMENT DENTURES

As their name suggests, immediate replacement dentures are those that are fitted at the time that one or several teeth are extracted. They are usually provided when a patient is to lose one or several anterior teeth and requires the extracted teeth to be replaced at the same time for aesthetics, rather than have visible, unsightly spaces for a while.

Although the aesthetic concerns of the patient are very understandable in these circumstances, it has to be accepted that the resulting denture will not be as accurate a fit as if it had been constructed conventionally – after the tooth extraction and following a suitable period of tissue healing.

Due to the usual event of bone resorption occurring after the extraction, the denture also becomes slack relatively quickly and requires relining or even remaking at some point.

As these alterations are expected to be required, the immediate replacement denture is always made from acrylic, which can be quite easily added to and adjusted.

When significant bone resorption has occured, usually after 4 to 6 months, a new denture can be constructed in chrome-cobalt if required.

DETAILS OF PROCEDURE – IMMEDIATE REPLACEMENT DENTURES

The appliance construction follows similar stages to that of a conventional acrylic denture, except that there may be no possibility nor requirement for a try-in if no other teeth are missing except those to be immediately replaced by the denture.

It is imperative that the completed denture is ready for fitting on the day that the patient is due to have the extractions carried out, and this must be checked (as well as that the correct teeth have been incorporated into the denture construction) before the patient's teeth are extracted.

TECHNIQUE:

- The dentist, nurse and patient wear personal protective equipment for each appointment
- The dental chair is kept upright for patient comfort and ease of access for the dentist
- Initial impressions are taken in alginate material, and sent to the laboratory for study model casting and possibly for special tray construction
- A special tray may not be necessary if only one tooth is to be immediately replaced, as the completed denture is expected to be less accurate than a conventional one anyway
- Similarly, wax bite rims may also not be necessary if the study models can easily be placed into the correct occlusion without them
- In these simple, one-tooth cases, it is usual to take a shade at the initial impression stage and proceed directly to the final acrylic construction of the denture
- Otherwise, the second accurate impression and occlusal bite recording are carried out at the next appointment, as usual
- The final decision on tooth shade is made by the dentist and the patient, and the technician copies the tooth shapes from the study models

TOOTH REPLACEMENT WITH DENTURES

- At the next appointment, a waxed try-in of any teeth already missing is provided, but of course the teeth to be immediately replaced cannot be present at this stage
- The try-in is checked for accuracy of fit, occlusion and aesthetics as far as possible, and any minor adjustments are carried out at the chairside
- Once the try-in and study models are returned to the laboratory for completion of the denture, the technician carefully removes the teeth to be extracted from the model and replaces them with suitable denture teeth, ensuring that the occlusion is not altered during the process
- The flasking process is carried out to replace the wax base with the permanent acrylic of the denture
- At the final appointment, the teeth to be replaced are extracted under local anaesthesia, and once haemostasis has been achieved, the denture is inserted into the patient's mouth
- The aesthetics are checked, and the fit and occlusion are checked as far as possible, bearing in mind the patient is still numb from the local anaesthetic
- Post-operative verbal and written care and cleaning instructions are given to the patient, and a review appointment is provisionally made so that any problems that become apparent once the local anaesthetic has worn off can be corrected

AFTERCARE OF DENTURES

Any type of denture is designed to be a removable appliance, one that the patient can take out of the mouth for cleaning purposes as well as to leave out overnight. Acrylic partial dentures are designed to fit around any standing teeth, and these areas allow plaque to accumulate and cause either localised caries of standing teeth or periodontal disease if the plaque is not removed promptly.

As chrome dentures are usually designed to cover less oral soft tissue, they tend to allow less plaque accumulations to develop. Plaque is still produced in patients with no natural teeth of their own and once mineralised into tartar, deposits can often be seen as a yellow crusty layer in the centre of lower full dentures or at the sides of upper full dentures. Tartar forms in these areas as they are close to the openings of various salivary glands in the mouth, and saliva provides the minerals for plaque to harden into tartar.

Dentures should be cleaned at least twice daily, using either a specific denture paste or ordinary toothpaste with a toothbrush. They are best cleaned over a bowl of water to avoid breakages if dropped, and should be rinsed well before reinserting.

The important surface of the denture to be cleaned is that which covers the oral soft tissues – the roof of the mouth with upper dentures or the bony ridge of the lower jaw with lower dentures. These areas are in contact with the soft tissues whenever the dentures are worn, and any food debris or plaque that is left in these areas allows microorganisms to flourish, in particular a fungus which causes oral thrush and denture stomatitis ('denture sore mouth').

Tiny perforations and scratches in the acrylic elements of dentures that occur over time also allow staining to develop, especially with products such as tea, coffee and red wine.

Various denture soaking agents are available for use overnight to assist with cleaning and stain removal (Figure 9.8), but care should be taken with bleach-based ones which are not suitable for chrome dentures, as they cause metal corrosion with time.

TOOTH REPLACEMENT WITH DENTURES

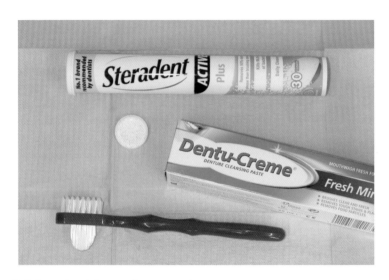

Figure 9.8 Examples of denture cleaning products

Chapter 10

Tooth replacement with implants

REASON FOR PROCEDURE

Missing teeth can be replaced using bridges, dentures or implants. Each technique has its own advantages and disadvantages, but they are all required for the same reasons – to provide adequate masticatory function and to improve aesthetics.

Implants are the most advanced technique of tooth replacement, although their use has been developing over at least the last 30 years. They involve the surgical placement of a threaded titanium cylinder (implant) into the jaw bone, which then has an abutment screwed into its top end to project into the oral cavity. This abutment then forms the attachment for either a crown replacing a single tooth, a bridge retainer replacing several teeth, or an overdenture replacing many if not all the teeth in a dental arch.

The advantages that implants have over other methods of tooth replacement are that they can be used in patients without having to cut into adjacent teeth to construct bridgework, and in patients with very poor retention for conventional dentures.

However, these more complicated cases can involve all of the following:

- Oral and/or periodontal surgeon
- Specialist in prosthetics
- Advanced computerised radiographic techniques
- Specialist implant laboratory

The procedure described is for the more simple replacement of a single tooth only.

BACKGROUND INFORMATION OF PROCEDURE – SINGLE TOOTH IMPLANT

Even when a single tooth is to be replaced, a detailed dental and radiographic assessment of the patient must be carried out by the dentist beforehand. This determines the feasibility

Basic Guide to Dental Procedures, Second Edition. Carole Hollins.
© 2015 John Wiley & Sons, Ltd. Published 2015 by John Wiley & Sons, Ltd.

of placing the implant and its likelihood of success, as well as the suitability of the patient for the procedure and likelihood of complying with the long term care of the restoration.

The initial placement of the implant cylinder is a full surgical technique, and is usually left *in situ* for up to 6 months while the jaw bone grows around it to anchor it firmly. Only then is the abutment attached and the single tooth crown constructed and placed.

During the interim period, the patient is provided with either a temporary denture or a temporary etch retained bridge, to replace the missing tooth and sit comfortably over the implant head.

However, more recently, a technique is being developed whereby the implant cylinder is placed at the time of tooth extraction, and then a single temporary crown is fitted over the top. This can only be done when the replaced tooth is kept free from occlusal loading, so that the bony attachment between implant and jaw bone can occur.

DETAILS OF PROCEDURE – SINGLE TOOTH IMPLANT

Only those dentists who have been suitably trained to provide implants undertake the procedure, as the technique is a specialised field that is not covered by undergraduate training.

In a normal situation, the patient has an anterior tooth already missing and replaced either by a denture or an acid etch retained bridge. The latter is removed intact before the implant placement, and then adjusted as necessary and reattached while the healing process occurs. All necessary radiographs and study models are taken and assessed beforehand.

Specialist surgical instruments and equipment are required, and the dental nurse provides good moisture control throughout the procedure.

An example of an implant kit containing various items such as bone drills, locators, and various sizes of implant cylinder is shown in Figure 10.1.

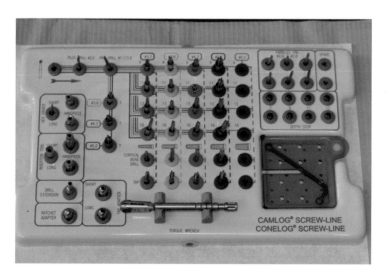

Figure 10.1 Example of implant kit

TOOTH REPLACEMENT WITH IMPLANTS

TECHNIQUE:

- Current radiographs of the implant site are available for reference by the dentist, and the implant dimensions and required angulation of insertion previously determined
- The dentist, nurse and patient wear personal protective equipment at each appointment
- As the implant placement technique is a full surgical procedure, the dentist and nurse wear sterile gowns over their uniforms, as well as sterile hair covers and sterile (surgical grade) gloves (Figure 10.2)
- The patient drapes are also single-use and sterile, rather than the usual clinical (non-sterile) type
- The dental chair is placed at an angle to allow easy and comfortable access for the dentist and nurse, as well as full visibility of the operative site
- Local anaesthetic is administered to all the surrounding oral soft tissues and allowed to take full effect
- The dentist cuts the surrounding gingiva with a scalpel blade and peels it back from the underlying bone, using surgical instruments (see Figure 7.4a, b, and d)
- The dental nurse carefully retracts the soft tissues and uses high speed suction to maintain a clear operative field, and provide copious irrigation during bone surgery

(continued)

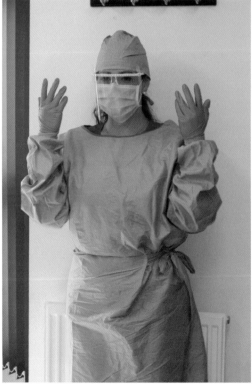

Figure 10.2 Personal protective equipment suitable for an implant procedure

TOOTH REPLACEMENT WITH IMPLANTS

TECHNIQUE: (Continued)

- The irrigation solution for the procedure is provided as a bag of sterile fluid which is connected to the specialised hand piece equipment (Figure 10.3)
- The jaw bone ridge is flattened at the point where the implant is to be inserted
- A hole is drilled into the jaw bone at the correct angulation and to the correct depth, using specialised implant drills (mill)
- The prepared depth is checked using a calibrated depth gauge
- The chosen implant is driven into the jaw bone using specialised insert instruments and a surgical hammer, and a radiograph shows its correct positioning (Figure 10.4)
- The gingival tissue flaps are repositioned to close the surgical site, with just the implant head projecting through (Figure 10.5)
- If the missing tooth requires replacement during the healing process, the implant head is covered with a plastic cap, and either a temporary denture or a temporary etch retained bridge is placed
- Full verbal and written post-operative instructions are given to the patient
- Following 3 months of healing and the natural attachment of the implant to the surrounding jaw bone, the plastic cap is removed and a suitable abutment is screwed into the implant cylinder

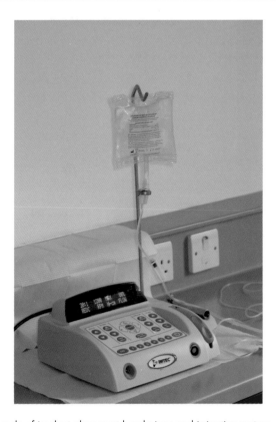

Figure 10.3 Example of implant placement hand piece and irrigation system

TOOTH REPLACEMENT WITH IMPLANTS

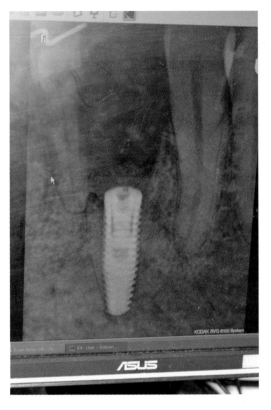

Figure 10.4 Radiograph showing position of implant cylinder

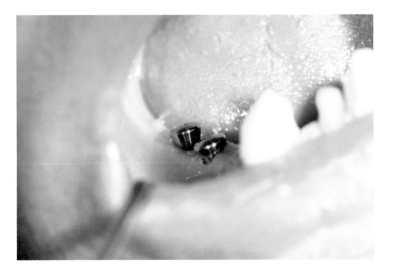

Figure 10.5 Implant head in place

TECHNIQUE: (*Continued*)

- Its shape is that of a conventionally prepared crown core, and its size is dictated by the adjacent tooth positions and the patient's occlusion
- An accurate impression is taken of the abutment and the adjacent teeth, using a silicone or polyether elastomeric material, and an opposing arch impression and occlusion are recorded in the usual way as for a conventional crown or bridge preparation
- The technician constructs the crown in the laboratory, using the same procedure as for a conventional crown
- At the final appointment, the crown is cemented onto the abutment after checking for fit, function and aesthetics and appears no different from a conventional crown cemented to a tooth (see Figure 6.5)
- Full verbal and written post-operative instructions are given to the patient

AFTERCARE OF IMPLANTS

Although the implant cannot be affected by caries, it can develop plaque accumulations around it and allow a periodontal infection to occur. Ultimately this can result in the formation of periodontal pockets around the implant, destruction of the bone-implant attachment, and loosening of the implant itself.

As with real teeth, the prevention of periodontal infection depends on a consistently high standard of oral hygiene being carried out by the patient. This should include correct toothbrushing, the use of interdental cleaning aids around the implant and the use of a good quality toothpaste and mouthwash.

Where bridges are supported by implants, the gingival ridge beneath any areas of missing teeth is cleaned using Superfloss in a similar way to that used for conventional bridges (see Figure 6.6).

Regular dental examinations should be carried out of both the real teeth and the implant, and regular oral hygiene reinforcement and scaling as necessary.

TOOTH REPLACEMENT WITH IMPLANTS

Chapter 11

Tooth alignment with orthodontic appliances

REASON FOR PROCEDURE

Although a patient's desire for straight teeth is usually based on aesthetics, there are several dental advantages to aligning uneven teeth. Crooked and crowded teeth provide lots of potential areas for plaque to accumulate that would not exist if the dental arch was well aligned. It takes a consistently high standard of oral hygiene for life in these cases to prevent any carious or periodontal damage from occurring with time, as each crooked tooth and crowded area requires individual attention during every toothbrushing session.

When teeth are severely crowded, they sometimes do not bite together well enough for the patient to chew food efficiently, and in very severe cases where the jaw sizes do not match, the patient may also experience speech difficulties. These severe cases often benefit from a combined approach of orthodontics and jaw surgery.

When the bottom jaw bites too far behind its normal position, the upper anterior teeth appear to project forwards quite prominently (proclined), and these upper teeth are vulnerable to trauma or even fracture by being so positioned (Figure 11.1).

Finally, the psychological well-being of the patient should be considered in severe cases, where the malocclusion is responsible for excessively low self-esteem and may be the cause of childhood teasing or even bullying.

The simpler techniques used for tooth alignment are:

- Removable appliances
- Conventional fixed appliances
- Short-term cosmetic fixed appliances
- Non-brace techniques – aligners

BACKGROUND INFORMATION OF PROCEDURE – REMOVABLE APPLIANCES

Removable appliances are made from an acrylic base with metal attachments to provide retention and are similar to acrylic dentures. They have additional metal components

Basic Guide to Dental Procedures, Second Edition. Carole Hollins.
© 2015 John Wiley & Sons, Ltd. Published 2015 by John Wiley & Sons, Ltd.

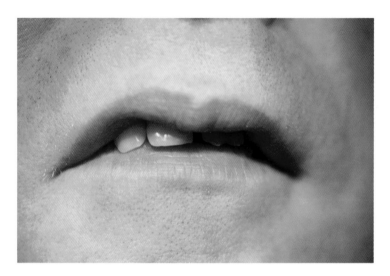

Figure 11.1 Proclined incisors with damage evident to the left tooth

incorporated as necessary to carry out the required tooth movement to be achieved, and these can be one of a variety of springs, screw devices, or adjustable metal bars (Figure 11.2).

These components are checked and adjusted by the dentist on a regular basis to effect tooth movement.

Where severe crowding is present in the dental arch, it may be necessary for tooth extraction to be carried out before an appliance is fitted. This creates the space required to reposition the other teeth and align the arch.

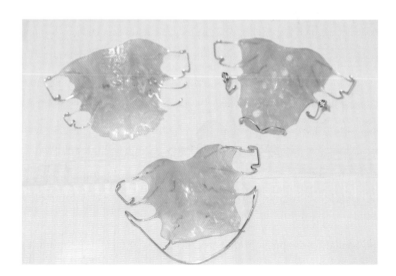

Figure 11.2 Examples of removable appliances

The amount of movement possible with a removable appliance is sufficient in many cases to fully correct malaligned teeth, but the force applied is limited by the appliance being removable – if too much force is applied, the brace is not stable in the mouth. It is then that a fixed appliance is required.

Whichever type of appliance is planned, many new plaque retention areas are created in the patient's oral cavity and it is imperative that a consistently good standard of oral hygiene and diet control are practised throughout the course of orthodontic treatment.

Poor oral hygiene is the main factor that prevents many patients from being offerred orthodontic treatment, no matter how great their need.

DETAILS OF PROCEDURE – REMOVABLE APPLIANCES

The dentist carries out an oral, photographic and radiographic assessment of the patient beforehand, and determines the orthodontic treatment required and the appliance necessary to achieve it by taking study model impressions and studying the casts produced. The need for any tooth extractions is decided, and then the full treatment course is put to the patient to decide whether to undergo orthodontic treatment. This includes the need for the appliance to be worn at all times except during meals, and the necessity of good diet control and oral hygiene throughout the full course of treatment.

If the patient is amenable to the propsed course of treatment, the removable appliance can be constructed.

TECHNIQUE:

- The dentist, nurse and patient wear personal protective equipment at each appointment
- Alginate impressions are taken of both dental arches for the technician to produce the working casts (see Figure 4.10)
- The written design of the appliance is sent with the impressions
- The patient receives oral hygiene instruction and dietary advice, usually from the dental nurse
- At the next appointment, the new appliance is checked for accuracy of its design and then tried in the patient's mouth (Figure 11.3)
- Once comfortably tight, any metal components involved in tooth movement are activated by the dentist and the treatment commences (Figure 11.4)
- Specific oral hygiene instruction is given for the appliance itself, as well as the wearing details
- At each appointment thereafter, the dentist checks the progress of the tooth movement against the original study casts to ensure it is progressing correctly
- Retentive cribs are tightened to ensure the appliance is not loose, and active components are adjusted accordingly
- Various instruments may be required during a removable appliance fit or adjustment procedure
- Once the tooth movement required is achieved, a retainer is provided to hold the teeth in their new positions until they have settled into alignment
- The retainer can either be the deactivated removable appliance itself, or a soft gum shield type, both of which are usually worn at night only

TOOTH ALIGNMENT WITH
ORTHODONTIC APPLIANCES

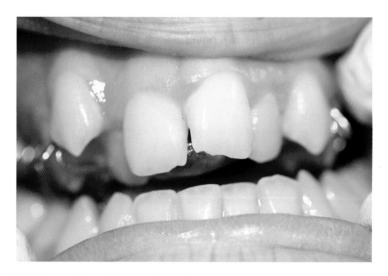

Figure 11.3 Removable appliance in the mouth

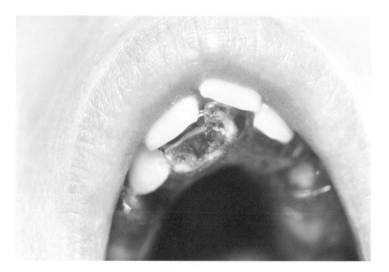

Figure 11.4 Activated spring on the right incisor

BACKGROUND INFORMATION OF PROCEDURE – CONVENTIONAL FIXED APPLIANCES

As their name suggests, fixed appliances are actually bonded onto the patient's teeth for the duration of the orthodontic treatment. In this way, greater force can be applied

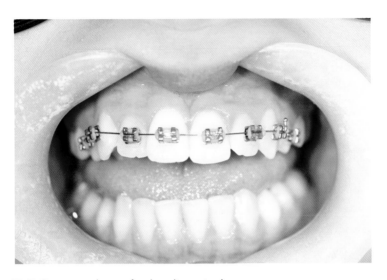

Figure 11.5 Conventional upper fixed appliance in place

and more severely malaligned teeth corrected than can be achieved with removable appliances alone.

However, greater care is needed by the patient during normal day-to-day activities so as not to dislodge any components of the appliance, as it cannot be removed for meals, cleaning or during sport sessions as a removable appliance can. Similarly, a low sugar and acid diet must be strictly followed, as the number of plaque retentive areas created by a fixed appliance is large, and caries can easily occur.

Conventional fixed appliances tend to be used in child and teenage patients rather than adults and aim to produce an 'ideal' occlusion in both arches, as well as aligning poorly positioned or crowded teeth.

The fixed appliance consists of individual metal brackets and bands that are harmlessly bonded onto each tooth in exactly the correct position, and joined together by tying a continuous archwire into each component (Figure 11.5). The wire carefully guides the movement of each tooth along it, gradually aligning the dental arch as it does so. The wire is changed on a regular basis by the dentist, using thicker, less flexible ones as the treatment progresses.

As with removable appliances, tooth extraction may have been required to create space in the dental arch first.

DETAILS OF PROCEDURE – FIXED APPLIANCES

The dentist carries out an oral, photographic and radiographic assessment of the patient beforehand, and determines the order and progression of the archwires required, using the initial study casts. The need for any tooth extractions is decided upon and discussed with the patient while presenting the treatment plan. The strict diet and oral hygiene

TOOTH ALIGNMENT WITH
ORTHODONTIC APPLIANCES

control necessary throughout the course of treatment is also explained, and then the patient decides whether to proceed with the full course of orthodontic treatment. If the patient is amenable to the treatment proposed, the fixed appliance can be fitted.

The components of a conventional fixed appliance are shown in Figure 11.6.

The instruments and materials required to bond a conventional fixed appliance are shown in Figure 11.7.

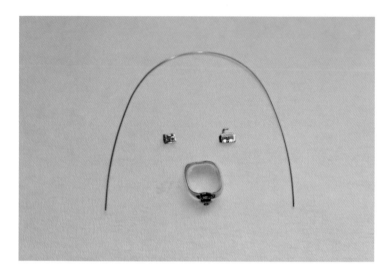

Figure 11.6 Components of a conventional fixed appliance

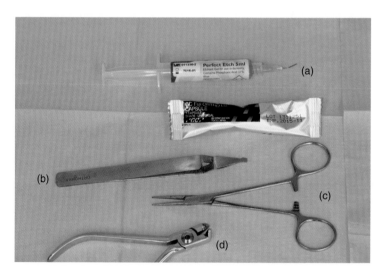

Figure 11.7 Examples of materials and instruments for fixed appliance procedures. (a) Acid etch and bonding material. (b) Bracket holders. (c) Elastic holders. (d) Archwire cutters

TECHNIQUE:

- The dentist, nurse and patient wear personal protective equipment at each appointment
- The dental chair is placed supine for ease of access, and good moisture control is provided throughout the bonding appointment using low speed suction and cotton wool rolls
- The decision is made previously with regard to whether just one or both dental arches are to be bonded at the same appointment
- The teeth are blown dry and a spot of acid etch is applied to the centre of the labial surface of each tooth in the dental arch
- The etch is washed off and carefully collected using high speed suction, then the teeth are dried again
- Individual brackets are then bonded one at a time to each tooth, in exactly the correct position and at the correct angulation for each tooth, using a special orthodontic material similar to either composite or glass ionomer materials
- Any bands required are sized on the tooth and then cemented firmly into place using any material that is used for crown cementation
- Once all the tooth attachments are firmly in place, the first archwire is positioned and tied onto each attachment using special elastic loops
- The first archwire is usually the thinnest and most flexible available, as it needs to be accurately distorted into each attachment, no matter how malaligned the teeth sit in the dental arch
- The archwire ends are trimmed to avoid sticking into the patient's cheeks
- Detailed oral hygiene instructions are given for the thorough cleaning of the appliance, without dislodging it
- This task may be carried out by a suitably trained dental nurse as an extended duty skill, and is discussed in detail in Chapter 13
- At each appointment thereafter, progress is checked against the original study casts to ensure the required tooth movement is proceeding correctly
- The archwire is replaced as necessary with a gradually thicker and less flexible successor, as the dental arch gradually aligns
- Once the tooth movement required has been achieved, a retainer is constructed for each dental arch to hold the teeth in their new positions until they have settled into alignment
- The retainer may be a soft gum shield type, to be worn at night only, or may be a fixed wire bonded to the backs of the teeth for a firmer method of retention
- In recent years it is the norm to provide post-orthodontic tooth retention for life to avoid any relapse, rather than just for a set period of time
- Both arches are then de-bonded, final models and photographs are taken, and the fixed retainers are cemented into place or the removable retainers are given to the patient
- If necessary, the teeth are scaled and polished to remove any residual plaque or tartar

BACKGROUND INFORMATION OF PROCEDURE – SHORT-TERM COSMETIC FIXED APPLIANCES

For adult patients, the concept of having to wear conventional fixed appliances for up to 2 years to align their teeth is usually enough to dissuade them from undergoing this type of treatment, but very often their only complaint is the appearance of their front teeth alone. Their posterior occlusion (the way their back teeth bite together) has developed and become stable years earlier, so there is often no requirement to adjust the back sections

TOOTH ALIGNMENT WITH
ORTHODONTIC APPLIANCES

of the dental arches, and consequently a second type of fixed appliance treatment has been developed for these patients, which has the following advantages over conventional treatment:

- As only the front teeth are to be re-positioned, the treatment time is greatly reduced and the technique is actually referred to as short-term orthodontics
- In carefully chosen cases, the treatment time is usually between 4 and 9 months, with an average of 6 months (hence the phrase 'six month smiles')
- The back teeth are not moved during the treatment so the occlusion remains stable, as it was before treatment began
- The space required to align the front teeth is provided by careful trimming and adjustment of individual tooth widths as the treatment progresses, and only in rare cases is tooth extraction required
- The components of the fixed appliance used in short-term orthodontcis are aesthetically acceptable to adult patients, as they are all tooth-coloured

However, not all cases are suitable to be treated with this technique and the dentist chooses those which are appropriate with great care. Children and teenagers are treated using conventional fixed appliance therapy so that the ideal occlusion is developed.

DETAILS OF PROCEDURE – SHORT-TERM COSMETIC FIXED APPLIANCES

The dentist carries out an oral, photographic and radiographic assessment of the patient beforehand and discusses with the patient the main complaint so that the treatment parameters are determined. Impressions are taken in alginate to provide a set of

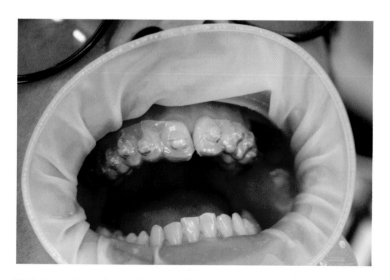

Figure 11.8 Prepared quadrant of short-term fixed appliance

TOOTH ALIGNMENT WITH ORTHODONTIC APPLIANCES

pre-treatment study models (see Figure 4.10), and a second set of impressions is taken using a more accurate material such as silicone. These are sent to a specialised laboratory where the working models are cast and used to construct the fixed appliance itself.

In the laboratory, the technician carefully places each bracket onto each model tooth in the same way as the dentist does when bonding a conventional fixed appliance in the surgery. Once placed, the brackets are secured into their positions with two warmed sheets of rubbery material that are drawn down over the models under vacuum. When cooled, these sheets are trimmed and split in the midline to produce a quadrant of the appliance for each area of the mouth to be treated: left and right upper arch and/or lower arch (Figure 11.8). These are then returned to the dentist so that they can be bonded to the patient's teeth.

The bonding technique is very similar to that used for conventional fixed appliances, as are the instruments and materials required (see Figure 11.7).

TECHNIQUE:

- The dentist, nurse and patient wear personal protective equipment at each appointment
- The dental chair is placed supine for ease of access, and good moisture control is provided throughout the bonding appointment using low speed suction, cotton wool rolls and a full mouth soft tissue retractor
- The teeth in one quadrant are blown dry and a spot of acid etch is applied to the centre of the labial surface of each tooth
- The etch is washed off and carefully collected using high speed suction and the teeth are dried again
- A thin layer of adhesive is then painted onto each etched tooth
- Meantime, the dental nurse applies the bonding cement to the brackets in the quadrant that is being bonded
- The tray is then seated onto the quadrant of teeth and the cement is set using a curing light
- Once all four quadrants have been bonded, the double trays are carefully peeled off the teeth, leaving the brackets in their correct positions on each tooth
- Excess cement is carefully removed, and any necessary tooth trimming is carried out to begin creating the space necessary to resolve the tooth crowding
- The archiwre is then tied into each bracket in a similar way to that of conventional fixed appliances
- The bonded appliance is shown in Figure 11.9
- In cases where the lower arch brackets interfere with the patient's full bite, small bumps of composite filling material are placed to prop the bite open slightly while the teeth move into better positions – these bumps are then removed once the bite has adjusted and the brackets are safe from being knocked by the upper teeth
- Detailed oral hygiene instructions are given for the thorough cleaning of the appliance, without dislodging it
- At each appointment thereafter, progress is checked against the original study models, any necessary tooth trimming is carried out to allow the crowded teeth to align, and new archwires are placed
- Once the tooth movement required has been achieved, both a fixed retainer and a removable soft gum shield retainer are provided for each arch, and is worn for life to prevent relapse of the tooth positions
- Both arches are then de-bonded, final models and photographs are taken, and the fixed retainers are cemented into place
- If necessary, the teeth are scaled and polished to remove any residual plaque or tartar

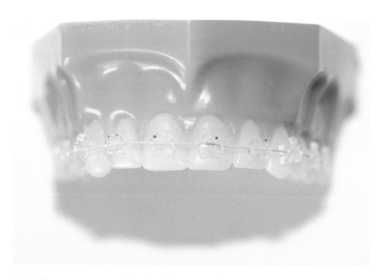

Figure 11.9 Short-term cosmetic fixed appliance in place on model

BACKGROUND INFORMATION OF PROCEDURE – ALIGNERS

For those adult patients who do not wish to wear any form of orthodontic appliance fixed to their teeth, even cosmetic ones, a technique of achieving tooth movement using a series of pre-formed, retainer-like appliances has been developed. These are called 'aligners'. In skilled hands, a wide range of tooth movement can be carried out with this technique, without the patients having anything bonded to their teeth, but movements such as de-rotation of twisted teeth are particularly difficult to achieve. Nevertheless, aligners are a useful alternative to fixed appliances for suitable adult patients.

DETAILS OF PROCEDURE – ALIGNERS

The dentist carries out an oral, photographic and radiographic assessment of the patient beforehand, and discusses the patient's treatment aims to determine the suitability of this type of orthodontic treatment.

Impressions are taken in alginate to provide a set of pre-treatment study models (see Figure 4.10), and a second set of impressions are taken using a more accurate material such as silicone. These second impressions are sent to a specialised laboratory where the working models are cast and used to produce the series of aligners required to straighten the teeth in each arch.

The working models are scanned in three dimensions into a specialised computer programme, which then automatically produces an image of the perfectly aligned arches. The computer then determines the tooth movements required to go from the initial arches to the aligned arches, and produces a set of gum shield-like aligners which must be worn in sequence over a set period of time to produce the aligned arch results. These are then sent back to the dentist, who ensures that the patient can insert and remove the first aligner correctly, and so the treatment begins.

Some patients are capable enough to have the full set of aligners handed over at this appointment, knowing the sequence to follow and how long each one must be worn for before moving onto the next one, but the majority re-attend to have the aligners fitted sequentially by the dentist.

No special oral hygiene techniques are required as the aligners are removed for cleaning and tooth brushing, but the patients must ensure that they clean their teeth after each meal before re-inserting the current aligner so that food debris is not inadvertently trapped beneath it and does not cause tooth cavities to develop.

At the end of the treatment, the final aligner acts as the retainer.

AFTERCARE OF ORTHODONTIC BRACES

As with acrylic dentures, removable appliances are cleaned with a toothbrush and fluoride toothpaste over a bowl of water after each meal. This is especially important at bedtime as the orthodontic appliance must be worn over night. The patients must also clean their own teeth thoroughly after each meal while the appliance is out, in the usual manner – see Chapter 2.

Fixed appliances have to be thoroughly cleaned *in situ* after each meal, using a combination of toothbrush, fluoride toothpaste, and interdental brushes used specifically to clean beneath the archwire itself – see Chapter 13 for details.

Some good quality electric toothbrushes have special orthodontic heads for use by the patient during the course of orthodontic treatment (Figure 11.10).

Patients with removable appliances are advised to store the brace in a rigid container while out of their mouth at mealtimes or during sport sessions, to avoid breakages. Fixed

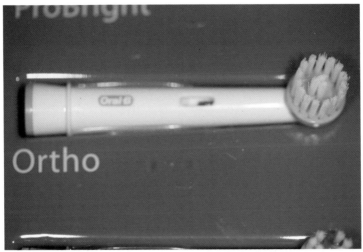

Figure 11.10 Orthodontic head for an electric toothbrush

TOOTH ALIGNMENT WITH
ORTHODONTIC APPLIANCES

appliances can be protected from damage during sport sessions using specially designed shields that fit over them in the mouth. These also prevent soft tissue trauma if the patient inadvertently receives a blow to the mouth; however, contact sports are best avoided during the course of the orthodontic treatment.

If the oral hygiene is not sufficiently maintained, or the diet correctly controlled, the patient risks developing caries in any tooth, but especially in those teeth in contact with the orthodontic appliance. In fixed appliance cases, this can result in unsightly cavities on the most visible part of each tooth that require permanent restorations for life.

Chapter 12

Tooth whitening

REASON FOR PROCEDURE

In an increasingly appearance-conscious society, tooth whitening is becoming a greatly popular treatment for patients to request. In the majority of cases it is carried out for aesthetic reasons only; however, some patients have unnaturally dark teeth that cause them great embarrasment and low self-esteem. As with some orthodontic patients, the dentist is in a position to improve the quality of those patients' lives by performing a relatively simple and non-invasive technique.

There are a variety of tooth whitening systems available, including over-the-counter products and whitening toothpastes on sale.

When used correctly, they are all perfectly safe and cause no damage whatsoever to the teeth. The alternative dental treatment to achieve tooth whitening is to undergo multiple veneer or crown preparations, and all of the long-term maintenance and care of these restorations that that would entail.

The procedures discussed are:

- Home whitening using trays
- In-house power whitening

BACKGROUND INFORMATION OF PROCEDURE – HOME TRAY WHITENING

This is a simple technique whereby the patient self determines the use of the product and the end result achieved. It involves the use of specially constructed trays – similar to thin gum shields or orthodontic retainers – that are worn at home by the patient with the whitening paste within them. The trays can be worn as often as the patient decides, and obviously the more usage produces the greater whitening effect, but a noticeable tooth shade improvement normally takes weeks to develop.

As long as the trays fit accurately around the teeth, the treatment course can be repeated as often as the patient wishes. The whitening paste has no effect on any restorations

Basic Guide to Dental Procedures, Second Edition. Carole Hollins.
© 2015 John Wiley & Sons, Ltd. Published 2015 by John Wiley & Sons, Ltd.

already present, such as white fillings or crowns, so these may require replacement at a later date if the shade difference is noticeably obvious.

DETAILS OF PROCEDURE – HOME TRAY WHITENING

Several home whitening products are available to the dental profession, but all rely on the use of custom-made trays to hold the paste on the surfaces of the teeth for long enough to have an effect. Other than the provision of the product and construction of the trays for each patient, the dentist has little input to the procedure.

TECHNIQUE:

- The dentist, nurse and patient wear personal protective equipment
- Alginate impressions are taken of one or both dental arches, for the working models to be cast
- Using a shade guide provided by the whitening paste manufacturers, the patient's tooth shade is recorded so that the degree of whitening achieved can be quantified
- A photograph may also be taken and kept in the patient's records for future reference
- The cast models are used to construct the customised, vacuum-formed trays for each patient, either in-house or at a laboratory
- The taking of the impressions and the production of the whitening trays are both tasks that can be carried out by a suitably trained dental nurse as extended duty skills – see Chapter 13 for details
- The teeth which are to be whitened (usually premolar to premolar) have a spacing agent placed over their front surface on the model which creates a 'well' area in the tray, so that the whitening gel is held in the correct position over each tooth while the tray is being worn (Figure 12.1)
- At the next appointment, the trays are checked for accuracy of fit and then the paste application into the tray is demonstrated to the patient (Figure 12.2)
- Excessive amounts of paste should not be used, as this is not only wasteful but the excess also spills onto the soft tissues and may cause irritation
- Each consignment of whitening paste has patient information details enclosed, and these are explained verbally, then given to the patient for reference, as various products are available for either daytime or nightime use, with varying concentrations of whitening agent
- The patients can request more whitening paste as necessary, and can carry out the whitening procedure at home whenever they wish
- Some patients use the technique continually, especially those who smoke and therefore tend to be more susceptible to tooth staining
- Others home-whiten sporadically for special events such as holidays, weddings, parties and other special occasions

BACKGROUND INFORMATION OF PROCEDURE – POWER WHITENING

As the name suggest, this is a whitening technique that provides an instant result for the patient after just one application. It relies on the use of an intense light source to

TOOTH WHITENING

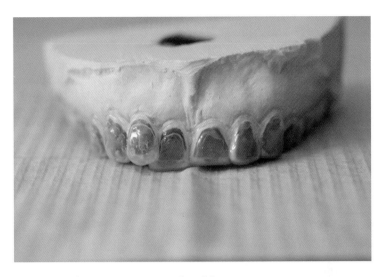

Figure 12.1 Home whitening tray on spaced model

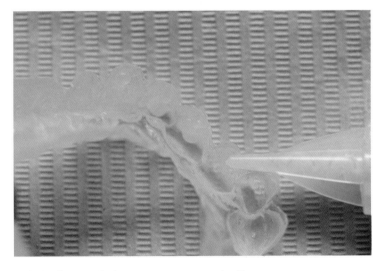

Figure 12.2 Application of whitening agent into tray 'well'

TOOTH WHITENING

chemically activate the whitening process of the paste after it has been applied to the teeth, and must be done in a controlled environment at the practice.

As the activated paste is so intense, all the soft tissues of the oral cavity must be protected from contact with it during the procedure to avoid soft tissue irritation or burns. Similarly, the patient's face and lips should be protected from the light source by being covered in total block suncream and lip balm.

DETAILS OF PROCEDURE – POWER WHITENING

Suitable patients are chosen carefully, as the intense nature of the procedure can cause temporary tooth sensitivity, sometimes intense in nature. This is prevented in the majority of cases by the patient's use of a high concentration fluoride toothpaste for several weeks before the whitening procedure is carried out. Also, some medications and even some herbal products can cause the patient to be over-sensitive to the light source used, causing sunburn or sunstroke-like symptoms. Careful pre-operative questioning identifies any likely problems.

Patients who have anterior tooth restorations (fillings, veneers or crowns) are advised that these are likely to require replacement after the whitening procedure, as they are not affected by the process and are in contrast with the whitened teeth.

The shade guide is used to determine the pre-treatment tooth shade, and should be photographically recorded.

TECHNIQUE:

- The dentist, nurse and patient wear personal protective equipment throughout the procedure, especially orange-tinted safety glasses whenever the light source is in use
- The patient is made comfortable in the dental chair, angled at 45°, as the procedure can take up to 2 h once started
- Suncream and lip balm are spread liberally over the patient's facial soft tissues
- The special lip and tongue retractor is carefully placed in the mouth so that all the oral soft tissues are held away from the teeth
- The inner sides of the lips, cheeks and the surface of the tongue are fully covered with cotton gauze to give full protection and moisture control (Figure 12.3)

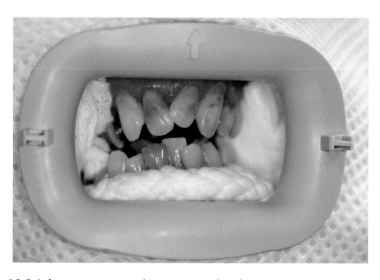

Figure 12.3 Soft tissue retraction and moisture control in place

TOOTH WHITENING

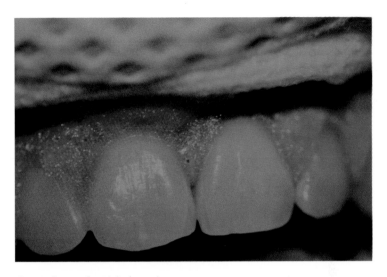

Figure 12.4 Isolation of teeth before whitening

- The protective paste ('liquid dam') is carefully run across all the exposed gingival tissues up to the necks of the teeth, then set hard so that it provides a light-proof barrier for the underlying tissues (Figure 12.4)
- The whitening paste is mixed and carefully applied to the labial surfaces of all anterior teeth
- The power light is positioned directly over these teeth and locked in position for each of the three 15-min cycles of exposure required (Figure 12.5)
- The teeth are washed, dried and fresh whitening paste is reapplied before each exposure
- At the end of the procedure the new tooth shade is recorded, and the soft tissues are checked for any signs of irritation and a soothing balm placed if necessary
- The patient is given full post-operative instructions with regard to avoiding smoking and highly coloured foods and drinks for 48 h, to avoid staining of the teeth, as the teeth are very porous during this initial period
- Any tooth sensitivity is temporary and easily alleviated using a desensitising gel provided in each whitening kit

AFTERCARE OF WHITENED TEETH

Any restorations previously present may need replacement, especially with the power whitening technique. Some patients may choose to continue the initial shade improvement achieved with the in-house procedure by using customised trays and home-whitening pastes, and the process is as previously described.

The length of time the whitening effect lasts (Figure 12.6) with no further treatment depends upon the smoking and dietary habits of the patient. In particular, tea, coffee and red wine are all notorious for causing tooth staining in any patient, and advice should be

TOOTH WHITENING

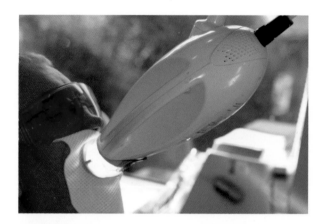

Figure 12.5 'Zoom' light in use

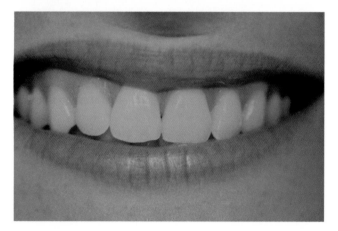

Figure 12.6 End result after power whitening of upper teeth

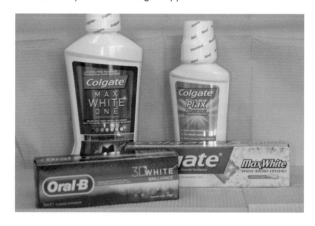

Figure 12.7 Examples of whitening oral healthcare products

TOOTH WHITENING

given on reducing their consumption for a lasting effect after whitening. The use of one of the many whitening tooth pastes and mouthwashes available also helps to maintain the whitening effect when used regularly (Figure 12.7)

As any tooth whitening technique is non-invasive, no special care and maintenance instructions are necessary, except to carry out a good daily oral hygiene programme.

TOOTH WHITENING

Chapter 13

Extended duties of the dental nurse

REASON FOR INCLUSION

This chapter is relevant in the United Kingdom, where dentists and dental care professionals (including dental nurses) are regulated by the General Dental Council (GDC).

Extended duties are those skills which may be developed by registrants after their initial qualification to enhance the scope of their practice, following appropriate training to a suitable level of competency, and with suitable indemnity insurance in place. It involves undergoing appropriate training in the workplace, which is delivered by a team member who is already trained and competent in the same skills, rather than by attending a formal training course elsewhere. This training is often referred to as being delivered 'in house', meaning that it has occurred on the workplace premises.

Details of the 'in house' training must be retained to prove that it has actually been given, and the most suitable format is as a mini hand-out which lists the information that has been passed on to the registrant. Records should be kept of each time that the registrant then carries out the supervised extended duty (including in the patient's records where the skill is used directly on a patient) until the registrant is deemed to be competent – this should also be recorded. Ideally, the workplace can develop and use assessment sheets to provide a record of the supervised tasks, and examples are given for some of the extended duties available to dental nurses in the Appendix.

Once deemed competent, the registrant's indemnity insurance should be arranged to include cover for extended (or extra) duties, rather than cover just for basic duties.

At all times, all GDC registrants must carry out their duties in accordance with the Council's standards document 'Standards for the Dental Team' and ensure that they never attempt to provide care or carry out tasks which fall outside their scope of practice.

The standards and scope of practice documentation is available to download at www.gdc-uk .org

BACKGROUND INFORMATION ON BASIC DUTIES

In the United Kingdom, all dental nurses must be qualified in their basic duties and registered with the GDC to legally work at the chairside, or they must be a student on

Basic Guide to Dental Procedures, Second Edition. Carole Hollins.
© 2015 John Wiley & Sons, Ltd. Published 2015 by John Wiley & Sons, Ltd.

an approved training course working to gain their basic register-able qualification. The basic duties of a dental nurse are those which they are expected to carry out to provide clinical and other support to registrants and patients, and are described as follows:

- Prepare and maintain the clinical environment, including the equipment
  - Set up the surgery area and equipment for a range of dental procedures
  - Maintain the surgery area and equipment between procedures so that it is safe to be re-used for several patients
  - Close down the surgery area and equipment at the end of a work session so that it is safe to be left, and safe to be re-used at a later date
- Carry out infection prevention and control procedures to prevent physical, chemical and microbiological contamination in the surgery or laboratory
  - Carry out full decontamination and sterilisation procedures to prevent cross infection
  - Dispose of contaminated items by the correct waste segregation category and method
  - Use all accepted methods of preventing contamination of equipment and items in the surgery and laboratory
- Record dental charting and oral tissue assessment carried out by other registrants
  - Tooth charting
  - Periodontal charting
  - Soft tissue assessment
  - Orthodontic and occlusal assessment
- Prepare, mix and handle dental bio-materials
  - Filling materials (temporary and permanent)
  - Impression materials
  - Luting cements
  - All accessory materials
- Provide chairside support to the operator during treatment
  - Readying the patient
  - Having all the relevant equipment, instruments and materials to hand
  - Assisting during the procedure
  - Monitoring the patient throughout the procedure
- Keep full, accurate and contemporaneous patient records
- Prepare equipment, materials and patients for radiography
  - Switch the equipment on
  - Have the correct film packet, cassette, sensor plate and holder to hand
  - Have the correct patient identified and ready for the radiographic procedure
- Process dental radiographs
  - Use automatic and manual processing equipment correctly to produce radiographs
  - Maintain automatic and manual processing equipment correctly
  - Replace and dispose of processing chemicals correctly
  - Accurately record quality assurance ratings of radiographs
  - Recognise common exposure, handling and processing faults of radiographs
- Monitor, reassure and support patients
- Give appropriate patient advice
  - Administration advice
  - Basic dental emergency advice
  - Basic treatment advice
  - Basic oral health advice

- Support the patient and their colleagues if there is a medical emergency
  - Recognition of signs and symptoms of various medical emergencies
  - Resuscitation skills
  - Maintain up-to-date medical emergency knowledge and skills
- Make appropriate referrals to other health professionals
  - Refer patients to an appropriate colleague for advice when information required is outside their own knowledge and capabilities

BACKGROUND INFORMATION ON EXTENDED DUTIES

Once the dental nurse has qualified in the basic duties shown above and become a GDC registrant, additional skills that could be developed during appropriate 'in house' training include the following;

- Further skills in oral health education and oral health promotion (see later)
- Assisting in the treatment of patients who are under conscious sedation (see later)
- Further skills in assisting in the treatment of patients with special needs
- Further skills in assisting in the treatment of orthodontic patients (see later)
- Intra- and extra-oral photography (see later)
- Shade taking
- Pouring, casting and trimming study models
- Tracing cephalographs

All these skills can be carried out without direct intervention from another registrant once the required level of competence has been achieved. Throughout the working career, the registrant should then attend suitable and verifiable continuing professional development activities in those areas of extended duties which involve direct access to patients (especially the first four duties listed above), so that their knowledge and skills are maintained. Regular monitoring of their competence in the final four duties can be carried out in the workplace by other, suitably trained and knowledgeable colleagues.

Further additional skills can also be developed in the following areas but only when on prescription from another registrant – so a more senior registrant has made the decision that the task is a necessity for a particular patient, and has delegated its completion to a suitably trained and competent dental nurse:

- Taking radiographs – specifically, pressing the exposure button when instructed to do so
- Placing rubber dam
- Measuring and recording plaque indices (see later)
- Removing sutures after the wound has been checked by the dentist (see later)
- Applying topical anaesthetic to the prescription of the dentist
- Taking impressions to the prescription of the dentist or a clinical dental technician (CDT) (see later)
- Constructing occlusal registration rims and special trays
- Constructing mouth guards, bleaching trays and vacuum-formed retainers to the prescription of the dentist (see later)
- Repairing the acrylic component of removable appliances
- Application of fluoride varnish to the prescription of the dentist, or directly as part of a structured dental health programme

FURTHER SKILLS IN ORAL HEALTH EDUCATION AND ORAL HEALTH PROMOTION

The two main oral diseases – dental caries and periodontal disease – are both caused by an accumulation of plaque, either on the tooth surface or within the gingival crevice or periodontal pockets (when present) respectively. Instruction from the dental team in how to remove this plaque effectively, as well as appropriate dietary advice, is the mainstay of good oral health promotion to prevent dental disease in patients.

Only the most dedicated of patients are likely to maintain a high standard of oral hygiene without any intervention or advice from the dental team, so it is likely that many patients will require regular reinforcement of key oral health messages throughout their time with the practice. As this patient support is often best delivered in one-to-one sessions and can be time consuming, a dental nurse with appropriate training in these extended duties is a huge benefit to the workplace, by allowing the dentist and other dental care professionals to provide treatment to some patients while the dental nurse delivers personal oral health education to others.

SIMPLE BRUSHING, FLOSSING AND INTERDENTAL CLEANING INSTRUCTIONS

The aim of conventional tooth brushing is to remove plaque from the gingival crevice area around each tooth, and from the labial, buccal, lingual, palatal and occlusal surfaces of the teeth. Conventional tooth brushing will not clean the interdental areas unless a sonic brush is used, or an electric brush with an interdental adaptation (see Figure 2.15).

Flossing (or the use of dental tape) and the use of interdental brushes are recommended for thorough interdental cleaning of the mesial and distal contact points of teeth.

To ensure that the patient learns from the oral hygiene advice and is willing and able to carry out the instructions given by the dental nurse at home afterwards, the instruction session must achieve all the following:

- Be delivered at a level of understanding suitable for each individual – this involves the use of terminology relevant to each patient, as well as the use of good communication skills; this topic is covered in detail in both text books dedicated to dental nurse training: 'Levison 11th edition' and 'Level 3 Diploma in Dental Nursing' ('NVQ 3rd edition')
- Be sensible in the advice given – this will involve giving valid reasons for the actions explained and the points made so that the patients can understand why the advice is relevant to them
- Be easily remembered by the patient – this will involve helping the patient to develop a systematic approach to their oral hygiene regime, one that they can follow each day without having to think about it
- Be reinforced appropriately – this will involve the use of relevant patient information leaflets and hand outs which the patient can take home and refer to at a later date
- Be recorded in the patient's notes – this allows the advice given to be re-evaluated at a later date by the dental nurse (or other team members) and adjusted accordingly, to ensure that the patient achieves a consistently good level of oral hygiene

EXTENDED DUTIES OF THE DENTAL NURSE

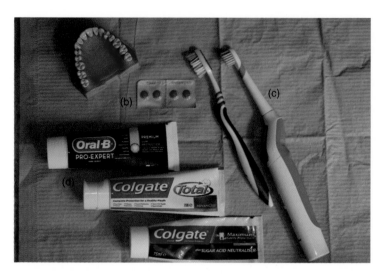

Figure 13.1 Examples of aids and products for use during OHI session. (a) Demonstration model. (b) Disclosing tablets. (c) Tooth brushes. (d) Toothpastes

Tooth brushing

Simply chatting to the patient about tooth brushing techniques will have little effect in improving their skills; they need to be able to see what is being discussed, and ideally to be able to 'have a go' themselves while being advised by the dental nurse (a typical 'tell; show; do' learning experience). A good supply of relevant oral hygiene products and aids is therefore essential to the success of the session (Figure 13.1), as well as a large mirror so that they can watch themselves while brushing. When discussing a child's brushing techniques with a parent, the dental nurse should demonstrate on the child so that the parent learns how to correctly supervise the child's brushing until the child is of an age to carry it out successfully without supervision (Figure 13.2).

TECHNIQUE:

- Briefly discuss the aims of adequate tooth brushing to the patient, with particular reference to any problems already identified with the current technique (such as missing the lower teeth by keeping the mouth closed, taking too little time, and so on)
- Demonstrate the required tooth brushing technique on a dental arch model, so that the patient can see the correct tooth brush manipulation and which areas are to be cleaned
- Allow the patient to 'have a go' at tooth brushing on the model, so that the correct brush angulation and speed and force of brushing are achieved
- Using the model, divide each dental arch into three sections: left side, right side and front, and then divide each section further into actual tooth surfaces

- Refer to these areas in terms the patient can understand – cheek side, tongue side, biting surface, and so on
- Ask the patients where they normally start and finish their tooth brushing, and then develop a systematic routine of including each of the eight tooth surface areas in both arches into that regime, so that no surface is missed
- Provide the patients with a waterproof bib and then use a disclosing tablet to expose their plaque retention areas – these can be viewed in the large mirror
- Allow the patients to 'have a go' at brushing the disclosed plaque off their teeth using the new regime that has just been discussed, reinforcing and updating the advice as necessary if they keep missing certain areas
- By the time the disclosed plaque has been fully removed, the patients should have developed a methodical approach of their own to brush all tooth surfaces in their mouth, which they can then repeat at home on a daily basis so that it becomes a subconscious routine
- Effective full mouth brushing should take around 2 min, and patients can be advised to use an egg timer or alarm call to help them learn to pace themselves accordingly
- The patients should be instructed not to rinse their mouth after spitting out the excess toothpaste at the end of the brushing session – any toothpaste remaining around the teeth is an important source of topical fluoride
- A small headed, multi-tufted medium nylon bristled tooth brush is suitable for the vast majority of patients, and is likely to need replacing every 3 months or as soon as the bristles show signs of wear (see Figure 2.6)
- The dentist will have recommended a suitable toothpaste for the patients to use, depending on whether they require a good quality fluoride toothpaste or one with additional additives for a particular dental problem (see Figure 2.4)
- Good quality, re-chargeable electric tooth brushes can also be recommended, especially those that use a sonic method of cleaning, as these take the hard work out of the task for the patient
- The vibratory action of the electric brushes, especially when accidently caught on other teeth as they are moved around the mouth, does take time and perseverance by the patient to get used to them – the dental nurse should encourage this perseverance, as the level of cleaning is likely to be far better than that achieved manually for the vast majority of patients
- The patient should also be instructed to clean the teeth over a sink and with the lips closed around the electric tooth brush during use – this limits the amount of 'dribbling' of the tooth paste solution that always occurs with their use, and avoids spillages onto clothing
- The benefits of electric tooth brushes should be reinforced to suitable patients whenever necessary:
  - More effective cleaning than manual tooth brushing
  - Sonic effect allows some interdental cleaning to occur
  - Head adaptations allow a variety of uses, including specific interdental cleaning
  - Many have 2 min timers incorporated, to ensure brushing occurs for long enough
  - Many have 30 s beeps to remind patients to move to the next quadrant; this ensures full mouth cleaning
  - Many have sensors to detect excessive pressure during use; this stops the brush from working briefly and helps teach the patient to use the correct brushing force
  - Heads are interchangeable, so one base unit can be used for several patients within a family, each with their own tooth brush head
  - Heads tend to last longer than manual brushes
- A similar demonstration session to that described for manual brushes can be carried out by the dental nurse for patients new to the use of electric tooth brushes

EXTENDED DUTIES OF THE DENTAL NURSE

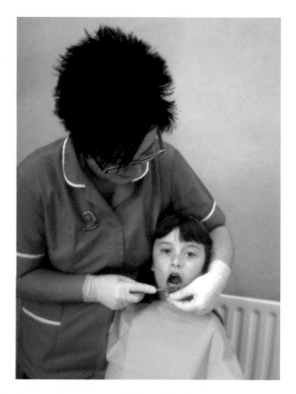

Figure 13.2 Dental nurse demonstrating child tooth brushing techniques

Flossing and interdental cleaning

These skills are required to assist the patient in removing interdental plaque on a regular basis, where regular tooth brushing alone is ineffective. Again, a clear demonstration of the correct techniques, assisted by good aids and products, is the key to engaging the patients in learning these skills and enabling them to carry them out at home (see Figures 2.8, 2.9 and 2.12).

TECHNIQUE:

- The technique used to clean interdentally will depend to a large extent on the dexterity of the patient, the options being;
  - Use of conventional dental floss or tape
  - Use of pre-threaded 'flossette' type devices
  - Use of interdental or interspace brush (Figure 13.3)
  - Use of electric brush adaptations
- Wood sticks are not recommended for routine interdental cleaning as they are designed more for occasional use to dislodge food particles that have become stuck interdentally

- A discussion of any prior attempts by the patients to clean interdentally will help to determine the technique that may be suitable for them
- With conventional dental floss and tape, many patients find the use of waxed tape more successful than of floss, as the wax allows the material to slide more easily into the interdental areas without forcing it through and risking cutting into the gums, and the tape then provides a larger surface area for tooth cleaning
- A demonstration is given of how to wrap the floss/tape around the fingers to provide a suitable length which can be guided into the interdental area and manipulated across the tooth surfaces using the thumbs (see Figure 2.10)
- Once proficient, the patients can be supervised to insert the floss/tape into an interdental area and wrap it around one of the tooth surfaces (mesial or distal), and then use a sawing action to clean the tooth surface as the floss/tape is withdrawn from the area (see Figure 2.11)
- They then unwrap a small section of floss from one finger and wrap it onto the other finger so that a clean section becomes available – this is then guided back into the same interdental area and used to clean the opposing tooth surface in the same way
- Patients who struggle with this technique for their posterior teeth can be instructed in the use of 'flossette' type devices in the same way to clean these interdental areas (see Figure 2.8)
- It may take several devices to clean the interdental areas fully, as the floss/tape is secured in the prongs and cannot be changed once soiled – the patients should be discouraged from continuing to use a heavily soiled 'flossette' as they are merely transferring plaque and food debris from one interdental area to another, rather than cleaning the tooth surfaces
- Suitably sized interdental brushes will be the method of choice for interdental cleaning for some patients
- Determine the size necessary for the patient (see Figure 2.13), and demonstrate how the brush end can be angled to access posterior interdental areas more easily (Figure 13.4)
- Allow the patients to 'have a go' at inserting the interdental brush in various areas of their mouth, and then using a brushing and twisting action to clean the tooth surfaces before withdrawing it (see Figure 2.14)
- The brush can also be used with a smear of toothpaste, so that fluoride and cleaning agents are also introduced into the area
- Large interdental brushes or interspace brushes are more suitable where large gaps are present between teeth, such as where a tooth is missing from the arch
- The brushes can be rinsed clean and re-used, but must be discarded when the bristles show signs of wear
- For those patients who routinely use an electric brush to carry out their oral hygiene regime, or those who are suitable to be advised to do so, various interdental and interspace head adaptors are available with good quality varieties, which are used to simulate the manual techniques described

DIET ADVICE

Regular and efficient plaque removal will help prevent caries and gingival and periodontal problems from developing, but the incidence of caries is also greatly influenced by the patient's diet. A diet containing regular non-milk extrinsic sugars and dietary acids will always have the potential to allow caries to occur, no matter how effective the oral hygiene regime.

EXTENDED DUTIES OF THE DENTAL NURSE

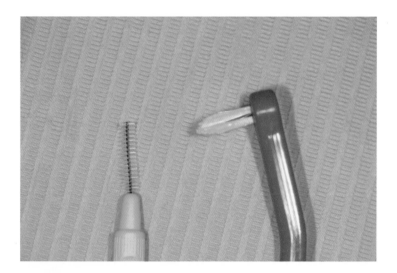

Figure 13.3 Interdental and interspace brushes

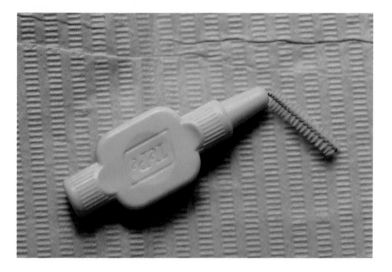

Figure 13.4 Interdental brush angled to aid use

The vast majority of patients are aware of the potential for obvious foods and drinks to cause caries, such as chocolates, cakes, carbonated drinks, biscuits, and so on. What many are unaware of are the 'hidden sugars' in many foods and drinks, the role that acidic products have in causing caries, and the importance of frequency and timing of the consumption of these products in the development of caries. Dietary advice should be geared around these areas.

To give effective diet advice, the patient's dietary contents and habits first need to be known, and the most effective way of discovering this information is to have the patient complete a diet sheet like the one shown below. The aim is to have an accurate record of the following points on a daily basis:

- What food and drink is consumed
- When they are consumed throughout a 24-h period
- When any oral hygiene procedures are carried out during the same time cycle
- What variations there are from day to day, with both the products consumed and the oral hygiene procedures undertaken

To be effective, the patient has to be totally honest – and this must be emphasised before proceeding with a dietary recording and analysis, otherwise there is little point in continuing. The desire to help the patient avoid future restorative dental treatment (and its cost) and to maintain a healthy smile should be stressed from the outset by the dental nurse.

A selection of packaging from various food and drink products containing hidden sugars may be used as 'props' to help convince the patient that the advice is given on a non-judgemental, purely helpful basis by the dental nurse. Again, good communication skills are required if the patient is not to be alienated by the whole procedure.

Once the diet sheet (or sheets if there is a large variation between week days and weekends, for example) has been completed and returned to the practice by the patient, it should be carefully analysed to determine the answers to the four questions set above. The dental nurse may discuss the findings with the dentist or another competent dental care professional, making notes of the relevant points to discuss with the patient. The patient then attends an oral hygiene instruction and promotion session with the dental nurse.

Tuesday	Food or drink	Oral hygiene
6 a.m.	Cereal with sugar, orange juice	—
7 a.m.	—	Tooth brushing, fluoride tooth paste
8 a.m.	—	—
9 a.m.	—	—
10 a.m.	Biscuit, coffee with two sugars	—
11 a.m.	—	—
12 p.m.	Pizza, chocolate muffin, diet coke	—
1 p.m.	—	Chewing gum, not sugar free
2 p.m.	—	—
3 p.m.	Diet coke, chocolate biscuit	—
4 p.m.	—	—
5 p.m.	Cheese and onion crisps	Chewing gum, not sugar free
6 p.m.	—	—
7 p.m.	Chicken burger and chips with side salad, glass of white wine	—
8 p.m.	Glass of white wine	—
9 p.m.	Glass of white wine	Tooth brushing, fluoride tooth paste and general use mouthwash
10 p.m.	—	—
11 p.m.	Glass of diet lemonade	—
12 a.m.	—	—

The information contained in the diet sheet example shown above, and to be discussed with the patient, is as follows.

Food and drink consumed in this scenario;

- Several obvious sugar and acid episodes
  ○ Sugar in cereal and in coffee
  ○ Orange juice and carbonated drinks
  ○ Biscuits and muffin
  ○ Wine
- Several hidden sugar episodes;
  ○ Cereal – even plain examples such as whole wheat cereal and corn flake style products contain sugar
  ○ Pizza – the tomato paste base contains sugar, as do most tomato sauce or paste products
  ○ Chewing gum – unless stated as 'sugar free' these products will contain sugar
  ○ Chicken burger – if additions such as mayonnaise or relish are used

Time of consumption in this scenario;

- The sugar and acid 'hits' occur frequently throughout the day
- This allows potentially harmful levels of food debris and plaque acids to lie in direct contact with tooth surfaces for prolonged periods of time, causing demineralisation

Time of oral hygiene procedures in this scenario;

- Tooth brushing occurs within the hour after breakfast, so some food debris and plaque will be removed
- No other oral hygiene measures occur for the following 14 h
- This allows all sugars and acids consumed in that time to potentially cause some caries, especially interdentally where no cleaning technique has been carried out for the whole 24-h period
- The beneficial effects of the bedtime tooth brushing and mouth washing procedures will be cancelled out by the consumption of the carbonated drink less than 2 h later
- This acidic drink then has the following 7 to 8 h to lie undisturbed and erode the tooth enamel overnight

Any variations between completed diet sheets for different days can be analysed in a similar manner.

Armed with all this information, the dental nurse can give the necessary dietary advice to the patients in an effort to educate them in reducing the potential harm that their dietary habits may cause. It is unrealistic to expect the patients to change their diet completely, and it is highly unlikely that an average diet would avoid all sources of hidden sugars. Consequently, the advice given should focus on reasonable and achievable goals for that particular patient, including the following suggested points.

Food and drink consumed:

- Can healthier alternatives be used, such as
  ○ Artificial granulated sweetener on the cereal and in the coffee
  ○ Savoury biscuits and cheese (although there is likely to be a hidden sugar content)

- º Fruit or yogurt instead of crisps (although the yogurt may contain hidden sugar)
- º Limit the carbonated drinks, or have squash drinks instead – even 'diet' drinks are potentially harmful if they are fizzy, because they are acidic
- º Plain water instead of any other overnight drink
- White wine contains less sugar than many other alcoholic drinks such as ciders, sherries and mixers with spirits, but it is still acidic, so the length of drinking time should be monitored by the patient

Time of consumption:

- Frequency?
  - º The same foods and drinks consumed in two or three set meals rather than spread over the 14 h period will cause less tooth damage, as there are less sugar and acid 'hits' on the teeth
  - º Can the orange juice be taken before the cereal at breakfast, so that the acid is much reduced before tooth brushing is carried out – the combination of softened enamel from acid exposure and tooth brushing can cause increased enamel loss
  - º In particular, the overnight drink of lemonade has the potential to cause massive demineralisation if carried out on a regular basis, and should be replaced by plain water

Time of oral hygiene procedures:

- Frequency?
  - º Much plaque develops in the mouth overnight, so can the teeth be brushed both before breakfast (to remove that already present) and after breakfast (to remove that developing from the food just consumed) – this will remove the maximum amount of harmful plaque
  - º Can a lunchtime oral hygiene procedure be carried out – ideally tooth brushing with a fluoride toothpaste, or the use of a good quality mouth wash
  - º If not, sugar free chewing gum will stimulate saliva flow to wash away some debris, and physically pull some particles off the teeth As a last resort, swilling the mouth with plain water after a meal will have some beneficial effect
- Procedures?
  - º If acids are likely to be consumed on a regular basis, advise on the use of enamel repair products to minimise the erosive effect
  - º Avoid brushing immediately after finishing acidic drinks, including alcohol – wait for at least 20 min to allow the acids to be neutralised, or use a mouth wash
  - º Introduce an interdental cleaning procedure into the regime – bedtime may be ideal as the patient is likely to have more time than in the morning before work
  - º If time is an issue, advise the use of a good quality sonic electric tooth brush that will clean interdentally on a regular basis
  - º Use sugar free chewing gum as a cleaning aid when other procedures are not possible, but do not chew gum excessively as this will encourage tooth wear on the biting surfaces of the teeth

In summary, any amount of this information and these oral health instruction and promotion techniques can be developed by the dental nurse into personalised oral health

EXTENDED DUTIES OF THE DENTAL NURSE

education sessions with the patient. The information here covers the basics of oral health instruction and promotion techniques, and can be used in total or as a starting point for the development of a suitable training programme.

To be successful in this extended duty, the dental nurse must be adequately trained to become competent in all the following skills;

- Tailor the information to the direct needs of each patient
- Ensure the information is correct and in line with the policies and beliefs of the work place
- Communicate effectively so that the oral health messages are correctly delivered
- Maintain an up-to-date level of knowledge of the topics likely to be discussed with patients
- Know the limits of one's knowledge and understanding, and be willing to ask a senior colleague for inputs when necessary

A post-registration qualification in Oral Health Education is available for dental nurses in the United Kingdom, which trains students to a much greater depth of knowledge in this topic and provides them with a recognised qualification. Further details are available at www.nebdn.org

ASSISTING IN THE TREATMENT OF PATIENTS WHO ARE UNDER CONSCIOUS SEDATION

Conscious sedation is an anxiety control technique used to allow fearful (or phobic) patients to undergo routine dental procedures, as well as to allow regular patients to undergo fearful or traumatic dental procedures. The two techniques most frequently used in general practice are

- Single drug intravenous sedation
- Inhalation sedation (previously referred to as relative analgesia)

As an extended duty where both techniques are used, the role of the dental nurse may include any or all of the following skills:

- Be able to set up the equipment and materials to carry out intravenous sedation
- Be able to read a pulse oximeter machine
- Be able to take the patient's blood pressure
- Be able to carry out basic safety checks on the inhalation sedation machine
- Be able to monitor the patient during a conscious sedation session, and record the vital signs when necessary

In workplaces where only one or the other technique is used, the level of competency of the dental nurses is limited to that technique alone, and to the specific tasks that they have been trained to carry out only. The role of gaining informed consent in written form before a conscious sedation procedure is a regulatory requirement, and is the responsibility of the dentist rather than a duty for the dental nurse to carry out.

EXTENDED DUTIES OF THE DENTAL NURSE

Intravenous sedation

This is a technique of conscious sedation for adult patients where a single drug is injected intravenously into them so that

- Their anxiety of dental treatment is significantly reduced
- They are willing to receive dental treatment
- They remain conscious throughout and therefore do not require intubation

Examples of the equipment and materials required to be set out for the induction procedure are shown in Figure 13.5, and the function of all the potential items required are as follows:

- Midazolam (Hyponovel) ampoule – the drug that is injected intravenously to produce the sedation
- Flumazenil (Anexate) ampoule – the reversal drug to bring the patient out of the sedation in case of emergency
- 5 mL syringes and long needles – to draw up the Midazolam (and Flumazenil when required)
- Cannula – either a venflon or a butterfly to administer the Midazolam

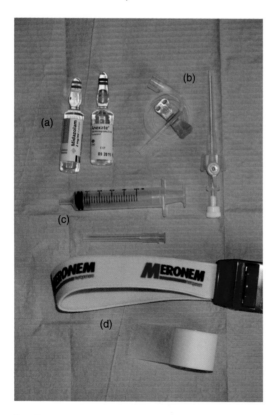

Figure 13.5 Example of items to set out for intravenous sedation. (a) Intravenous drug and antidote. (b) Selection of cannulas. (c) Syringe and needle to draw up agents. (d) Tourniquet and tape

- Alcohol wipe – to clean the injection site before the cannula is used
- Tourniquet – to fasten around the upper arm or wrist to raise the vein
- Arm splint – to keep the arm straight throughout the procedure if a butterfly is used in a vein in the arm, as the needle remains in the vein and may cause damage if the patients bend their arm (a venflon has a plastic tube which remains in the vein and the arm can therefore safely be bent)
- Micropore tape – to secure the cannula in the vein throughout treatment, and to hold a cotton wool roll over the site after the cannula has been removed (alternatively a plaster may be used)
- Pulse oximeter (Figure 13.6a) – the machine connected to the patient throughout the procedure by a finger probe, which reads their oxygen levels (as a %) and their pulse rate (as a number counted per minute)
- Blood pressure machine – either a dedicated device or as part of the pulse oximeter (see Figure 13.6b), which is used to record the patient's blood pressure both before and after the procedure
- Oxygen cylinder and nasal cannula – to administer oxygen to the patients during the procedure if their oxygen level is at 90% or below for more than a minute, or if their oxygen level keeps dipping
- Mouth props – for use during the procedure to keep the patients' mouth open wide, otherwise they will keep closing it while in a relaxed state

The nurse's role during the induction procedure is to

- Assist with taking the patient's blood pressure before starting the induction, or actually take the blood pressure using an automated machine
  - Place the cuff around the upper arm in the correct location (this is usually marked on the cuff itself, for both the left or right arm)
  - Use the Velcro strip to secure the cuff in place
  - Ensure the cuff tubing is connected to the machine correctly
  - Press the start button to inflate the cuff
  - Follow the deflation of the cuff and make a note of the automatically recorded blood pressure reading, writing the systolic pressure over the diastolic pressure on the monitoring sheet (see below)
- Help to keep the patient as calm and relaxed as possible during the induction by talking quietly but encouragingly to them, by holding their hand if possible (or getting someone else to do so)
- Assist the dentist by passing the necessary items to carry out the induction, in the correct order
- The order is: tourniquet → alcohol wipe → cannula → Midazolam syringe → micropore tape
- Close the vein with a finger while the needle is removed, if a venflon is used
- Attach the syringe end to the butterfly tubing, if a butterfly is used
- Release the tourniquet when told to do so
- Apply the micropore tape to secure the cannula
- Assist with applying the arm rest when a butterfly is used in a vein in the arm
- Attach the finger probe correctly to the patient – the diode window side is usually marked with a finger nail pictogram on the probe, so that it is not placed upside down
- Switch on the pulse oximeter and ensure the alarm is on and is automatically set at 90% – this level can be raised if necessary but only on the direction of the dentist
- Record the first oxygen and pulse readings, and the time they were taken on the monitoring sheet

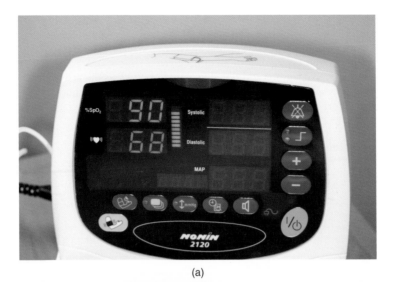

(a)

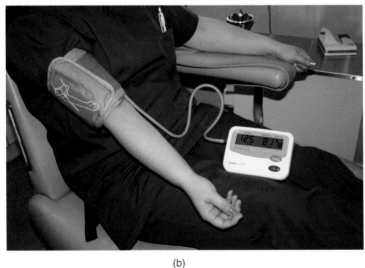

(b)

Figure 13.6 (a) Example of a combined pulse oximeter and blood pressure machine (b) Dedicated blood pressure machine in use

Monitoring the patient during the procedure

The patient must be monitored throughout the procedure, with a written record kept of the oxygen levels and pulse rate readings at 10 min intervals.

- Use the monitoring sheet provided and complete all sections (example shown in Figure 13.7)
- The information to be recorded is as follows:
  - Pre- and post-operative blood pressures

EXTENDED DUTIES OF THE DENTAL NURSE

- Oxygen levels
- Pulse rate
- Drug used, amount given, time of first and last increments
- Batch number and expiry date of all drugs given
- Details of any problems or additional information, such as the provision of oxygen
- The level of responsiveness of the patient at discharge, and the time of discharge
- Patient's escort

IV SEDATION PROCEDURAL RECORD

PATIENT NAME: DATE:

ASA: RELEVANT MH?   YES   NO

IV DRUG	EXPIRY DATE	BATCH NUMBER	INCREMENTS		TOTAL DOSE
			FIRST	LAST	

VENOUS ACCESS?	SITE	CANNULA
YES DIFFICULT NO		

MONITORING TIME	OXYGEN SATURATION	PULSE	BLOOD PRESSURE

RECOVERY SITE	SURGERY		
FIT FOR DISCHARGE	WALK	TALK	LISTEN
POST-SEDATION INSTRUCTIONS	TO ESCORT–VERBAL/WRITTEN		
TIME OF DISCHARGE			
CLINICIAN			
NURSE			

Figure 13.7 Example of an intravenous sedation monitoring sheet

In addition, the patients should be monitored visually to notice the following:

- Their colour, especially any blueness which indicates lack of oxygen
- Their chest movements, especially whether they are regular and steady or not, which indicates a possible respiratory obstruction
- Their level of responsiveness, especially whether they respond to verbal commands or not, which indicates their level of sedation may be too deep and they are at risk of passing into unconsciousness
- Whether they are tapping their finger or clenching their hand with the finger probe on, as this will send false readings to the pulse oximeter, as well as setting off the alarm
- Whether they are bending their arm with a butterfly inserted, as this will pierce the side of their vein and cause bruising

Sedation patients are understandably anxious before the induction session begins, and will appreciate the presence of a friendly and empathetic dental nurse to 'hold their hand' – whether physically or emotionally. During the session the patients will be relaxed and will often have to be given the same instructions several times before they respond (turn their head, open their mouth wider, breathe through their nose, and so on) – it is important that they are spoken to pleasantly and calmly, and that they are constantly reassured by the dental nurse throughout the session.

Although midazolam does cause a period of amnesia (memory loss) during its use, the patient is not deaf, so no inappropriate comments or personal chatting should occur during the session – the dental nurse should be wholly focussed on the welfare and comfort of the patient throughout.

The dental nurse's role during the recovery period is to

- Remain with the patients and monitor their visible signs
- Talk to the patients to help their recovery
- Assist with, or take, a post-operative blood pressure reading
- Assist with the removal of the cannula and place a dressing
- Ensure the monitoring sheet is fully completed when the patient is ready to be discharged
- Check with the escort that the post-operative instructions are understood and will be followed
- Report any problems to the dentist
- Assist the patient safely from the premises

Inhalation sedation

This is a conscious sedation technique suitable for child and adult patients, where they inhale a variable mixture of gases so that

- Their anxiety of dental treatment is significantly reduced
- They are willing to receive dental treatment
- They remain conscious throughout and therefore do not require intubation

The equipment to set out for the procedure is as follows:

- Inhalation sedation trolley which is connected to the oxygen and nitrous oxide gas supplies – the gas flow and percentage of nitrous oxide delivered is controlled with the machine dials

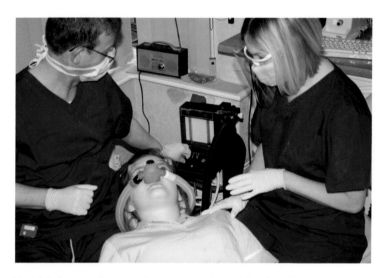

Figure 13.8 Inhalation sedation machine in use with nasal hood in place

- Nasal hood with tubing – this is placed over the patient's nose to inhale the gas mixture during the session without impeding access to the mouth (Figure 13.8)
- Scavenger tubing – taking away exhaled air from the operative area so that waste gases do not build up, as the dental team will be affected by the sedative gas mixture otherwise

The pulse oximeter and blood pressure machine do not have to be used with inhalation sedation, but it is good practice to do so and record the readings as for IV sedation.

Pre-operative checks

The inhalation sedation machine must be checked prior to every use on a patient to ensure that it is working correctly, and this is carried out as follows:

- Check the oxygen and nitrous oxide cylinders are switched on and that the gas is flowing (Figure 13.9)
- The level of nitrous oxide in the cylinder can only be determined by weighing the cylinder, so it cannot be assumed that the dial reading is accurate
- The pin index system on the pipe connections prevents the incorrect connection of the gas cylinders to the delivery machine when the colour coding is followed
  - Oxygen – white
  - Nitrous oxide – blue
- On the machine, the reservoir bag is filled and checked for any leaks by listening for a gas escape and by squeezing the bag to ensure it does not deflate
- The oxygen flush button is checked for its correct working, so that the patient can be given 100% oxygen in an emergency (Figure 13.10)
- The nitrous oxide cut-off ability is checked to ensure the flow switches off automatically if the oxygen flow stops, so the machine will not operate without a minimum oxygen flow

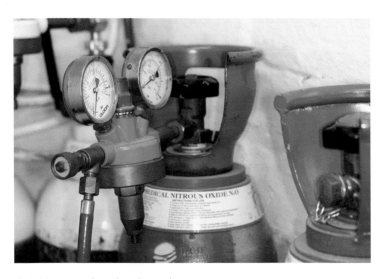

Figure 13.9 Nitrous oxide tank, valve and gauge

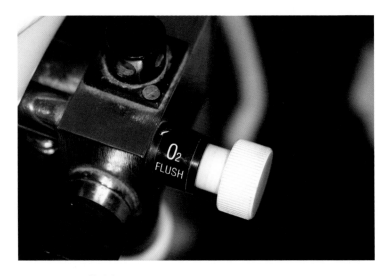

Figure 13.10 Oxygen flush button

- The minimum flow is set at 30% oxygen, and this is also checked to ensure the flow cannot be reduced any further – so the maximum nitrous oxide delivery can only be 70%
- The flow dial calibrations are checked to ensure they work correctly, so if 30% oxygen is given the nitrous oxide should read 70%, if 50% then 50%, and so on

If any of these are not working, the machine is not safe to be used and the matter must be reported to the dentist.

EXTENDED DUTIES OF THE DENTAL NURSE

The role of the dental nurse during induction and treatment is as follows:

- During induction, the nasal hood is placed on the patient and the gas mixture is gradually altered to increase the percentage of nitrous oxide in use until a suitable level of sedation is achieved
- The patient may need to be reminded to breathe through the nose and not to talk during induction
- The technique allows the patient to respond well to a degree of hypnotic suggestion, and it is important not to interrupt the induction during this phase, but still help to keep the patient calm by hand holding, for example
- During the session the patient should be visibly monitored as for IV sedation
- Keep a note of the maximum % of nitrous oxide given to the patient, and whether active or passive scavenging was used (ideally, scavenging should always be active so that the waste gases are physically drawn away from the area and expelled)
- The patient must be given a minimum of 2 min of 100% oxygen at the end of treatment before removing the nasal hood and disconnecting the machine, otherwise they will develop diffusion hypoxia
- Nitrous oxide does not cause patient amnesia, so no inappropriate comments must be made throughout the session
- The gas does have some analgesic properties, but it is unlikely to be enough for undergoing dental treatment without local anaesthetic
- The patient should be able to leave the premises within 15 min of the end of the inhalation session, and adult patients do not need an escort
- The machine must be closed down correctly, by switching off the cylinders, flushing out the machine, and disposing of the single-use liner of the nasal hood

A post-registration qualification in Dental Sedation Nursing is available for dental nurses in the United Kingdom, which trains students to a much greater depth of knowledge in both techniques. The qualification awarded is a usual employment requirement for those wishing to work with conscious sedation techniques in the dental hospital setting. Further details are available at www.nebdn.org

FURTHER SKILLS IN ASSISTING IN THE TREATMENT OF ORTHODONTIC PATIENTS

Most orthodontic treatment is carried out in specialist practices or clinics in the United Kingdom, so many dental nurses have little or no access to the speciality in general practice. Of those dental nurses who do work within the orthodontic speciality, one with extended duties in this area of dentistry is a valuable member of the team in delivering this treatment, along with the dentist and the orthodontic therapist. The extended duties that can be developed include any or all of the following:

- Recognition and laying out of the specialised orthodontic instruments and materials – although this area of dentistry is included in the dental nurse curriculum of the register-able qualification, the knowledge required is only to a basic level
- Setting up of brackets and tubes for the bonding of fixed appliances
- Specific oral hygiene instruction for orthodontic patients

- Measurement and recording of plaque indices before, during and after treatment (this skill can be gained as a separate extended duty – see later)
- Tracing cephalographs (this skill can be gained as a separate extended duty)

Laying out instruments and materials

The vast majority of orthodontic treatments carried out in the United Kingdom involve the use of removable or conventional fixed appliances (see Chapter 11 for further details). Many of the instruments and materials required for the fitting/bonding, adjustment, and removal of these appliances are unique to this speciality and are therefore unlikely to be familiar to many dental nurses. The table below lists the most likely instruments to be required for removable appliances (see Figure 11.2) and conventional fixed appliances (see Figure 11.5) and their functions. Those to be laid out will be determined by the appliance involved and the stage of the treatment that is being undertaken.

Item	Function
Adam pliers	Removable appliance – to tighten cribs, adjust springs and retractors
Straight hand piece with acrylic bur	Removable appliance – to trim the acrylic base plate of the appliance
Measuring ruler	Removable and fixed appliances – to take accurate measurements of tooth movements, such as the overjet
Bracket holders (see Figure 11.7b)	Fixed appliance – to pick up, hold and position individual brackets during their bonding onto the teeth
Alastik/elastic holders (see Figure 11.7c)	Fixed appliance – ratcheted design to pick up and tightly grip alastiks and elastics as they are used to tie in the arch wire to the bracket (alastik) or to provide traction to teeth (elastics)
Arch wire (end) cutters (see Figure 11.7d)	Fixed appliance – angled wire cutters to trim off the excess ends of the arch wire from directly behind the molar band or tube, often with a self-gripping attachment so that the cut piece of wire can be safely removed from the mouth
Wire cutters (Figure 13.11a)	Fixed appliance – straight wire cutters to trim off the ends of wire ties or ligatures
Bracket removers (Figure 13.11b)	Fixed appliance – chisel-ended pliers to remove brackets from the teeth at the end of treatment or when a bracket needs removing and repositioning
Band removers (Figure 13.11c)	Fixed appliance – chisel-ended blade and a plastic stopper to remove bands at the end of treatment; the stopper rests on the occlusal surface of the tooth while the other blade is located at the gingival rim of the band, and then the pliers are squeezed together to dislodge the band from the tooth

The materials that may be required to be laid out are as follows;

- Alginate impression material and water for pre- and post-operative study models, and for the working model when a removable appliance is to be constructed (see Figure 4.11)

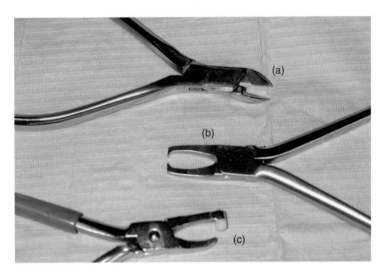

Figure 13.11 Fixed appliance instruments. (a) Wire cutters. (b) Bracket removers. (c) Band removers

- Acid etch and a suitable bonding agent when a fixed appliance is to be placed (see Figure 11.7a)
- Luting cement for the cementation of molar bands (see Figure 6.4)

Setting up for a bonding procedure

Bonding a conventional fixed appliance to an upper, lower or both arches is a fiddly and sometimes time-consuming procedure, and forward preparation is a key element in the smooth running of the appointment, for both the patient and the dentist.

The dental nurse can assist greatly by being trained to set out the brackets and molar tubes beforehand. This is best done using an orientation card with a sticky backing on which the brackets and tubes can be firmly located, ready for the procedure. Each bracket and tube is designed for use on a specific tooth only and great care must be taken in orientating each one correctly. Brackets have coloured dots placed on their disto-gingival wing by the manufacturers to assist in their identification, but the colours used may vary between suppliers, so bracket sets should not become mixed together. The exception is lower incisor brackets which have a rounded base that follows the gingival margin of the tooth, but can otherwise be used on any of the lower incisors. Canine brackets can also have disto-gingival hooks placed by the manufacturer for use with elastic traction. Molar tubes have distally orientated hooks which are set gingivally, so upper right molar tubes can also be used on lower left molars, and upper left molar tubes can also be used on lower right molars.

When placing the brackets, the dental nurse should use the bracket holders so that they become familiar with their use and handling.

A correctly laid out orientation card for an upper and lower bonding is shown in Figure 13.12.

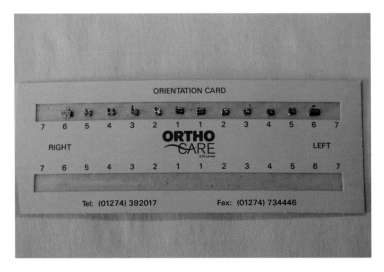

Figure 13.12 Orientation card ready for upper bonding

Orthodontic oral hygiene instruction

Both removable and fixed appliances provide many more stagnation areas in the patient's mouth than would exist without the appliance *in situ*, and the high level of oral hygiene that must be maintained throughout the treatment is imperative if tooth damage and localised gingival problems are to be avoided. The patient must be taught how and when to clean adequately around the appliance, as well as any necessary dietary controls to be followed during the treatment phase – this oral hygiene instruction can be delivered by a suitably trained dental nurse.

Over and above any general oral hygiene advice and instruction which is relevant to all patients, that specific to those wearing removable appliances is as follows:

- Food and drink must be confined to mealtimes rather than having snacks throughout the day, as the teeth will need cleaning every time something has been consumed so that food debris is not held against the teeth by the appliance
- The quantity of food and drink containing non-milk extrinsic sugars and acids must be kept to an absolute minimum, to reduce the potential of causing cavities during treatment
- The appliance must be removed and cleaned twice daily with a tooth brush and toothpaste, taking care not to damage any springs or clasps while doing so
- Cleaning should be carried out over a sink of water so that if dropped, the appliance will not break
- Both fluoride mouthwash and toothpaste should be used during the treatment phase on a daily basis, to provide maximum protection against caries to the teeth
- Patients should be encouraged to self-disclose their teeth on a weekly basis to ensure their oral hygiene regime is adequate
- If extraction spaces are present in the dental arch, the patient should be instructed in the use of an interspace brush to clean the area effectively until space closure occurs

EXTENDED DUTIES OF THE DENTAL NURSE

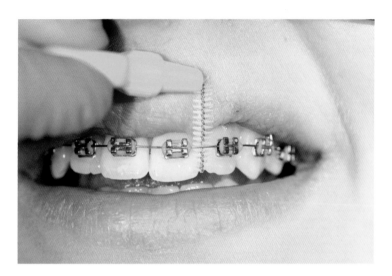

Figure 13.13 Use of interdental brush to clean beneath the arch wire

Over and above any general oral hygiene advice and instruction which is relevant to all patients, that specific to those wearing fixed appliances is as follows:

- The quantity of food and drink containing non-milk extrinsic sugars and acids must be kept to an absolute minimum, to reduce the potential of causing cavities during treatment
- Both fluoride mouthwash and toothpaste should be used during the treatment phase on a daily basis, to provide maximum protection against caries to the teeth
- Patients should be encouraged to self-disclose their teeth on a weekly basis to ensure their oral hygiene regime is adequate
- Patients should be instructed in the use of interdental brushes to clean around each bracket where the arch wire passes over, as this is a particular stagnation area where ordinary manual tooth brushing alone is not sufficient (Figure 13.13)
- Alternatively the patient can be instructed in the use of an electric tooth brush with an orthodontic head attachment to clean these areas (see Figure 11.10)

In either form of orthodontic treatment, if a less than adequate level of oral hygiene is being maintained by the patient, the dental nurse can provide a one-to-one disclosing and cleaning session, to emphasise the problem areas and help the patient to improve plaque removal.

Measurement and recording of plaque indices

A plaque index is a method used to measure the amount of plaque present in the patient's mouth at any time, and when carried out repeatedly at further visits it provides a record of a patient's progress in oral hygiene standards. So it allows a numerical value to be placed on the level of oral hygiene at that point, which can then be used to monitor progress over a period of time – and the use of a numerical value makes the information more

understandable to the patients; they can quantify their own progress. Plaque indices are particularly useful with potential and ongoing orthodontic patients because they provide information that can be used in the following ways:

- A high plaque index in a potential orthodontic patient prevents the start of treatment until improvement is seen – it 'weeds out' unsuitable patients who are most likely to develop caries if treatment proceeds
- It gives the patient something to aim for if they desire treatment – to reduce the numerical value to an acceptable level
- It monitors the compliance of the patient during treatment – if problems are identified, they can be resolved before tooth damage occurs
- If problems continue, the treatment can be abandoned with a recorded (and therefore irrefutable) good reason, and hopefully before tooth damage occurs
- When treatment has been successfully completed, a lowered index provides a retrospective record of the need for the treatment initially – the patient's oral hygiene has improved as cleaning became easier with well-aligned teeth

Two established methods are available for measuring and recording the amount of plaque present in the patient's mouth – one method involves every tooth present, while the other involves just six teeth as a representative sample of the mouth as a whole, and is therefore a speedier procedure.

METHOD 1:

- Assume each tooth is divided into six sites – mesial, mid and distal on both the buccal and lingual/palatal sides
- Multiply the number of teeth present in the patient's mouth by six – a typical teenager is likely to have all but their third molars present, so 28 teeth $\times$ 6 = 168
- The presence or absence of plaque at each site is determined by running a blunt probe along the gingival margins of each tooth, or by thoroughly disclosing the patient and looking directly at the teeth
- Total the number of sites (out of 168) where plaque is present – so say 102 sites out of 168 had plaque present, 102/168
- Multiply this fraction by 100 to give a percentage plaque index = 60.7%

A plaque index this high indicates the patient has a poor standard of oral hygiene and is not suitable for orthodontic treatment until the plaque index has been much reduced and then maintained at a reduced level consistently. So the quantified information can be used to motivate a keen patient to improve oral hygiene, or to justify the denial of treatment to an insistent patient who has little interest in improving oral hygiene, but wants treatment anyway.

METHOD 2:

- Six teeth are chosen as a representative sample of the mouth – the upper right first molar (UR6, 16) and lateral incisor (UR2, 12), and the upper left first premolar (UL4, 24); the lower left first molar (LL6, 36) and lateral incisor (LL2, 32), and the lower right first premolar (LR4, 44)

(continued)

METHOD 2: (*Continued*)

- The presence or absence of plaque is determined on four sites of each tooth – mesial and distal of both the buccal and lingual/palatal sides
- The plaque is scored as follows;
  - No plaque = 0
  - Plaque present by probing = 1
  - Visible plaque = 2
  - Extensive plaque = 3
- The average plaque scores of each tooth are added together and then divided by six (the number of teeth that have been recorded) to give a single figure which is taken as a representative average for the mouth as a whole – this is the patient's plaque index
- So using the following example;
  - UR6 = 2
  - UR2 = 0
  - UL4 = 2
  - LL6 = 3
  - LL2 = 3
  - LR4 = 2
- Total = 12 ÷ 6 = plaque index 2
- Using this qualitative and quicker method, the plaque index will range from 0 (excellent) to 3 (poor), so again this patient is currently unsuitable for orthodontic treatment

---

The plaque index can be calculated by the dental nurse at any point during treatment and compared with the pre-operative scores to monitor the oral hygiene progress of the patient, and highlight any potential problems as they occur and before any tooth damage is likely to have happened. The plaque index can be recorded at the examination or recall appointment of any patient, not just those considering orthodontic treatment, and is a useful method of monitoring routine oral hygiene standards and the patient's compliance with any previous oral hygiene instruction given.

Methods of recording the information to determine the plaque index vary widely, but probably one of the simplest ways is to use a variation of a standard periodontal diagnosis and treatment plan chart (Figure 13.14a). The chart has the buccal, lingual, and palatal surfaces of each tooth pre-printed onto it, and plaque can be recorded as either a coloured dot at each site (method 1) or as a numerical value at each site (method 2). Alternatively, a pre-printed dental arch diagram (Figure 13.14b) can be used in a similar fashion.

A post-registration qualification in Orthodontic Dental Nursing is available for dental nurses in the United Kingdom, which trains students to a much greater depth in this speciality and is particularly useful for those dental nurses wishing to work in a specialist orthodontic workplace. Further details are available at www.nebdn.org

TAKING IMPRESSIONS

Alginate impressions are the most frequently taken and widely useful of the impression materials available. They are used to produce study models in various fields of dentistry, to produce opposing models and initial models in fixed and removable prosthodontics, and

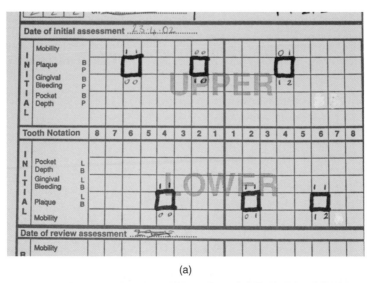

(a)

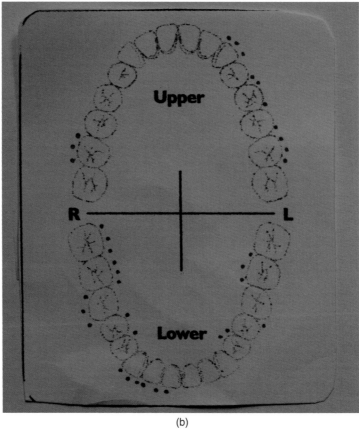

(b)

Figure 13.14 Examples of plaque index recording methods. (a) Variation of standard periodontal chart. (b) Pre-printed dental arches

to produce models for the construction of mouth guards, vacuum formed retainers, and whitening trays (see later).

A trained and competent dental nurse who is able to take consistently good quality and therefore useful alginate impressions is an asset to any dental workplace. The stages involved in taking alginate impressions are as follows:

- Selection of the patient – many patients are fearful of undergoing impression taking, as they believe they will choke, gag, or vomit, and excessively fearful patients are best left to the dentist to handle
- Selection of the trays
- Mixing of the alginate and loading of the trays
- Insertion of the loaded trays
- Removal of the trays after setting
- Monitoring and handling of the patient throughout

The equipment and materials required to take a set of study models are shown in Figure 4.11.

Selection of the trays

It is usual for single use, perforated box trays to be used for alginate impression taking, with the correct tray handle inserted before use. Tray handles should always be used, otherwise the trays may be difficult to remove once the alginate has set.

Suitably sized trays should just fit over the dental arch in either jaw, without being excessively wide (they will be difficult to insert through the oral aperture of the lips), without being excessively long (they need go no further posteriorly than the end of the dental arch), and without being excessively short (they must record the full length of the dental arch). A trial tray insertion must always be carried out on the patient before proceeding with the impression taking, to avoid poor quality impressions which will need to be retaken. When a chosen tray has been inserted, it should be lifted up and down over the dental arch – if there is any catching on the teeth, or any resistance to being fully seated, then the tray is too narrow (Figure 13.15a and b).

Usually upper trays are used for upper impressions, and lowers for lower impressions. However, on occasions when the palate does not need to be recorded (such as with retainers and bleaching trays) a suitably sized lower tray may be used in the upper arch, and this is also less likely to stimulate a gag reflex in some patients.

Mixing of the alginate and loading of the trays

All dental nurses are familiar with the correct mixing of alginate, and the technique is summarised below.

- Ensure the powder measuring scoop and the water measure are for the same material, otherwise the 1 : 1 powder to water proportions will be incorrect
- Shake the powder container to mix the contents
- Use full and levelled scoops of powder, usually two are required for each impression
- Make a well in the powder in the mixing bowl and pour the room temperature water into the centre of the well (Figure 13.16a)
- Fold the powder into the water initially then vigorously mix and spatulate the mixture against the sides of the bowl (Figure 13.16b)
- Ensure all of the powder is mixed in and that no air bubbles have been introduced into the mix – when fully mixed it should have a uniform consistency (Figure 13.16c)

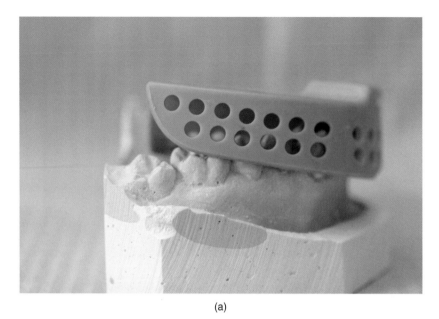

(a)

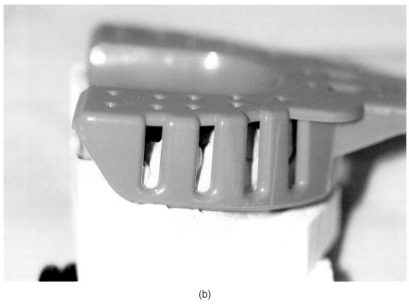

(b)

Figure 13.15 Sizing of tray for impression taking. (a) Tray catching molar teeth – too narrow. (b) Correct tray size, just covering the dental arch

EXTENDED DUTIES OF THE DENTAL NURSE

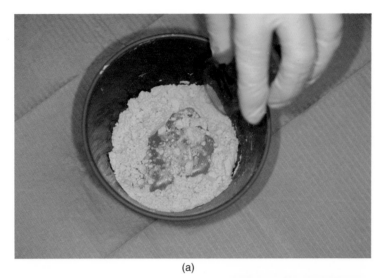

(a)

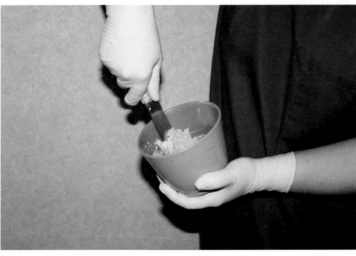

(b)

Figure 13.16 (a–e) Alginate mixing and tray loading

Upper trays are loaded with the full mix gathered on the spatula, and from the back of the tray forwards so that it is loaded uniformly across its whole width and length (Figure 13.16d).

Lower trays are loaded in two stages, with half the mix gathered on the spatula for each. The first half of the mix is loaded into one half of the tray from the inner side of the tray arch, and the second half into the other side (Figure 13.16e) so that the tray is equally filled with the impression material.

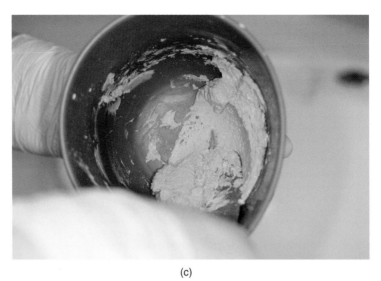

(c)

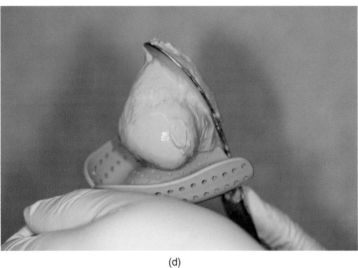

(d)

Figure 13.16 (*continued*)

Insertion of the trays

Each impression is mixed, loaded, inserted and removed one at a time. The insertion technique is as follows:

- The patient wears a waterproof bib, and sits upright in the dental chair
- The patient is instructed to relax the lips and to breathe at a normal rate through the nose while the impression is in the mouth

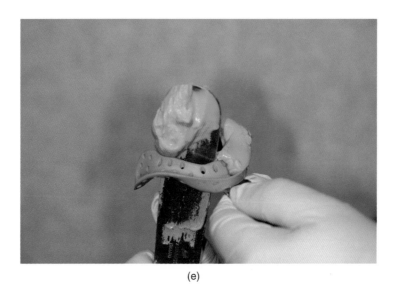

(e)

Figure 13.16 (continued)

- The lower impression is inserted while standing in front of the patient, by angling the loaded tray so one end passes through the oral aperture first and then swung over to that side of the dental arch – this brings the other side of the tray through the oral aperture and over the other side of the dental arch
- A right-handed dental nurse will find the process easier if the right side of the tray is inserted first, and the left hand is used to gently retract the lips as the left side is inserted later (and the opposite for a left-handed dental nurse)
- Once the full tray is hovering over the full lower arch it is gently pushed down onto the teeth, ensuring that the teeth are in the centre of the tray all around the arch (so not too close to either the buccal or lingual side of the tray)
- The lower lip may be pulled out and 'rolled' up over the front of the tray, to ensure the labial sulcus is fully recorded
- The tray is held evenly in this position with the fingers until setting occurs, in particular it must be held firm if the patient swallows as the tray would lift up otherwise
- The patient is asked to waggle the tongue from left to right, and then touch the outer surface of the upper lip with it – this moulds the inner edge of the impression and avoids the tongue being recorded in the impression, instead of the teeth
- The upper impression is inserted while standing behind the patient, to the right (for a right-handed dental nurse) or to the left (for a left-handed dental nurse)
- Again, the tray is inserted by angling first one side and then the other through the oral aperture while retracting the lips with the other hand (right side first for right-handed dental nurse, as previously)
- Once the full tray is hovering below the full upper arch, it is gently pushed up onto the teeth, from the back forwards to prevent material being pushed into the patient's throat
- Again, ensure that the teeth are in the centre of the tray all around the arch

- The upper lip may be pulled out and 'rolled' down over the front of the tray to ensure the labial sulcus is fully recorded
- The tray is supported evenly in this position with the fingers until setting occurs

Removal of the trays after setting

Any excess impression material can be squeezed to determine if setting has occurred – that in the patient's mouth will have set quicker still because the oral cavity has a warmer environment. Otherwise, the impression material lying in either labial sulcus can be touched to determine if it has fully set – it should feel firm and not leave any impression material on the gloves when the finger is pulled away.

Once set, the trays are removed by exerting a firm upward pressure on the tray handle of the lower tray, and a firm downward pressure on the tray handle of the upper tray. Sometimes, a finger run around the buccal and labial sulci will be necessary to break the suction force around the edges of the impression before it can be dislodged. The impression can then be gradually eased over the teeth and out of the mouth, reversing the angle and swing action of the insertion process so that the patient's soft tissues are not uncomfortably stretched.

On removal, the impression should be checked for accuracy before being sent for disinfection – if it is not adequate, then the impression taking must be repeated. For example, the impression shown in Figure 13.17 has well-rolled edges and no air blows, but the upper right molar tooth has not been fully recorded in the impression, and this may require a retake.

If the impressions are acceptable they are disinfected in the usual manner – rinsed, soaked, rinsed, packaged with damp gauze in a sealed bag, and correctly labelled.

Monitoring and handling of the patient

Suitable personal protective equipment must be provided and worn by the patient, and the dental nurse must wear clinical gloves throughout the whole procedure. The dental

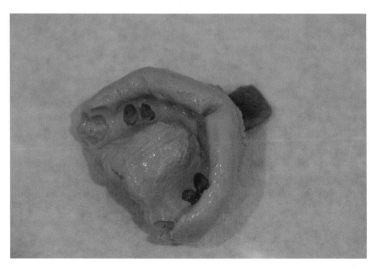

Figure 13.17 Example of an upper alginate impression

EXTENDED DUTIES OF THE DENTAL NURSE

nurse must always be aware of the fear and trepidation that some patients may exhibit when told they require impressions to be taken, and they should be empathetic to the patient's concerns. Any patient who is overly anxious should be referred to the dentist.

Some patients prefer to know what is involved in the procedure beforehand, others prefer not. Where possible a short and simplified explanation should be given to all patients; in particular the following points should be mentioned:

- The material sets relatively quickly, and the impressions will be removed as soon as possible
- Stay calm and breathe at a normal rate through the nose throughout the procedure
- If they begin to panic and try to remove the trays, their mouth will be covered in unset impression material which is difficult to remove – they must concentrate on their breathing and allow the procedure to continue
- Allow the lips to remain relaxed so that they can be retracted and manipulated as necessary by the dental nurse
- Follow the tongue instructions carefully
- Once the impressions are in place, they may tip their head forwards if they wish – this reduces the choking fear
- Do not worry if they begin dribbling while the impression is still inserted and setting – the waterproof bib will prevent any clothing damage
- Some considerable effort may be required to remove the impressions in some patients (because they have undercuts which 'lock' the impression in place), but it is *not* enough to pull their teeth out
- Give a distraction technique if necessary to overly anxious patients – for example, ask them to concentrate and count backwards from three hundred in 3s in their mind once the trays are in place (so 300, 297, 294, 291, and so on)

During the procedure, the dental nurse should also remain calm and in control of the situation. Make encouraging comments throughout ("you're doing really well", "we've nearly finished now", "well done", and so on).

Once the impressions are removed, help the patient to have a rinse and then check and remove any extra-oral impression material from their facial area – never send the patient away looking a mess. Also check if any impression tags are stuck between their teeth, and provide floss for the patient to dislodge it. Congratulate them on 'surviving' the ordeal and reiterate how well they did.

CONSTRUCTING BLEACHING TRAYS

Bleaching trays, mouth guards, and vacuum formed retainers are constructed in a similar process to each other, the difference being the material used for each one. The technique used to construct bleaching trays is described. These are devices made for patients to use at home when carrying out tooth whitening (see Chapter 12). Mouth guards are worn by patients who have a bruxing habit (tooth clenching and grinding habit) that is causing tooth wear and/or tooth fracture, or jaw joint discomfort, and vacuum formed retainers are the gum shield-type retainers worn by patients after completing a course of orthodontic treatment (see Chapter 11).

Each device is made by pulling a warmed sheet of varying thickness EVA tray material (Figure 13.18) over a stone model of the patient's dental arch, which is then sucked tightly

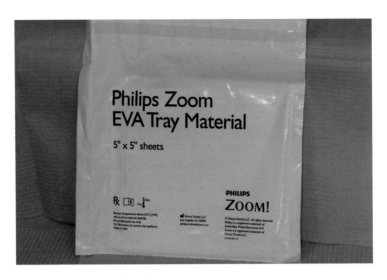

Figure 13.18 EVA tray material pack

onto the model under vacuum. Bleaching trays are made from very thin EVA sheets, while orthodontic retainers and mouth guards are constructed from thicker materials.

Once the tray has been removed from the model and carefully trimmed, a unique device is produced which is a perfect fit over the patient's own teeth. As the fit is so accurate, it cannot be placed into the mouth in any but the correct position (so it is easy for the patient to wear), it fits tightly but comfortably onto the teeth (so it does not fall out or become loose), and the material used is transparent so the device is not obvious.

An example of a vacuum machine used for the tray construction is shown in Figure 13.19.

The technique of producing the bleaching tray is as follows:

- The stone models of the dental arches to be bleached are provided by the laboratory, or cast up on site
- They are trimmed to remove the sulci areas, and upper models have the palate removed or a hole placed through so that the suction under vacuum can be applied to all sides of the model
- The teeth to be bleached (this varies between patients) have a spacer material present on the labial surfaces, so that a well is formed during tray construction for the application of the bleaching gel – the spacer in the images used is blue wax
- The model is placed on the base of the machine and a sheet of EVA loaded and locked into the tray reservoir above it (Figure 13.20)
- The heater above the material is switched on to warm the sheet – it is ready to be pulled over the model when the warmed sheet hangs about 1.5 cm below the reservoir (Figure 13.21)
- The tray reservoir is pulled sharply down to the bottom of the machine so that it lies over the model, and the vacuum is switched on immediately (the heater can be switched off at this point)
- The suction produced pulls the sheet tightly over the model to produce the tray – the vacuum should be left to run for a minimum of 30 s

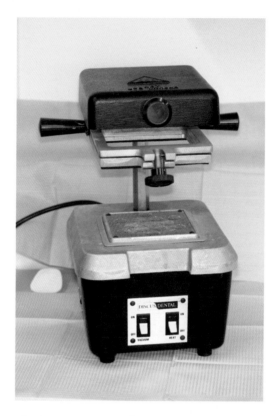

Figure 13.19 Example of a vacuum tray machine

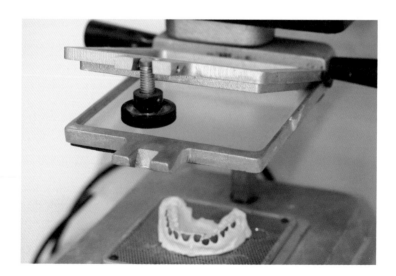

Figure 13.20 Machine loaded with model and tray material

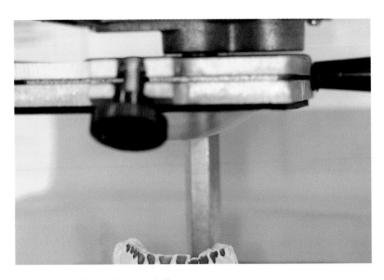

Figure 13.21 Warmed EVA sheet ready for use

- Once the construction is complete, the machine is switched off and the model and tray are left to cool before handling
- Bleaching trays are carefully trimmed to follow the gingival line of the teeth, producing a scalloped edge (Figure 13.22)
- Orthodontic retainers and mouth guards are trimmed to leave a 2 mm extension beyond the gingival margins, so that the tray edge lies on the gingivae
- The trimmed edges are smoothed to avoid any soft tissue trauma – an emery board or similar file is ideal

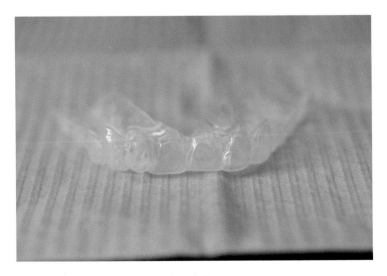

Figure 13.22 Bleaching tray trimmed and ready for use

EXTENDED DUTIES OF THE DENTAL NURSE

INTRA- AND EXTRA-ORAL PHOTOGRAPHY

Photographs are an important diagnostic and assessment tool for the clinician, as well as being a powerful method of convincing patients that a dental problem exists or of showing them the before and after appearance of suggested dental treatments. Digital images in particular are extremely useful when a second opinion is required about a case (especially potentially suspicious soft tissue lesions), as they can be securely emailed to a specialist. Away from the hospital environment, photographs are used a great deal to assist in orthodontic assessments and to provide before and after views once orthodontic treatment has been completed. A suitably trained dental nurse can be tasked to take both intra- and extra-oral photographs for these purposes.

Old style clinical photography involved the use of 'instamatic' type cameras, which produced a hard-copy 'polaroid' image within a few minutes. Digital imagery produces instant images without the need for film, and these can be loaded directly onto a computer and also downloaded as a hard copy if required. Once on the computer screen, they can be 'zoomed in' so that the image (or a section of it) can be enlarged, although the clarity of the picture deteriorates after a certain point.

An example of a suitable camera and attachments for clinical photography is shown in Figure 13.23.

The particular features of the camera and its potential uses are as follows:

- The camera body has interchangeable lenses, the one required for intra-oral (close up) photography is a macro lens

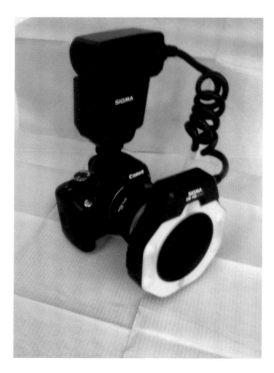

Figure 13.23 Digital camera and ring flash

- The ring flash shown provides sufficient diffuse light directly at the object, rather than a bright burst of intense light in the surroundings as produced by an ordinary flash – it is simply screwed onto the camera body top and to the lens with a ring adapter
- The mode dial on top of the camera body allows the camera to automatically set itself to take images in the selected mode – so on this camera, close-up shots are taken with the dial set to a flower pictogram, while portrait images are taken with it set to the head pictogram
- The lens focus mode switch on the side of the lens is used to change between automatic focus (AF) and manual focus (MF) – usually AF is used, but when intra-oral images are taken looking into the mouth, sometimes the camera automatically focuses onto the lip or an anterior tooth, when the image required is more posterior – in these cases MF should be used and the lens focused manually by the operator onto the required focal point
- When taking intra-oral images, the soft tissues often need retracting either by hand, with a mouth mirror, or using specific lip retractors (Figure 13.24)
- Difficult to see areas such as the upper arch or lingual to the lower incisors can be viewed more easily with the use of oral mirrors (see Figure 13.24) – these are best run under cold water before use to prevent them misting while the patient breathes
- Figure 13.25 shows a typical portrait style view, while Figure 13.26 shows an intra-oral view of a prepared cavity in a tooth – the lens focus mode was set to MF to avoid the camera automatically focusing on the anterior teeth
- Images can be viewed immediately on the camera viewer or loaded onto the computer for a larger and more detailed image
- The memory card from the camera is removed and inserted into the correct entry port of a card reader device – an adapter may be necessary for some card types (Figure 13.27)
- A USB cable connects the card reader to the computer and the images are present in the 'removable disk device' option – they can then be uploaded *en masse* as a file to the computer, or individually as a JPEG
- As the images are accessible immediately, any that require retakes can be carried out while the patient is still present

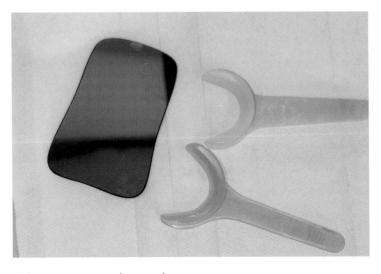

Figure 13.24 Lip retractors and intra-oral mirror

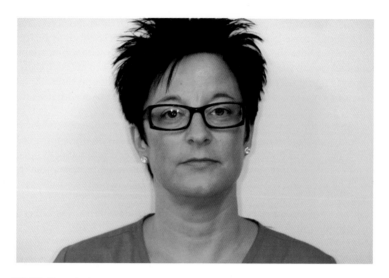

Figure 13.25 Portrait view

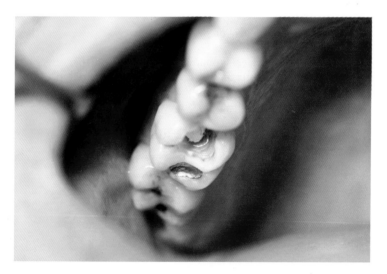

Figure 13.26 Intra-oral view

REMOVING SUTURES

Sutures are used to close a surgical site and hold the edges of a flap of soft tissue in position while the tissues heal, after surgery or trauma. Once the site has been checked by the dentist to ensure that full healing has occurred without any inflammation or infection present, the sutures can be carefully removed by a suitably trained dental nurse.

The procedure is often time consuming because care must be taken not to pull the healed surgical area as it will hurt the patient, and often there are several sutures to be removed.

EXTENDED DUTIES OF THE DENTAL NURSE

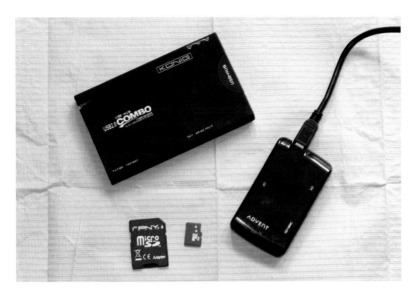

Figure 13.27 Examples of memory card readers and adapters

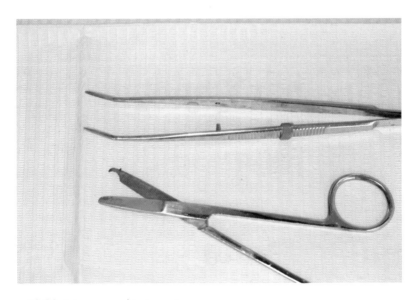

Figure 13.28 Suture removal instruments

The sterile instruments required for suture removal are a mouth mirror, a pair of college tweezers and a pair of suture removal scissors (Figure 13.28). The scissors have a half-moon cut out of one blade so that the suture loop can be located here and held while being cut (Figure 13.29) – with an ordinary pair of scissors the loop would ride along the blade during cutting and pull uncomfortably on the wound.

EXTENDED DUTIES OF THE DENTAL NURSE

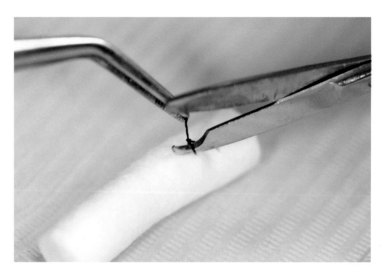

Figure 13.29 Holding suture end taut while cutting through the loop

The technique of suture removal is as follows:

- The dental nurse and the patient wear appropriate personal protective equipment
- Angle the dental chair and light to provide easy access to the sutures
- Use the mouth mirror to retract soft tissues if necessary – sometimes a second dental nurse may be required to carry this out when the sutures lie posteriorly
- Remove any food debris from the sutures with a small bore aspirator if necessary
- Count the number of sutures present and check with the procedure notes that they tally – if not, ask the patients if they were aware of losing any sutures (black braided silk is often used and may appear as a piece of black cotton to the patient) and refer back to the dentist for advice
- Gently find and hold one tied end of the suture with the tweezers, and then pull to hold it taut
- This should lift the top of the suture loop off the soft tissues, allowing the suture scissors to be placed beneath it with the cut out blade closest to the surgical tissues
- The suture loop needs to be located in the half-moon cut out of the blade so that the suture thread remains in place during cutting
- When correctly positioned, make the cut while holding the suture end with the tweezers
- Once cut through completely, the suture is removed from the mouth and placed on a tissue
- Repeat the process for all the sutures
- Count the number removed again, and then check that each one has been fully removed – they should each appear as a cut loop of thread with a knot and two tied ends present
- If any problems occur, seek the advice of the dentist – do not undertake any further tasks than the training allows

EXTENDED DUTIES OF THE DENTAL NURSE

Post-operative advice

The patient should be advised to continue hot salt water mouth washes for the next few days to assist the area to heal completely now that the sutures have been removed. They can carry out their routine oral hygiene techniques in this area without fear of catching the sutures, and they can eat and drink as normal. They should not touch the area with their fingers, as they may introduce infection.

Assessment sheet

Example of an impression taking assessment sheet

PATIENT IDENTIFIER	1963
DATE	4th February 2014
REASON FOR IMPRESSION(S)	Upper tooth whitening tray
MATERIALS USED	Alginate and water
TRAY(S) USED	Upper boxed single use tray – perforated
EQUIPMENT AND OTHER MATERIALS USED	Mixing bowl, spatula, water measure and scoop Tray handle, disinfection and packaging items
MIX DETAILS AND TRAY LOADING	Smooth mix with no residual powder Tray fully loaded from posterior edge forward, with full coverage and no excess material
ANY COMPLICATIONS	Pt wary of gagging, therefore nervous but compliant
QUALITY OF IMPRESSION	Correctly set throughout on removal, no air blows or defects Full arch recorded
ASSESSED BY	CH
POST-OPERATIVE CARE GIVEN	Pt congratulated Assisted with providing mouth rinse and carried out removal of material from around pt lips
DISINFECTION AND PACKAGING DETAILS	Rinsed in dirty sink Immersed in impression disinfectant solution for 10 minutes Rinsed and wrapped in damp gauze Sealed in air tight bag with completed laboratory docket, marked as 'disinfected'

Basic Guide to Dental Procedures, Second Edition. Carole Hollins.
© 2015 John Wiley & Sons, Ltd. Published 2015 by John Wiley & Sons, Ltd.

SATISFACTORY OR NOT YET SATISFACTORY	Satisfactory
NOTES	Fully prepared for procedure Good communication with pt throughout Good mixing and loading technique Correctly determined when impression had set Removed without tearing impression Good pt care afterwards Correct disinfection and packaging carried out

Example of a suture removal assessment sheet

PATIENT IDENTIFIER	1745
DATE	12th January 2014
PREVIOUS SURGICAL PROCEDURE	Surgical extraction of grossly carious UR6 (16) Flap raised
SITE CHECKED BY	CH
INSTRUMENTS SET OUT	College tweezers, mouth mirror Suture scissors
NUMBER AND TYPE OF SUTURES	3 black braided silk
PRESENTATION AT ROS APPOINTMENT	Site healed, no inflammation present Some food debris on suture ends
NOTES OF ROS PROCEDURE	Sutures aspirated with narrow bore to remove food debris and make ends clear End of each suture found and gently held taut while sutures cut and removed Assisted by second nurse to retract right cheek
ANY COMPLICATIONS	None once retraction assistance provided
POST-OPERATIVE INSTRUCTIONS GIVEN	Pt told to carry out HSWMW again today to prevent soreness Pt told to carry out routine OHI in the area from now, and return if any problems before the pre-set review appointment next month

ASSESSED BY	CH
SATISFACTORY OR NOT YET SATISFACTORY	Satisfactory
NOTES	No problems with set up Accurate observation of surgical area re; healing Handled instruments competently and realised assistance with retraction was required Did not proceed with ROS until happy with retraction and visibility

Glossary of terms

Abrasion cavity a self-inflicted worn area produced at the neck of a tooth by over-vigorous toothbrushing

Acid etch an acidic material used in dentistry on the enamel of a tooth to chemically roughen it, allowing greater adhesion of some fillings and cements

Acute infection an infection of sudden onset, and therefore associated with pain and swelling

Aesthetics relating to a pleasing appearance, as in the aesthetics of a veneer for instance

Aligners a set of pre-formed, gum shield-like orthodontic devices which are worn sequentially to gradually allow tooth movement to occur, resulting in well-aligned dental arches

Amalgam a malleable filling material used to fill cavities in posterior teeth, and composed of various metal powders mixed with liquid mercury

Apex locator an electronic device used during root treatment to determine the full length of a root canal, by giving off a signal when the apex has been located

Apicectomy the surgical removal of a root apex and any associated pathology, and involving access to the root via the jaw bone

Articulating paper thin carbon paper used to detect high spots on new restorations, by being placed between the teeth and leaving coloured marks when the patient occludes

Articulator a three-dimensional jig device that mimics occlusion and jaw movements when a set of study casts are accurately placed within

Bitewing radiograph a posterior intra-oral radiographic view, taken to show interdental caries or restoration overhangs

Bonding the technique of 'glueing' the brackets and tubes of a fixed orthodontic appliance to the patient's teeth using special adhesive dental materials

Bone resorption the natural process that occurs to the jaw bones after tooth extraction, so that a smooth ridge contour is produced

Bridge a dental device used to replace a missing tooth (or teeth) by the construction and insertion of a device made up of several crowns (units) joined together in a single span

Bruxism the habitual clenching and grinding of the teeth, often causing excessive tooth wear or tooth fracture

Calculus minerlised deposits of plaque that form at the gingival margins causing inflammation, it is also referred to as tartar

Caries a bacterial infection of the hard tissues of the teeth causing cavities, also referred to as tooth decay in lay terms

Cephalograph a specialist radiographic view used mainly in orthodontics to determine the severity of a patient's jaw discrepancies

Basic Guide to Dental Procedures, Second Edition. Carole Hollins.
© 2015 John Wiley & Sons, Ltd. Published 2015 by John Wiley & Sons, Ltd.

Chronic infection an infection of very slow but persistent onset, and therefore usually painless

Composite a malleable filling material used to fill cavities in anterior and posterior teeth, and which gives a tooth-like appearance to the completed filling

Conscious sedation an anxiety control technique using the administration of drugs to relax the patient sufficiently for treatment to proceed, while they remain conscious (awake) throughout the procedure

Crown a dental device used to cover the whole of a tooth with a pre-constructed 'cap' made of precious metals or porcelain, to strengthen the remaining tooth structure or to improve the aesthetics

Demineralisation the action of acids on the tooth enamel to produce weakened areas that are more prone to carious attack

Dental impression a device used to record the patient's tooth positions in the dental arch using an impression material in a tray, so that the set material remains accurate while a cast (study model) is made

Dental pantomograph (DPT) a radiographic view taken to show all of the teeth and their surrounding bony structures in one image, and used in orthodontics and complicated case diagnoses

Dentine the inner living tissue forming the bulk of the tooth structure, it contains nerve endings and therefore allows sensation in the tooth

Disclosing tablet a coloured tablet of vegetable dye which stains plaque when chewed in the mouth; it is used during oral hygiene instruction to show patients where their plaque has accummulated and to assist them in its full removal

Distal surface the surface of any tooth which lies furthest away from the midline of the dental arch (the 'back' of the tooth)

Edentulous the condition of having no natural teeth present

Enamel the outer surface of the erupted crown of a tooth, it is a mineralised, non-living tissue

Extended duties in the United Kingdom, those additional duties that may be performed by a dental nurse following appropriate and recorded training, over and above those skills acquired at basic certification

Extraction of a tooth, the procedure of permanently removing a tooth from its socket

Fissure a natural anatomical cleft in the occlusal surface of a tooth, between the cusps

Fissure sealant a resin-like material used to seal over the tooth fissures and prevent food debris from lodging there and causing cavities

Fluoride a compound of the chemical fluorine which is added to oral health products (tooth paste, mouth wash, and so on) to help prevent dental cavities from forming in the teeth

Gingival crevice a 2mm deep crevice around the necks of all healthy teeth, where plaque accumulates when oral hygiene standards are poor

Gingival margin the edge of a restoration (such as a crown) that lies at the gingival crevice

Gingivitis inflammation of the gingivae, or gums

Glass ionomer a malleable dental material which can be used to fill cavities or cement items such as crowns, veneers, and orthodontic brackets onto the teeth

Gutta percha point a natural rubber material used to root fill a tooth, and provided in various length and diameter points

Haemostasis the arrest of blood flow in an area, especially after tooth extraction

Immediate replacement denture a denture which is inserted at the time of tooth extraction, to replace missing teeth immediately

Implant a threaded titanium cylinder which is surgically screwed into the jaw bone to support an artificial tooth, teeth, or a denture; it is a method of tooth replacement

Inlay a solid dental device used to close a cavity in a tooth, using a material such as gold or porcelain and made out of the mouth by a technician

Intensifying screen a device used within extra-oral radiographic cassettes to reduce x-ray exposure to the patient

Interdental area the area at the point where two adjacent teeth touch together

Intra-oral radiograph one that is exposed to x-rays while within the patient's mouth

Labial surface the outer surface of an anterior tooth that lies against the lips

Lens focus mode switch a control button on a camera which allows the operator to choose between automatic focus (controlled by the camera) and manual focus (controlled by the operator) when taking intra- and extra-oral dental images

Lingual surface the inner surface of any lower tooth that lies against the tongue

Lining a material used in the base of a cavity before filling, to protect the underlying pulp tissue

Luting cement a cement mixed to a creamy consistency and used as an adhesive in crown and bridge cases

Malalignment the uneven, out-of-line positions of teeth in a dental arch, often caused by crowding

Mastication the correct term for the act of chewing of food

Matrix band a thin strip of metal or acetate used in a holder to separate adjacent teeth during filling

Mesial surface the surface of any tooth which lies closest to the midline of the dental arch (the 'front' of the tooth)

Minor oral surgery a variety of surgical procedures carried out in the mouth which do not necessitate hospital admission, and which are usually carried out under local anaesthesia

Mode dial a control dial on a camera which can be altered by the operator for different types of photographic view (portrait, landscape, close-up, action, and so on) which allows the camera to automatically set itself to take the ideal image for that particular setting

Moisture control the act of removing fluid contamination from the oral cavity during dental procedures, often involving the use of suction equipment and absorbent materials

Non-milk extrinsic sugars those sugars other than lactose which have been added to foods and drinks during food processing, and that are responsible for causing tooth decay

Non-vital tooth one that has died

Occlusal surface the biting surface of a posterior tooth

Occlusion the tooth positions achieved when the jaws are closed together and the upper and lower teeth are contacting

Overdenture a denture constructed to attach to and fit over the top of implant abutments

Periapical radiograph an anterior or posterior radiographic view, taken to show a full tooth including its root and the bone immediately surrounding it

Periodontal disease an infection of the supporting structures of a tooth in its socket, by one of several bacterial microorganisms

Periodontal ligament the tough connective tissue that holds a tooth in its socket

Plaque a sticky film of food debris and bacteria (biofilm) that forms on the teeth causing caries and gingivitis if not removed

Plaque index a numerical score given to the presence of plaque in the patient's mouth at the time of checking, which is used to help monitor their oral hygiene levels before, during, and after treatment

Pulp chamber the inner hollow chamber of a tooth, containing nerve tissue and blood vessels (pulp)

Pulpectomy the removal of the whole tooth pulp from the pulp chamber; it is also referred to as root canal treatment or root canal therapy

Pulp exposure the breaching of the pulp chamber and exposing its contents to the oral cavity

Pulpotomy the removal of the pulp tissue from the top of the pulp chamber only, leaving that in the root of the tooth intact

Pulse oximeter a machine used to help monitor a patient during conscious sedation therapy, which records their oxygen saturation and pulse, and sometimes their blood pressure

Refined sugar a sugar not naturally present in a food but added during manufacture, and highly cariogenic

Root apex the very tip of a tooth root, where nerves and blood vessels enter and leave the tooth

Rubber dam a sheet of rubbery material used to isolate a tooth during dental procedures to provide good moisture control

Saliva the watery fluid naturally produced by the salivary glands and emptied into the oral cavity to provide lubrication, amongst other functions

Scaler an instrument used to remove calculus from teeth and roots

Short-term orthodontics a type of orthodontic treatment carried out for cosmetic reasons and usually only involving the anterior teeth, which can be completed in a much shorter time frame than conventional orthodontics

Stagnation area any area in the oral cavity that allows the accumulation of plaque to occur, either occuring naturally such as the fissures of the teeth, or such as overhanging filling edges

Stock tray a plastic or metal standard shaped tray used for taking initial impressions or study model casts

Supine lying horizontal, as in the usual working position of the dental chair during procedures such as restorations

Suture the correct medical term for a 'stitch' – a piece of tied material (such as silk) which is used to hold the cut ends of a wound together while tissue healing takes place

Vasoconstrictor a chemical added to local anaesthetic solutions to prolong anaesthesia by constricting the surrounding blood vessels

Veneer a dental device used as a 'false front' to a tooth, usually to hide discolouration or to alter the shape of a tooth

X-ray cassette a specialised case containing intensifying screens, used for extra-oral radiography such as orthopantomographs

Index

Basic Guide to Dental Procedures, Second Edition. Carole Hollins.
© 2015 John Wiley & Sons, Ltd. Published 2015 by John Wiley & Sons, Ltd.

CRITICAL
CARE NURSING
The Humanised Approach

Edited by

SARA J. WHITE
& DESIREE TAIT

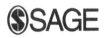SAGE

Los Angeles | London | New Delhi
Singapore | Washington DC | Melbourne

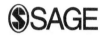

Los Angeles | London | New Delhi
Singapore | Washington DC | Melbourne

SAGE Publications Ltd
1 Oliver's Yard
55 City Road
London EC1Y 1SP

SAGE Publications Inc.
2455 Teller Road
Thousand Oaks, California 91320

SAGE Publications India Pvt Ltd
B 1/I 1 Mohan Cooperative Industrial Area
Mathura Road
New Delhi 110 044

SAGE Publications Asia-Pacific Pte Ltd
3 Church Street
#10-04 Samsung Hub
Singapore 049483

Editor: Alex Clabburn
Editorial assistant: Jade Grogan
Production editor: Martin Fox
Copyeditor: Mary Dalton
Proofreader: William Baginsky
Indexer: Elske Janssen
Marketing manager: Tamara Navaratnam
Cover design: Wendy Scott
Typeset by: C&M Digitals (P) Ltd, Chennai, India

Library of Congress Control Number: 2018943848

British Library Cataloguing in Publication data

A catalogue record for this book is available from the British Library

ISBN 978-1-4739-7850-8
ISBN 978-1-4739-7851-5 (pbk)

CRITICAL
CARE NURSING

Sara Miller McCune founded SAGE Publishing in 1965 to support the dissemination of usable knowledge and educate a global community. SAGE publishes more than 1000 journals and over 800 new books each year, spanning a wide range of subject areas. Our growing selection of library products includes archives, data, case studies and video. SAGE remains majority owned by our founder and after her lifetime will become owned by a charitable trust that secures the company's continued independence.

Los Angeles | London | New Delhi | Singapore | Washington DC | Melbourne

Contents

About the Editors and Contributors

EDITORS

Desiree Tait, DNSc, MSc, SFHEA, DNE, DN, RGN

Desiree is a Principal Lecturer and Programme Leader for the BSc Adult Nursing Programme at the Faculty of Health and Social Sciences, Bournemouth University. She has 40 years' experience in the practice, theory and education of caring for people with acute and complex critical conditions. She has a particular interest in the philosophical values that underpin humanised care and how this can influence clinical decision making. Her doctoral research analysed nurses' experiences of recognising and responding to clinical deterioration and critical illness and this has informed more recent studies in recognising the value base of student nurses and managing complex conditions.

Sara J. White, EdD., MA, SFHEA, BSc (Hons), RGN

Sara is Associate Dean Student Experience and acting Deputy Dean of the Faculty of Health and Social Sciences, Bournemouth University. She has nearly 40 years' experience in Intensive Care, Coronary Care and nurse education. As a nurse educator she has a particular interest in the student experience and how the care they provide is humanised. She believes that the philosophical values that underpin the humanised care philosophy are critical to their way of being as they interact with each other, other health care professionals, the client's family and all they work with.

CONTRIBUTORS

Debbie Branney, RGN

Debbie is Project Manager, Acute Pain Team and Research Nurse, Royal Bournemouth and Christchurch Hospitals Foundation NHS Trust. Prior to this Debbie worked in both cardiothoracic and general critical care nursing, most recently as Deputy Clinical Leader, for over 20 years. Whatever role Debbie has worked in her ethos has never changed; the patient's needs always come first, and care must always be holistic.

Jonathan Branney PhD, MChiro, BN (Hons), FHEA, RN

Jonny is Senior Lecturer in Adult Nursing and Programme Leader for the PGDip Adult Nursing, Faculty of Health and Social Sciences, Bournemouth University. He has nearly 20 years' clinical and educational experience of caring for people with critical and long-term conditions and is passionate about teaching the biosciences that underpin safe and effective nursing care, using innovative teaching techniques wherever possible to engage students. His main research interests are in pain management, particularly towards improving the diagnosis and management of neck pain.

Mark Gagan LLM, PG diploma (Social research), RN, RNT

Mark is a Senior Academic and Programme Leader at Bournemouth University Faculty of Health and Social Sciences. His clinical background was as a nurse in critical care areas including Neonatal Intensive Care (NICU). His main interests include developing nursing strategies that promote a humanised approach to negotiating solutions to legal and ethical issues in the critical care environment.

Fleur Lowe, PGCE, BSc (Hons) Clinical Leadership, Dip HE, RGN, EN(G)

Fleur is a Senior Nurse and Educational Lead in the critical care outreach team at Salisbury NHS Foundation Trust hospital. She has 33 years' experience, 27 of which are in critical care. She has a particular interest in developing healthcare professionals in clinical practice, encouraging a humanistic approach to care both individually and collectively in their interactions with others.

Publisher's Acknowledgments

On behalf of the authors, SAGE would like to thank the academics who reviewed the content of the book, helping to shape and influence it for the better:

Julie Douglas, Keele University

Sue Faulds, University of Southampton

Jane Harden, Cardiff University

Cheryl Phillips, University of South Wales

Introduction

SARA J. WHITE AND DESIREE TAIT

Critical illness can occur at any age, but it is more often associated with middle age and beyond, often exacerbated by multiple co-morbidities. Commonly patients experience the physical symptoms of illness and disability before acknowledging them fully on an emotional level; denial is the most obvious example of this. Likewise after a return to health, or learning to live with chronic conditions, patients still experience concerns and fears related to their critical illness. Sometimes the critical care unit is perceived as a place where fragile lives are vigilantly monitored, cared for and on the whole preserved. Understanding how critical illness impacts on, and what critical care means to, patients and their families can help nurses to provide individualised humanised care for these patients and their family. This book consequently explores how senior nurses can help junior nurses understand the care they offer from a humanistic perspective as they anticipate, assess, monitor and respond to illness. Maintaining full confidentiality throughout, the book explores real-life case studies with a view to recognising and supporting effective behaviours and minimising and redirecting ineffective behaviours to help the patient, their family and the nurses caring for them.

We start the book by exploring the relationship between patient-centred care and holism and how these can be considered within a humanising care philosophy. **Chapter 1** discusses how the humanising dimensions relate to the patient, family and critical care nurse. The humanising framework and dimensions are complex and we recognise that the constructs merge, but for ease of use and explanation, we have deconstructed them throughout the book. A key focus of this book is that the expert nurse explores care through the lens of the professional gaze and the factors that affect clinical decision making in practice. We assist how s/he can do this at the same time as using the humanising dimensions.

We then move on to explore the complex and interrelated nature of the triggers that lead to critical illness. We explore the factors that can influence the progression from acute to critical changes in a person's condition. Consequently, **Chapter 2** begins with an exploration of critical illness from a cellular level and how this relates to the body's stress response and behaviour and inflammatory response. It also explores how personal, cultural and structural factors can trigger and exacerbate critical illness, affect the progression of the patient's condition and impact on their rehabilitation.

Two case studies, of Anna and David, who have respiratory problems (Type I and Type II Respiratory Failure), are used in **Chapter 3** as we explore the links between the humanising health care dimensions and issues related to culture, sepsis, acute delirium and critical illness and the impact of enforced isolation.

Chapter 4 explores the case study of Joseph who has acute myeloid leukaemia and is haemodynamically unstable. It takes the stance of the expert critical care nurse and how s/he works with and supports a junior member of staff who is newly qualified. The chapter also considers the clinical decision making and support needed for the family during Joseph's stay in ICU.

The complex patient journey of Michael as he progresses through a multifaceted myocardial infarction involving an intra-aortic balloon pump and Non-Invasive Ventilation (High Flow Nasal Oxygen and CPAP) is explored in **Chapter 5**. Here we discuss the predicaments experienced by his wife, those experienced by the Coronary Care Unit (CCU) staff and the Critical Care Outreach Team (CCOT). It also explores the role of the senior nurse in relation to humanising the care of a client in a complex situation and associated leadership and management of staff.

Chapter 6 discusses the experiences of Brian who has acute kidney injury. It explores factors of how nurses looking after him use their influence in the clinical decision making and the 'clinical gaze' as they risk assess him and how this may impact on patient outcome. It also explores the concept of hope as Brian clinically deteriorates.

Rebecca is the focus of **Chapter 7** where we explore how she manages her multiple health needs with her partner Simon. We explore Rebecca's admission for a gastric disorder and how multiple ward transfers had the potential for missed care. We also explore how sleep disturbances can have a detrimental effect on Rebecca, and consider the impact of her critical illness on Simon as her caregiver.

In **Chapter 8,** we discuss the case study of Conner who has multiple co-morbidities of Diabetes, pancreatic cancer and gastric exocrine problems. It offers a discussion regarding how pathophysiology of one condition can cause complications when trying to manage another. It explores the role of specialist nurses and how they can be vital in reducing ambiguity, distrust and family fear and how they can help humanise the care needs of Conner, his next of kin and family.

In **Chapter 9**, we draw on the two case studies of Richard and Steven as we discuss how the past medical history of the patient can hinder care, delay treatment and lead to dehumanised care. It also explores how a HEART choice model can be used to help humanise care for both the patient and the family at a time of critical illness. It explores how leadership and humanising care relates to sudden catastrophic illness, and in turn how this affects patients and their families' lives.

The practical and ethical challenges of providing safe and effective humanised nursing care in the contemporary critical care environment are offered in **Chapter 10**. It encourages analysis and critical reflection of the challenges of delivering humanised care to people who are critically ill in a highly technical and busy clinical environment. The chapter consequently examines and discusses concepts such as emotional labour, moral distress, and feelings of powerlessness and oppression and the effects these can have on those who deliver the care. It briefly also outlines how the use of ethical, legal and professional frameworks can enhance and encourage the humanisation of care for the benefit of patients, their families and significant others and for healthcare professionals too.

In **Chapter 11** we explore the case study of Fred, a 74-year-old man who had a Road Traffic Collision (RTC). We explore the underlying myopathy and physiology and consider how critical illness can lead to the complexity of delirium and how this can lead to Post-Traumatic Stress disorder. We visit how the senior nurse humanises the care of a complex situation as s/he leads and manages staff.

In the **Conclusion**, we situate this book as a text for nurses with critical care experience who are developing their humanising care, management, leadership, clinical wisdom and clinical decision making skills. Having explored triggers to critical illness, critical illnesses, the humanising care framework and different dimensions to help staff caring for the critically ill we hope you can incorporate the humanising framework into your own clinical areas of practice. By the end, you should have developed your professional gaze and feel confident in understanding and practising humanised clinical decision making.

CHAPTER 1

Humanised Care and Clinical Decision Making in Critical Care

SARA J. WHITE AND DESIREE TAIT

CHAPTER AIMS

1 To understand the relationship between person-centred care and a humanising philosophy.
2 To discuss how the humanising dimensions can relate to the patient, family and critical care nurse.
3 To explore the professional gaze of the critical care nurse and how this relates to effective clinical decision making.

INTRODUCTION

This chapter explores the relationship between patient-centred care and holism and how these can be explored within a humanising care philosophy. The complex way of being of the expert nurse is then explored through the lens of the professional gaze (*the professional practice of engaging in scanning, selective perception, recognition, diagnosis of and response to clinical deterioration*) and factors that affect clinical decision making in practice.

Humanising health care and the role of the expert critical care nurse in identifying and managing any shortcomings are a key feature of each chapter.

WHAT IS PATIENT-CENTRED CARE?

Patient-centred care (PCC) has a long tradition in nursing practice and is recognised as a core concept in health care and in quality improvement. It derived from the humanistic psychologist Karl Rogers in the 1940s (Rogers 1951) when he wrote about client centred therapy. Here he spoke of the bio-psychological perspective and that a person is shaped by their biological, psychological and social perspectives and as such clinicians needed to think beyond biology. Since Rogers's work scholars have offered many definitions and concepts for PCC which will now be explored and will show that it is the delivery of care that respects patient needs, preferences, and values and that this is not specific to situation or location.

Slatore et al. (2012: 411) identified that 'PCC has 5 domains, these being the bio-psychosocial perspective, with a focus on information exchange; the patient as a person; sharing power and responsibility; the therapeutic alliance; and the clinician as a person'. They highlight that information exchange, and effective accurate risk communication are at the centre of the bio-psychosocial perspective; that addressing patient concerns and listening to the patient about their concerns is treating the patient as a person. To treat a patient as a person involves shared decision making and ensuring the patient is involved in the planning of care and the sharing of power and responsibility.

Patient-centred care became more prominent as changes in nurse education occurred, as new advanced nursing roles and as new technologies were more evident. The evolution of PCC resulted in several dimensions and frameworks being produced for use in specialist areas, such as Kitwood's (1997) exploration of Dementia; Mead and Bowers (2000) on the medical model development of a medical framework; and Nolan et al.'s (2001) perspective on gerontology. Many studies have identified core elements of PCC in nursing and medicine. For example Hobbs (2009) offered a dimensional analysis of PCC and Rauta et al. (2012) explored PCC in the preoperative setting. Manley's (1989) research offered proposals for introducing Primary Nursing in ICU, as a method of work organisation in ICU, where the same nurse cared for clients from admission to discharge and by doing this a therapeutic relationship developed which led to greater PCC and job satisfaction for nurses. Whilst PCC continues to strive in practice today Primary Nursing, despite being valued, tends not to have a strong presence. Indeed today PCC, and not Primary Nursing, is central to UK and international political policy (see Box 1.1 below).

BOX 1.1

UK Policy That Supports Patient-Centred Care

- Department of Health (2000) National Service Framework for Coronary Heart Disease; Modern Standards and Service Models.
- Department of Health (2001) National Service Framework for older people.
- Department of Health (2006) Dignity in Care Campaign.
- Department of Health (2012) NHS England: Compassion in Practice. Nursing, Midwifery and Care Staff, Our Vision and Strategy.
- Health Improvement Scotland (2017) People at the Centre of Health Care. Person-Centred Health and Care.

- NHS Wales (2015) Health and Care Standards.
- World Health Organisation (2015) Preparing a Health Care Workforce for the 21st Century: The Challenge of Chronic Conditions.

Furthermore, patient involvement in delivery and design of services is at the forefront of modern health care and healthcare reform (Forbat et al., 2009; Angood et al., 2010; Mockford et al., 2011). Here literature discusses how PCC requires that people are treated as individuals, that care is centred on the person and not the disease, that autonomy is fostered and there is respect of the rights of the person. It explores how that person has a choice in the planning of their care which is derived from their explicit requirements rather than the requirement of the health professional; and enabling these components requires the building of mutual trust and understanding in order to find a common agreement about care which is contextually and culturally defined. This concordance requires the development of therapeutic relationships and McCormack and McCance (2010) believe this is achieved through expert communication and continuity of care. Key to this is quality care, which according to the Institute of Medicine (2001) is the provision of safe, timely, effective, equitable care, and in our evolving world needs to be culturally competent, appropriate and 'uniquely tailored to care to patients with diverse values, beliefs and behaviours' (Johnson, 2015: 87).

DOES PATIENT-CENTRED CARE IMPROVE PATIENT OUTCOME?

Berwick (2009), Hobbs (2009) and Radwin et al. (2009) report on the positive correlation between PCC and desirable health outcomes. Indeed Wolf et al. (2008), Hobbs (2009) and Epstein et al. (2010) report how PCC results in improved patient satisfaction because it improves time allocation for care delivery, lowers the treatment costs and decreases the period of time in hospital as patients are discharged earlier. However, while the frameworks for providing PCC exist and indeed the benefits have been highlighted, how is it defined?

Like others Stewart (2001) feels that patient-centred care is difficult to define and therefore is easier to recognise when care is not patient centred and this was shown in Mid-Staffordshire (Francis 2013) where reports of task-centred, function-focused, poor quality care and the dehumanising of experience, with a lack of care and compassion offered by healthcare professionals, led to the scrutiny of care. This highlighted that, amongst other things, continuity of care, good communication, quality care, management and leadership and clinical decision making were lacking. Slatore et al. (2012) explore how having a therapeutic alliance means that staff must determine what the patient desires and that they understand the proposed care plan, and to provide this staff must know the limitations of their own knowledge and involve other professionals when required. If positive patient and family outcomes and satisfaction are to be achieved staff must have a high level of quality communication and interpersonal skills (see Bite Size Knowledge 1.1) which are trustworthy, compassionate and respectful. The mastery of these skills can help the nurse understand the patient's world and 'treat' the whole person.

━━━ BITE SIZE KNOWLEDGE 1.1 ━━━━━━━━━━ ━━━━

A well-balanced repertoire of interpersonal skills

Verbal communication: this includes effective speaking and listening and questioning with clarity and confidence.

Non-verbal communication: this includes body language, facial expressions, eye contact, positioning, posture, voice, gestures.

Listening: this is active mindful listening.

Questioning builds upon listening and may initiate a conversation. Well-constructed questions demonstrate knowledge about issues or problems and enable the answers needed.

Manners are key to interpersonal skills and a basic understanding of etiquette and how it translates to other cultures and their expectations is important.

Problem solving is a skill and key to clinical decision making – the examination of all options and possible solutions; setting up systems, strategies and objectives to solve the problem; executing the plan and monitoring its progress.

Empathy is a complex skill; timing is critical and speaking genuinely and naturally is vital.

Social awareness and being aware of others' emotions is a vital interpersonal skill and putting a strategy in place to help that individual requires a high level of social awareness.

Self-management of our emotions and behaviour and exuding calm in times of high stress is undeniably necessary for the expert critical care nurse.

Responsibility and accountability are part of the NMC code (2015) but the expert nurse also offers counsel and assistance. S/he also manages conflict and if things go wrong operates a 'no blame culture' but explores the situation fully and responds in a way that addresses the issue comprehensively. In critical care this means tactfully standing up for what you believe the patient needs and defending that with confidence.

Patient-centred Care and Holism

Nurses believe that to provide PCC a holistic view is required. A simple definition of holism is that the whole is greater than the sum of its parts (Owen and Holmes, 1993);

however the expert nurse (see Bite Size Knowledge 1.2) will see holism as more than this. Holism is seeing individuals as a whole and that the parts of a whole are in intimate interconnection, such that they cannot exist independently of the whole, or cannot be understood without reference to the whole. A holistic view of the patient therefore focuses on all of the patient's and their family's needs and to provide this nurses need up-to-date knowledge, the ability to foster relationships on a personal, professional and organisational level and the ability to make informed clinical decisions (Epstein and Street, 2011; Esmaeili et al., 2014). However, some nurses offer *simple holism* which can be one-dimensional because of the way the parts of the whole are reduced (Stiles, 2011). The nurse who offers this simple holism tends to focus on the immediate proximity of factors (Cave, 2000) rather than complex issues that surround the factors. Woods (1998) understood this to be a pragmatic theory of holism.

BITE SIZE KNOWLEDGE 1.2

The expert nurse

Benner (1984, p84) states that 'The Expert nurse has an intuitive grasp of each situation and zeroes in on the accurate region of the problem without wasteful consideration of a large range of unfruitful, alternative diagnoses and solutions. The Expert operates from a deep understanding of the total situation. His/her performance becomes fluid and flexible and highly proficient. Highly skilled analytic ability is necessary for those situations with which the nurse has had no previous experience.'

Carper (1978) stated that there are four fundamental ways of knowing and the expert nurse engages with all of these as they have a critical understanding of patient requirements:

- Empirical knowledge: comes from science, or other external sources and can be empirically verified.
- Aesthetic knowledge: awareness of the immediate situation and the immediate practical action but also, being aware of the patient and their circumstances as a unique individual, and the combined wholeness of the situation.
- Personal knowledge: this is derived from personal self-understanding and empathy, including imagining oneself in the patient's position.
- Ethical knowledge: this is derived from an ethical framework and includes moral awareness and individual choices.

Rolfe et al. (2001) explore how making sense of our experience helps influence our present and future practice and is key to nursing but the expert nurse uses critical self-evaluation, critical reflection and reflexivity and has the ability to challenge long established practice traditions.

The expert nurse however is capable of offering *complex holism* (Stiles, 2011) or strong holism (Woods, 1998). Complex holism is to offer care that has a worldview of the patient and which does not reduce the multiple complexities of that patient care to simplistic aspects of care. For example, the complexity of individuals enables us to use a variety of ways of knowing our world and we have multiple perceptions of our world in order to create our worldview. However, Drury and Hunter (2016) highlight that essential elements of holistic care can disappear, such as spirituality. The American Holistic Nurses Association (2013: 1) acknowledges this and highlights that 'identifying the interrelationships of the bio-psycho-social-spiritual dimension of the person, recognises that the whole is greater than the sum of its parts'.

Indeed patient-centred nursing interventions are a response to the needs of the patients, and the family, and individualisation of care needs skill and expertise in team coordination (Esmaeili et al., 2014). It is the expert nurse who identifies and manages any shortcomings. Here s/he will ensure team coordination, which if unmanaged can lead to concerns related to the achievement of quality care and failure to receive essential information in a timely fashion (Audet et al., 2006). Hasse (2013) also believes that staff need time to ensure that clinical decisions are guided by the patient values.

Patient-centred holistic care tends to assume that patients have the time and knowledge to make best-valued decisions based on their own preference. However, patients in ICU often present with life-threatening illnesses and frequently, and inescapably, the nurse must focus on the immediacy of sustaining life. Indeed Ball and Stock (1992) examine how the work of nurses and technicians in high care area's overlap; and Farrell (2001) highlight that much of nurses' work centres on rules and task imperatives and that these are ingrained in the nurses' psyche; and Kelly (2007) stated that the reductionist, mechanistic and dehumanising medical model of 'cure' rather than 'care' dominates healthcare provision. Consequently whilst patient allocation and one nurse to one patient tend to be practised it is not always humanised.

SO HOW CAN CARE MOVE FROM BEING REDUCTIONIST AND MECHANISTIC TO HUMANISED?

McLean et al. (2016:.126) highlight that 'more experienced practitioners move between different ways of thinking with rapidity, ease and fluidity, whilst less experienced nurses became "stuck" in ways of thinking". Farias et al. (2013) found that whilst professionals were aware of the importance of humanised care, and its contribution to the recovery of the critically ill patient, technical care was still prevalent in intensive care. Nonetheless whilst the intensive care routine requires excellent technical and scientific education the expert nurse remembers that critical illness is not only about physiological alteration but also an alteration in the psychosocial and spiritual domains. Undeniably as health care becomes increasingly technical the need for humanisation is increasingly essential. Certainly since the idea of grouping the sickest patients together and the introduction of critical care medicine in the late 1960s, there have been significant developments in critical care, leading to critical care being recognised as a speciality in the UK in 1999. This recognised the vast advances in understanding of pathophysiology and organ failure, advances in technology, pharmacology and procedures in both medicine and nursing and how these were leading to greater critical illness survival. But have nurses lost the ability to offer patient-centred holistic care? Or is there another framework that moves beyond patient-centred holistic care? Whilst critical illness needs to be explored more (see Chapter 2), first we will explore the lifeworld philosophy and its approach to care.

LIFEWORLD APPROACH TO CARE

The lifeworld philosophy is a pre-epistemological stepping stone for phenomenological analysis (see Bite Size Knowledge 1.3) with the philosophical question of what it means to be human. Lifeworld relates to the 'world' in which we each live and how this is different for every person depending on their experience, their background and the meaning it has for us (Dahlberg et al., 2001). Lifeworld philosophy therefore is both personal and intersubjective and recognises the complexity of human life.

────── BITE SIZE KNOWLEDGE 1.3 ══════════════ ══════

Phenomenology

Phenomenology in its most basic form attempts to create conditions for the objective study of subjective topics such as consciousness and conscious experiences such as judgements, perceptions, and emotions. Through systematic reflection it tries to determine the essential properties and structures of people's experiences. Phenomenology offers possibilities for understandings of experiences which may be forgotten or overlooked. Existential phenomenology is a philosophical theory, or approach, which emphasises the existence of the individual person as a free and responsible agent who through their own will determines their own development.

In the context of lifeworld the expert nurse moves from offering patient-centred care which adopts a simple holistic approach to offering a more ontological humanistic lifeworld approach to the care (Todres et al., 2009) and one which is agreed by patients, practitioners and policy makers. Lifeworld refers to our own world that we live in and the everyday experiences that we have and what they mean to us to make us human and to live as a human being in the world; this encompasses wellbeing. Dahlberg et al. (2009) discuss how without a clear understanding of individual wellbeing, and how it includes the existential dimensions of freedom and vulnerability, healthcare practitioners may be in danger of assuming that absence of illness alone equates to health. However an existential view of wellbeing involves seeing it before it is divided into different domains (such as social wellbeing, political wellbeing) and that encompasses seeing wellbeing as a complex whole.

Dahlberg et al. (2009) went on to critique how this could be missing from PCC and developed a conceptualisation of lifeworld-led care. This they felt included 'three dimensions: a philosophy of the person; a view of wellbeing... [freedom of illness]... and not just illness and a philosophy of care that is consistent with this' (p.265). Integral to this is to practise a 'head, hand and heart' philosophy and is supported by Galvin and Todres (2007) and Galvin (2010). To adopt a 'head, hand and heart' philosophy is to practise humanly sensitive care and to do this a nurse should consider the worldview of the patient and the complex interconnected elements of the patient's world in a collaborative and meaningful way.

Galvin (2010) describes how an interconnected worldview has several dimensions that are intertwined and these are: intersubjectivity, embodiment, spatiality and temporality (see Table 1.1). Satisfaction of care and quality of care are strictly related to the concepts of humanisation of health care. The term 'humanisation of care' has gradually been used more and is informed by core dimensions of what it means to be human. So how can we take this worldview forward and apply it to critical care?

Table 1.1 The interconnected worldview - application to practice

Definition	Application to practice example
Intersubjectivity: all of our experiences and how they relate to one another	Use of patient diaries written prospectively, and the retrospective sharing of experience with patient and family. Exploring with the patient their missing time and experiences that the family cannot comprehend - i.e. noises that CC nurses understand but relatives may not.
Embodiment: experiencing the world through our bodies	Offering comfort and Presencing - what these mean from the patient's perspective and how the CC nurse can support this.
Spatiality: our experiences of objects and places that give us meaning	Understanding where you are and what has happened and is happening to you and reinforcement of this understanding.
Temporality: our experience and perception of time - past, present and future	Sharing of rituals and patterns occurring in the critical care environment (i.e. why it is necessary to have some lighting on at night and why observations are continually being undertaken).
	Sharing what is occurring outside of the CC environment (i.e. what is occurring in the news).

Humanising Conceptual Framework

Humanisation is to uphold what it means to be human as we move from past to present and aspire to the future by living within the fragility of our bodies whilst developing and preserving our values, our human characteristics and attributes, and what it means to us both personally and in relation to others. For a healthcare practitioner to offer humanised care they need to have knowledge of care which focuses on the insider perspective and Todres et al. (2009) proposed a humanising conceptual framework to help with this. The framework provides eight bipolar constructs each of which presents both the humanising and dehumanising features of care. Thus by using the dimensions, which aid understanding and application of humanised care, the nurse can enhance their practice by offering holistic person-centred care which has been informed by gaining a greater insight into the world of the patient, thus moving towards human-centred approaches to health care.

Todres et al. (2009) state that the humanising and dehumanising dimensions are touchstones for awareness when considering the complexity of living situations and are not to be seen as 'ideal' types and that in some respects they overlap. The dimensions they offer are:

1 insiderness and objectification
2 agency and passivity
3 uniqueness and homogenisation
4 togetherness and isolation
5 sense making and loss of meaning
6 personal journey and loss of personal journey
7 sense of place and dislocation
8 embodiment and reductionist body.

Todres et al. (2009) derived their humanising framework, a value base for guiding care, from lifeworld philosophy and existential phenomenology and were also influenced by sociological perspectives. Their framework emphasises a state of affairs in which the world is experienced and lived by the individual. Qualitative research has contributed to caring practice and understanding the 'insider' perspective is a key strength of qualitative research. However, for the caring professions the concepts of 'insiderness', or the 'the body as "me"' (Sakalys, 2006: 17), and 'caring' are equally important and Todres et al. (2014) discuss how 'caring for insiderness' can guide practice as nurses become familiar with the patients' feelings, moods, and emotions that help them live in their personal world.

However, despite the research on humanisation of care there is increasing evidence from the media that human dimensions of care, such as compassion and kindness, are being obscured by technology and specialisation of care. Galvin and Todres (2013) suggested that health care today gives little attention to what makes us feel human and what appears to be missing is enabling clients to feel secure and valued and be involved in their care but instead, dehumanising dimensions are prominent. In intensive care situations one might suggest that patient and family often accept the need to focus on the techno-logical elements of the current situation and the particular aspect of treatment (Todres et al., 2000), yet humanisation of care can be achieved albeit this is sometimes hard to accomplish. Morse (2012) supports this argument and proposes that the humanising framework can be used to guide further qualitative enquiry in order to explore, under-stand and meet the requirements of holistic care. The dimensions of humanised care will be explored throughout this book and Table 1.2 offers a description of the humanising dimensions and their practical application for the patient and for the nurse.

Table 1.2 Humanising dimensions for person-centred care

Humanising dimensions	Description	Practical application for the patient	Practical application for the nurse
Insiderness/ objectification	Recognising / not recognising their view of the world	Feeling that the nurse has a sense of who they are as a whole even in situations when the patient may not be able to use their usual communication strategies	Enhancing connectedness through learning about the person. This can come from the patient, their family, friends and carers; from their healthcare records; from documents such as 'This Is Me'
Agency/passivity	The ability / loss of ability or removal of opportunity to make your own choices and decisions and take responsibility for them	Sharing choices in their journey and being involved in decisions however small	Enabling patients to make their own choices throughout their critical illness however small their choice is
Uniqueness/ homogenisation	The human's unique view of the world / loss of recognition of their uniqueness	Understanding who they are and their perceptions of their life situation	Recognising uniqueness of each individual patient and their situation and their perception of their uniqueness and view of the world they live in
Togetherness/ isolation	A human's sense of belonging and kinship / loss of feeling of belonging leading to isolation	Feeling part of something and being able to share that with who they choose. Avoiding fear of isolation and not knowing what's happening	Recognising that belonging and kinship are part of the recovery process and this needs to be empowered in many different ways that make the patient feel human

Humanising dimensions	Description	Practical application for the patient	Practical application for the nurse
Sense making/ loss of meaning	A human's ability to see and understand the patterns and structure that make up their life / loss of this when the patterns and structure are changed or removed	Making sense of their situation and the patterns and routines they are experiencing. Not feeling disorientated and lost in time	Enabling patients to understand their critical illness, how it occurred, the treatment and management – past, present and future – e.g. by the use of patient diaries
Personal journey/ loss of personal journey	A human's personal life plan and aspirations / loss of goals and direction	Being aware of and understanding short- and long-term goals of care and the impact this will have on their personal journey and aspirations	Enable individuals to plan short-term and long-term goals which may require revisiting of their life plan and future aspirations. Involve specialist nurses and other healthcare practitioners
Sense of place/ dislocation	A sense of place (home) where they feel safe and relaxed / loss of feelings of safety and security	Feeling safe and secure in a highly technical environment	Ensure the patient feels safe and relaxed by understanding what has occurred / what is occurring and the environment (including equipment) surrounding them to enable this
Embodiment/ reductionist body	A human's experience of who they are and how they exist / loss of recognition of who they are as a human	Being able to be. Keeping a sense of self	Respect the patient's experience and what it means to them and how their perception is different from others and what one finds stressful another may not

MID-CHAPTER SUMMARY

We have identified that:

- Person-centred care is both a professional and a political driver for improved health care.
- Effective person-centred care is synonymous with excellent interpersonal skills and the ability to incorporate complex holism into clinical care.
- Expert nursing requires critical and reflective thinking, knowledge and skills, clinical experience, and the ability to analyse and challenge established practice.

- One way of understanding care in this context is to hold an interconnected worldview that supports:

  o intersubjectivity
  o embodiment
  o spatiality
  o temporality.

- Galvin and Todres's eight dimensions of humanisation offer a conceptual framework for understanding how humanised care can be central to nursing and healthcare practice.

In the next section we will explore how an understanding of lifeworld, humanised care and person-centred care can inform and enhance the process and activity of clinical decision making.

NURSES' CLINICAL DECISION MAKING IN CRITICAL CARE: MODELS AND PROCESS

The study of nurses' clinical decision making (CDM) in critical care has a history that began in the 1970s around the time that the first critical care units began to emerge (Ford, 1979; Ridley et al., 2003). The interest in clinical decision making at that time was influenced by the continued expansion of specialist critical care centres in the UK that led to the development of nationally based post-registration courses to offer nurses the opportunity to formally specialise in critical care and to develop the knowledge and skills required to make clinically effective decisions. The General Intensive Care Course was cited as being one of the most popular courses running at that time (Allan and Jolley, 1982). In as little as ten years nurses had formally established a specialist role in the care of the critically ill and in 1977 founded the British Association of Critical Care Nurses, the aims of which were to promote the art and science of intensive care nursing and to provide opportunities for education and exchange of ideas in critical care practice (Atkinson, 1986). Internationally the critical care environment provided researchers and theorists with an opportunity to explore and analyse nurses as they made rapid and complex decisions, often involving life and death situations.

During this period two core theories have emerged to explain the processes and patterns nurses and other healthcare practitioners use to make clinical decisions. These include: the information processing or hypothetico-deductive reasoning model (Tanner et al., 1987; Carnevali et al. 1984; Aspinall, 1979); and the intuitive-humanist model (King and Macleod Clark, 2002; Rew, 2000; Cioffi and Markham, 1997; Benner et al., 2011; Benner, 1984). A summary of the two approaches is included in Bite Size Knowledge 1.4 and 1.5. A critical analysis of these models reveals that as individual approaches each model has some strengths as well as limitations and these will be considered in the context of nurses' work in critical care and factors that affect clinical decision making.

The Hypothetico-deductive Model

The information processing or hypothetico-deductive model is based on the assumption that human short- and long-term memory are separate components of the decision making process. According to Carnevali et al. (1984) and Hamers et al. (1994), the short-term memory houses the information required to unlock the factual and experimental knowledge stored in long-term memory. The interface between the two components of memory leads to what Hamers et al. (1994) describe as a four stage process and Carnevali et al. (1984) describe as a seven stage process of diagnostic reasoning that leads to a decision being made. More complex iterations of the use of information processing in nurses' clinical decision making, using Bayesian logic, have also been explored, where a developing hypothesis is tested against new evidence that may positively or negatively test the probability of the hypothesis being correct (Hammond et al., 1967; Aspinall, 1979). Critical analysis of the effectiveness of these models when tested in practice reveals that they are flawed, as nurses were found to frequently overlap the steps and to change the order according to the urgency of the clinical situation, cultural and contextual factors, education and experience, organisational factors and hypothesis testing (Hancock and Easen, 2006; Hoffman, Aitken and Duffield, 2009; Ramezani-Badr et al., 2009). In summary, clinical reasoning appears to involve a complex pattern of influences that impact on the process of clinical decision making and while a hypothetico-deductive approach is a necessary and valuable component of clinical reasoning it is not in itself sufficient to explain the whole process and pattern of clinical decision making.

═══ BITE SIZE KNOWLEDGE 1.4 ═══════════════ ═══

The key elements of the linear hypothetico-deductive reasoning model for clinical decision making

Carnevali (1984)

1 exposure to pre-encounter data
2 entry to the data search field and shaping the direction of data gathering
3 coalescing of cues into clusters or chunks
4 activating possible diagnostic explanations (hypothesis)
5 hypothesis and data directed search of the data field
6 testing diagnostic hypothesis for goodness of fit
7 diagnosis.

(Continued)

(Continued)

Radwin (1990); Hamers et al. (1994)

1 cue acquisition
2 initiation of tentative hypotheses
3 interpreting the cues to confirm or refute initial hypotheses
4 selecting the most appropriate hypothesis.

What does the hypothetico-deductive model offer to support humanised clinical decision making?

- It offers recognition of the importance of cue acquisition and cue clustering.
- It offers a process for analysis and interpretation.

The Intuitive-humanist Approach to Clinical Reasoning

If the hypothetico-deductive model does not represent the reality of clinical reasoning is the intuitive-humanist approach the answer? It can be argued that humanising care supports the concept of complex holism where the embodied whole becomes the focus of care and management. In this context the expert nurse develops sophisticated and complex skills in order to assess and plan care. Benner et al. (2011), building on previous work by Benner (1984) and Benner et al. (1999), propose that critical care nurses develop habits of thought and action that lead to clinically effective everyday practice in critical care. Benner et al. (2011: 2) describe these habits of thought and action as:

- clinical grasp and clinical inquiry
- clinical forethought.

Benner's (1984) understanding of intuition is influenced by the philosophy of Heidegger (1962) and she utilises the six key aspects of intuitive judgement as interpreted by Dreyfus and Dreyfus (1986) as a tool to measure the presence of intuitive knowing. These can be summarised as: pattern recognition, similarity recognition, common-sense understanding, skilled know-how, a sense of salience and deliberative rationality. Standing (2010) argues that what Benner, in her 1984 work, provides is a favouring of intuition over analysis although this perspective is something that Benner et al. (1999) challenge in their later view of clinical wisdom.

Benner (1984) contends that adopting Heideggerian phenomenology allows consideration of the question of what it is to be human and the interpretation of human as 'being–in–the–world'. In this sense she argues that by observing expert nurses in practice and then interviewing those nurses in order to map the process of clinical decision making, evidence of intuitive knowing can be illustrated. In her phenomenological research the critical care nurses studied are able to act quickly and efficiently but can only give a vague explanation of the evidence or thought processes used in order to arrive at the appropriate clinical judgement (Benner 1984; Benner et al., 1999; 2011). In this sense, Benner et al. (1999) see intuition as a definable process of practical knowing that facilitates clinical decision making and *not* reasoning based on wild guesses or extrasensory perception. Other authors describe intuition as a non-rational process, based on feelings, sensing, or an awareness that emerges from subconscious data (Agan, 1987; Schraeder and Fischer, 1987; Meerabeau, 1992) A summary of these interpretations is identified in Table 1.3.

BITE SIZE KNOWLEDGE 1.5

The key elements of intuitive-humanist knowing

Table 1.3 Intuitive-humanist reasoning and knowing

Benner and Tanner (1987: 23)	'Understanding without rationale'
Rew and Barron (1987: 60)	'Knowledge of a fact or truth, as a whole; immediate possession of knowledge; and knowledge independent of the linear reasoning process'
Benner et al. (2011: 3)	'Thinking in action ... the patterns and habits of thought and action directly tied to responding to patients and families. The craft, situatedness and engaged thinking-in-action ... that does not supplement or replace evidence based use of knowledge'
Benner et al. (2011: 27)	'... embodied tacit knowledge'
Benner et al. (2011: 67)	'... pattern recognition, a sense of salience, and a sense of concern or heightened attentiveness based upon experiential learning in whole past concrete situations ... The clinician knowing more than he or she can say ... common sense'

Hassani et al. (2016: 35)	Understanding intuition as:
	 A feeling:
	      Internal feeling
	      Inspiration feeling
	      Personal feeling
	      Sixth-sense feeling
	      Trust feeling
	
	 Thought:
	      Quick thought
	      Obsessive thought
	
	 Receiving signs:
	      Psychological and physical signs
	
	 An alarm:
	      Imminent danger
	      Death prediction
	      Patient recovery

After proposing a place for intuition in the development of clinical wisdom, Benner et al. (1999) go on to argue that intuition based on many years of experience is frequently but not always correct; intuition may nevertheless act as an early warning sign and subsequently influence the focus and speed of clinical decision making. This argument is reinforced in a study by Hassani et al. (2016) of Iranian nurses who describe intuition as feelings, thoughts, signs and alarms that trigger increased attention to the patient's condition and early identification of clinical deterioration.

Herbig et al. (2001) further highlight the complexity and ambiguity associated with intuition, particularly in relation to experience-guided working. They describe intuition as being tacit knowledge that is acquired by the person during experiences in a special domain. Such knowledge is therefore personal, holistic, heavily influenced by context, and by processes and decisions made by the person and others during repeated experiences. These experiences may lead to knowledge development that is based on conflicting ideas or bad judgements and as such may not always offer the most appropriate insight or trigger to the clinical decision that has to be made. This argument is reinforced by Reischman and Yarandi (2002) who in a study of both expert and novice critical care cardiovascular nurses, found that the development of diagnostic expertise is dependent on pattern recognition (intuition) associated with the necessary domain-specific or context dependent knowledge.

Similarly a critical review of the intuitive-humanist model reveals that its use is not necessarily reliant on an evidence based algorithm of information processing but rather on the individual expertise and experience of the expert nurse (Thompson, 1999). This begs the question that if knowledge lies with the individual and is associated with automatic knowing, how can this knowledge be shared and validated? (Cioffi and Markham, 1997; Banning, 2008) Furthermore if intuition is not always correct can such 'knowing' be justified as nursing knowledge? As such, can those clinical judgements and actions based on intuition always be seen as appropriate and justified?

What does the intuitive- humanist model offer to support humanised clinical decision making?

- It recognises the importance of context.
- It acknowledges the significance of holistic and embodied understanding based on situational knowing.

So far we have seen that while both approaches offer necessary elements of complex expert decision making, neither provide a sufficient description of what is involved. The answer according to O'Neill et al. (2005) is to utilise a multi-dimensional model of clinical decision making based on hypothetical deduction and pattern recognition as the basis for decision making. She argues that this process is not linear and relies on:

- the use of patient specific pre-encounter data, anticipating and controlling the risk, prioritising nursing interventions (normative judgements)
- clinical protocol utilisation (prescriptive judgements)
- situational and client modifications in the context of practice (descriptive judgements)
- hypothesis generation, assessment of the clinical situation, pattern recognition (normative and descriptive judgements)
- implementation and evaluation of nursing action.

While this approach incorporates three theories of judgement and decision making described by Thompson and Dowding (2002) as: normative-rational and logical decision making; descriptive – processes involved in decision making; prescriptive – guidelines used to improve decision making, what this approach does not do is recognise the human, professional, ethical and contextual factors that influence clinical decision making in the realities of practice.

According to Standing (2005: 34) clinical decision making in nursing involves:

A complex process involving observation, information processing, critical thinking, evaluating evidence, applying relevant knowledge, problem solving skills, reflection and clinical judgement to select the best course of action which optimises a patient's health and minimises any potential harm. The role of the clinical decision-maker in nursing is, therefore to be professionally accountable for accurately assessing patients' needs, using appropriate sources of information, and planning nursing interventions that address problems and which they are competent to perform.

In her study she uses a phenomenological approach to understand the experiences of student nurses as they acquired their skills in nursing clinical decision making. Some of the key factors identified as influencing CDM were: listening and being there, experience, confidence, knowledge and understanding, self-confidence (Standing, 2010). What Standing is describing is a combination of subjective and objective reasoning which come together to optimise CDM. Other factors she identifies include knowledge, experiential, contextual, interpersonal, and human issues that individually or collectively influence how nurses prioritise, respond to and evaluate the effectiveness of the outcomes.

Standing's (2010) perspective offers a useful insight into how students learn and develop clinical reasoning skills in nursing but it does not offer a structure for understanding how experienced nurses working in acute and critical care environments make clinical decisions and what conditions are required for effective CDM to take place. The next section focuses on Tait's (2009) analysis of the process and conditions necessary for effective clinical decision making when recognising and responding to clinical deterioration in acute and critical care environments.

The process of recognising clinical deterioration began to emerge as a problem area for study in the 1990s when a number of international studies identified evidence of deficiencies in the clinical assessment and interpretation of life threatening dysfunction of a patient's airway, breathing and/or circulation leading to an increase in related patient morbidity and mortality following diagnosis and treatment of their condition (Buist et al., 2004; McQuillan et al., 1998; Goldhill et al., 1999; McGloin et al., 1999; Franklin and Mathew, 1994). In the UK and elsewhere the findings from these studies have led to the development of algorithmic risk assessment tools for recognising the early physiological signs of clinical deterioration, the development of critical care outreach teams and the recognition that critical care exists without walls – wherever a critically ill person exists (Audit Commission, 1999; Smith et al., 2013; Gao et al., 2007). While the clinical effectiveness of these approaches continues to be tested, a deeper understanding of how nurses make clinical decisions in these situations in both acute and critical care settings can offer insight into the conditions necessary for safe and effective CDM.

WHAT IS THE PROFESSIONAL GAZE AND CONDITIONS NECESSARY FOR RECOGNISING AND RESPONDING TO CLINICAL DETERIORATION?

Professional gaze is defined by Tait (2009: 232) as:

> The professional practice of engaging in scanning, selective perception, recognition, diagnosis of and response to clinical deterioration.

The concept of the clinical (professional) gaze is not new and according to Foucault ([1973] 1989) is how the medical profession developed a professional knowledge and power base through the objectification of the subject. Foucault refers to a point of defining change in the language and style of medical practice that occurred towards the end of the eighteenth century. He argues that this focused on the juxtaposition between clinical observation as an objectification of the clinical gaze and the scientific nature of medical knowledge. The emergence of what we understand as the medical model led to the visualisation of disease as an objective, measurable, systematic and scientific element of the subjective body and established the source of unique professional medical knowledge (Shawver, 1998; Parker and Wiltshire, 1995; Henderson, 1994). This knowledge included clinical signs and symptoms, clinical examination, medical language and the structure of the case. The object of the exercise was to access all the elements of the case that together made the unique diagnosis and led to a strategy for treatment. A diagnosis could not be made until all the elements had been considered and measured against alternative diagnoses. According to Foucault ([1973] 1989: 147), 'the clinical gaze is a gaze that burns things to their furthest truth'.

The clinical gaze/medical model therefore represents a pure hypothetico-deductive approach to clinical reasoning and incorporates a distinctly scientific process of assessment, history taking, and examination, reaching a diagnosis and prescribing treatment. Based on this approach if nurses follow the medical model, supported by physiological track and trigger tools such as NEWS (Royal College of Physicians, 2012) and ask for the support of outreach teams will this ensure safe practice and provide effective clinical decision making? Unfortunately the evidence suggests that both nursing and medical teams continue to provide suboptimal decision making in these situations (Odell et al., 2009; Tait, 2009). Both authors argue that the processes nurses, in particular, use to recognise and respond to clinical deterioration are highly complex and context dependent and therefore involve more factors than can be accommodated within the medical model.

For example in the study by Tait (2009), CDM or the nurses' professional gaze went beyond the objective clinical characteristics of the hypothetico-deductive model to reveal a process that incorporated a mixture of subjective and objective reasoning that when used by skilled practitioners working in a team and led by supportive management, had a positive impact on the patient's outcome. However, when the conditions for this process were limited by factors such as lack of experienced practitioners, poor communication and teamwork, there was evidence of suboptimal care.

The notion of the clinical gaze has been applied to nursing previously and the concept developed as a framework for nursing practice described by Ellefsen et al. (2007) as a theoretical framework for sharing ways of knowing within the nursing handover (Parker and Wiltshire, 1995); and in relation to nursing observation in an acute psychiatric inpatient unit (Hamilton and Manias, 2007). In Tait's study the professional gaze begins with the requirement to watch the patient for cues which may trigger the first signs of concern. This implied a professional responsibility for assessing and monitoring the patient situation. The second feature was concerned with the nature of the nurses' watchfulness and included the play of movement between the 'professional scan', 'focused observation' and 'waiting and balancing' leading to a clinical response. A conceptual framework for the professional gaze is illustrated in Figure 1.1.

Professional Scan

The professional scan describes vigilance in the process of watching and scanning for potential problems. In Tait's study (2009, p235) this is referred to as 'having sideways vision while at the same time concentrating on the particulars of practice . . . the visual thing'. Nurses in acute and critical care settings referred to utilising their senses of perception, sight, hearing, smell and touch and selectively attended to changes in the patient's behaviour, appearance, temperature and smell while listening to the patient as part of the

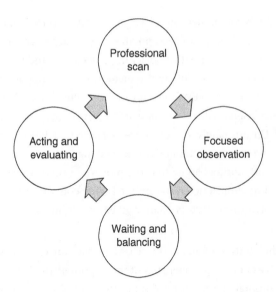

Figure 1.1 Summarising the continuous processes of the professional gaze

interpersonal process. The concept of professional scan is also found in work by Hamilton and Manias (2007) and Parker and Wiltshire (1995) who describe nurses relying on their sight and other senses to inform the scanning process. According to Tait (2009) the conditions necessary for optimal utilisation of the professional scan included: clinical, historical and experiential knowledge of the patient's conditions and/or situation; clinical assessment skills related to the subjective, contextual and objective elements of the patient situation; knowledge of clinical cues and patterns of cues; and knowing the patient. Interestingly in a review of literature by Zolnierek (2014) she found that knowing the patient resonates strongly with nurses and is a necessary condition of expert practice; in acute care settings, however, the literature reviewed showed that opportunities to know the patient are not supported and thus challenge opportunities to achieve an effective professional scan.

Focused Observation

Focused observation refers to the process whereby the cues and their relationship to each other trigger concern and the requirement to look further in order to interpret and diagnose the problem. Here the validity of their concerns is tested by the further evidence collected. In this process, the nurse enters a play of movement by questioning what was before him/ her, involving cycles of surveillance, data collection, talking to the patient/ family, reviewing the patient's history, their personal professional knowledge and experience of situations, the patient's clinical observations and investigations, and discussions with colleagues. If some of the conditions for focused observation are missing this can then impact on the speed of processing and lead to suboptimal care.

Waiting and Balancing

This process occurs as the nurse weighs up the evidence until s/he has the evidence to support the call for help. In her study Tait (2009) identified that the process of 'waiting and balancing' was influenced by the historically affected consciousness of the participants, described by Gadamer (1989 [1975]) as the subject's unique experience of history that informs how they interpret and understand their world. This included previous experience of having success when calling for help and their relationship with the medical team. Other necessary conditions for successful waiting and balancing include: prioritising skills; skills that facilitated teamwork; knowledge of and mutual respect within the team; and self-confidence in their professional role. Both focused observation and waiting and balancing can be supported and informed by the National Early Warning Scores (RCP, 2017) and tools such as Sepsis Screening (Sepsis Trust, 2016), but they alone are not sufficient to trigger action if, for example, the nurse's self-confidence or communication skills are impaired according to Tait (2009).

Acting and Evaluating

This process occurs when the nurse decides that help is required and action needs to be taken. This does not stop the process however and the cycle continues as the nurse continues with the professional scan and so on, repeating the cyclical process for the duration of the shift.

Tait's (2009) study does illustrate that there are a number of conditions necessary to support recognition and response to clinical deterioration and these are:

1 Knowledge:
   o theoretical – empirical and theoretical knowledge that supports professional practice
   o clinical guidelines – evidence based prescriptive guidance to support decision making
   o clinical – clinical nursing knowledge
   o situational – local and specialist knowledge of the clinical environment
   o experiential – clinical experience gained within nursing practice
   o the person – the patient and their family, evidenced by continuity of care.

2 Perception and memory:
   o cues – knowledge and understanding of clinical cues
   o pattern recognition – a memory of clusters of cues that lead to pattern recognition and a provisional diagnosis.

3 Professional and ethical practice – codes of practice that support safe and person-centred care, a duty of care.

4 Managing emotional work:

- o resilience – the ability to manage the stress and balance the challenges and benefits of nursing.

5 Feeling in control:

- o self-confidence – feeling empowered to act
- o personal and professional power – feeling empowered to act without ridicule, to have confidence in personal and professional knowledge
- o resources – to be able to manage effectively with the resources available.

6 Emotional intelligence – the ability to demonstrate effective interpersonal skills.
7 Mutual respect and reciprocity – the ability to identify individual and team strengths and weaknesses and to work together with mutual respect. To be listened to.

Figure 1.2 provides a summary of the professional gaze and the conditions necessary for effective decision making.

When considered together these factors highlight Galvin's (2010) interconnected world-view of humanised critical care practice including intersubjectivity, embodiment, spatiality and temporality. These conditions or factors have also been highlighted by other authors including Odell et al. (2009); Massey et al. (2016) and Wu et al. (2016) and while all of these authors have focused on the process of nurses recognising and respond-ing to clinical deterioration, what the findings do support is that in order to promote effective, patient-centred and humanised care nurses need to recognise the complexity of factors informing, not just the process of clinical decision making but also the knowl-edge, contextual, professional, situational and personal factors that influence clinical reasoning in practice.

FACILITATING LEARNING

Please consider the following:

1 Is person-centred care a method of organising nursing care or a way of promoting shared decision making in partnership with the patient?
2 How can we foster humanised team working?
3 Reflect with your team on the care that is delivered on your unit and question how humanised it is.
4 Reflecting on a recent example from practice:
- **i** think about how you made your decisions and the factors that influenced your decision making
- **ii** using the same example and Figure 1.2 explore whether the conditions necessary for your professional gaze were met, and if not why not?

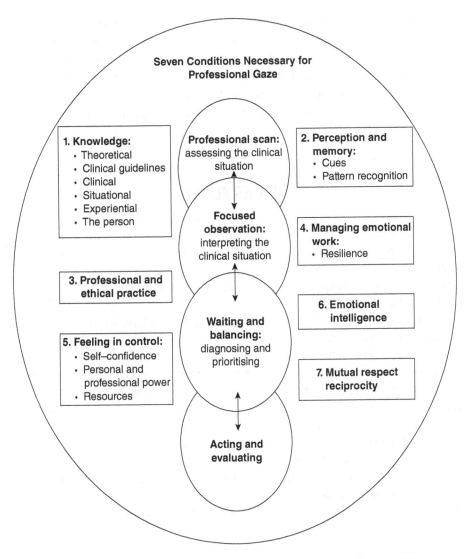

Figure 1.2 The process of clinical decision making highlighting the conditions necessary for effective recognition and response to change (Tait, 2009)

CHAPTER SUMMARY

Within this chapter we have explored the philosophical, theoretical and evidence based factors that inform acute and critical care nursing and clinical decision making for current and future practice. We have identified the significance of person-centred care and the notion of complex holism when exploring the work of expert nurses. The concept of lifeworld has been explored together with the humanising framework devised by Galvin and Todres (2013). The complexity of nurses' clinical decision making has been examined and a model offered (Figure 1.2) which supports the core elements of humanised care. In Chapter 2 we explore the nature of critical illness and the factors that trigger critical illness as well as the influence critical illness has on morbidity and mortality. In the following chapters the theories and models explored in Chapters 1 and 2 will be used to inform the analysis of case studies regarding the care and management of critically ill people.

FURTHER READING

Dahlberg, K. and Drew, N. (1997) A lifeworld paradigm for nursing research, *Journal of Holistic Nursing, 15*(3): 303–17.

Dahlberg, K., Drew, N. and Nystrom, M. (2001) *Reflective Lifeworld Research*. Sweden: Studentlitteratur.

Draper, J. (2014) Embodied practice: rediscovering the 'heart' of nursing, *Journal of Advanced Nursing, 70*(10): 2235–44.

Galvin, K. and Todres, L. (2009), Embodying nursing openheartedness: an existential perspective, *Journal of Holistic Nursing, 27*, 141–9.

Galvin, K. and Todres, L. (2011) Research based empathetic knowledge for nursing: a translational strategy for disseminating phenomenological research findings to provide evidence for caring practice, *International Journal of Nursing Studies, 48*(4): 522–30.

Holm, A.L. and Severinsson, E. (2016) A systematic review of intuition – a way of knowing in clinical nursing? *Open Journal of Nursing, 6*: 412–25.

Nursing and Midwifery Council (2015) *The Code: Professional Standards of Practice and Behaviour for Nurses and Midwives*. London: NMC.

World Health Organisation (2005) *Preparing a Health Care Workforce for the 21st Century: The Challenge of Chronic Conditions*. Geneva: WHO.

Zanotti, R. and Chiffi, D. (2016) A normative analysis of nursing knowledge, *Nursing Inquiry, 23*(1): 4–11.

REFERENCES

Agan, R.D. (1987) Intuitive knowing as a dimension of nursing, *Advances in Nursing Science, 10*: 63–70.

Allan, P. and Jolley, M. (1982) *Nursing, Midwifery and Health Visiting since 1900*. London: Faber & Faber.

American Holistic Nurses Association (2013) Holistic Nursing: Scope and Standards of Practice: AHNA and ANA. Silver Spring, MD

Angood, P., Dingman, J., Foley, M.E., Ford, D., Martins, B., O'Regan, P., Salamendra, A., Sheridan, S. and Denham, C.R. (2010). Patient and family involvement in contemporary healthcare, *Journal of Patient Safety, 6*(1): 38–42.

Aspinall, M. (1979) Use of decision making to improve accuracy of nursing diagnosis, *Nursing Research, 28*: 182–5.

Atkinson, B. (1986) The British Association of Critical Care Nurses, *Care of the Critically Ill, 2*(3): 111.

Audet, A.M., Davis, K. and Schoenbaum, S.C. (2006) Adoption of patient-centred care practices by physicians: results of a national survey, *Archives of Internal Medicine, 166*, 754–9.

Audit Commission. (1999) *Critical to Success: The Place of Efficient and Effective Critical Care Services within the Acute Hospital.* London: Audit Commission.

Ball, J. and Stock, J. (1992) *Nurses and Technicians in High Technology Areas: A Report Prepared for the Department of Health.* Brighton: Institute of Manpower Studies.

Banning, M. (2008) A review of clinical decision making: models and current research, *Journal of Clinical Nursing, 17*: 187–95.

Benner, P. (1984) *From Novice to Expert: Excellence and Power in Clinical Nursing Practice.* Menlo Park, CA: Addison-Wesley.

Benner, P. and Tanner, C. (1987) Clinical judgement: how expert nurses use intuition, *American Journal of Nursing, 87*(1): 23–31.

Benner, P., Hooper-Kyriakidis, P. and Stannard, D. (1999) *Clinical Wisdom and Interventions in Critical Care.* Philadelphia: W.B. Saunders Company.

Benner, P., Hooper Kyriakidis, P. and Stannard, D. (2011) *Clinical Wisdom and Interventions in Acute and Critical Care – a Thinking in Action Approach* (2nd edn) New York: Springer.

Berwick, D.M. (2009) What patient-centered should mean: confessions of an extremist, *Health Affairs, 28*(4): 555–65.

Buist, M., Bernard, S., Nguyen, T.V., Moore, G. and Anderson, J. (2004) Association between clinically abnormal observations and subsequent in-hospital mortality: a prospective study, *Resuscitation, 62*: 137–41.

Carnevali, D., Mitchell, P., Woods, N. and Tanner, C. (1984) *Diagnostic Reasoning in Nursing.* Philadelphia: Lippincott Company.

Carper, B.A. (1978) Fundamental patterns of knowing in nursing, *Advances in Nursing Science, 1*(1): 13–24.

Cave, P. (2000) The error of excessive proximity preference – a modest proposal for understanding holism, *Nursing Philosophy, 1*: 20–5.

Cioffi, J. and Markham, R. (1997) Clinical decision making by midwives: managing case complexity, *Journal of Advanced Nursing, 25*: 265–72.

Dahlberg, K., Drew, N. and Nyström, M. (2001) *Reflective Lifeworld Research.* Studentlitteratur, Lund.

Dahlberg, K., Todres, L. and Galvin, K. (2009) Lifeworld-led healthcare is more than patient-led care: an existential view of well-being, *Medical Health Care and Philosophy, 12*: 265–71.

Department of Health (2000) *National Service Framework for Coronary Heart Disease: Modern Standards and Service Models.* London: The Stationery Office.

Department of Health (2001) *National Service Framework for older people.* London.

Department of Health (2006) *Dignity in Care Campaign.* London: The Stationery Office.

Department of Health (2012) *NHS England: Compassion in Practice. Nursing, Midwifery and Care Staff, Our Vision and Strategy*. Available at: www.england.nhs.uk/wp-content/uploads/2012/12/compassion-in-practice.pdf

Dreyfus, H.L. and Dreyfus, S.E. (1986) *Mind over Machine. The Power of Human Intuition and Expertise in the Era of the Computer*. Oxford: Blackwell Science.

Drury, C. and Hunter, J. (2016) The hole in holistic patient care, *Open Journal of Nursing, 6*: 776–92.

Ellefsen, B., Kim, H.S. and Han, K.J. (2007) Nursing gaze as a framework for nursing practice: a study from acute care settings in Korea, Norway and the USA, *Scandinavian Journal of Caring, 21*: 98–105.

Epstein, R.M. and Street, R.L. (2011) The values and value of patient-centred care, *Annuals of Family Medicine, 9*: 100–3.

Epstein, R.M., Fiscella, K., Lesser, C.S. and Strange, K.C. (2010) Why the nation needs a policy on patient-centred health care, *Health Affairs, 29*(8): 1489–95.

Esmaeili, M., Mohammad, A.C. and Salsali, M. (2014) Barriers to patient-centered care: a thematic analysis study, *International Journal of Nursing Knowledge, 25*(1): 2–8.

Farias, F.B.B., Vidal, L.L., Farias, R.A.R. and Pereira de Jesus, A.C. (2013) Humanized care in the ICU: challenges from the viewpoint of health professionals, *Journal of Research: Fundamental Care on Line, 5*(4): 635–42.

Farrell, G.A. (2001) Fall tall poppies to squashed weeds: why don't nurses pull together more? *Journal of Advanced Nursing, 35*(1): 26–37.

Forbat, L., Hubbard, G. and Kearney, N. (2009) Patient and public involvement: models and muddles, *Journal of Clinical Nursing, 18*: 2547–54.

Ford, J. (1979) *Applied Decision Making for Nurses*. St Louis, MO: Mosby.

Foucault, M. ([1973]1989) (Translated by Sheridan, A.M.) *The Birth of the Clinic*. London: Routledge Classics.

Francis, R. (2013) *Report of the Mid Staffordshire NHS Foundation Trust Public Inquiry*. London: The Stationery Office.

Franklin, C. and Mathew, J. (1994) Developing strategies to prevent inhospital cardiac arrest: analysing responses of physicians and nurses in the hours before the event, *Critical Care Medicine, 22*: 24.

Gadamer, H. (1989 [1975]) *Truth and Method*. Translated and edited by Weinsheimer, J. and Marshall D.G. (2nd revised edition). London: Sheed and Ward.

Galvin, K. (2010) Revisiting caring science: some integrative ideas for the 'head, hand and heart' of critical care nursing practice, *British Association of Critical Care Nurses. Nursing in Critical Care, 15*(4): 168–75.

Galvin, K. and Todres, L. (2007) The creativity of unspecialisation: a contemplative direction for integrative scholarly practice. *Phenomenology and Practice, 1*: 31–46.

Galvin, K. and Todres, L. (2013) *Caring and Wellbeing: A Lifeworld Approach*. London: Routledge.

Gao, H., McDonnell, A., Harrison, D.A., Moore, T., Adam, S., Daly, K., Esmonde, L., Goldhill, D. R., Parry, G.J., Rashidian, A., Subbe, C.P. and Harvey, S. (2007) Systematic review and evaluation of physiological track and trigger warning systems for identifying at-risk patients on the ward, *Intensive Care Medicine, 33*(4): 667–79.

Goldhill, D., White, S.A. and Sumner, A. (1999) Physiological values and procedures in the 24 hours before ICU admission from the ward, *Anaesthesia*, *54*: 853–60.

Hamers, J., Huijer Abu Saad, H. and Halfens, R. (1994) Diagnostic process and decision making in nursing: a literature review. *Journal of Professional Nursing*, *10*(3): 154–63.

Hamilton, B.E. and Manias, E. (2007) Rethinking nurses' observations: psychiatric nursing skills and invisibility in the acute inpatient setting, *Social Science and Medicine*, *65*: 331–4.

Hammond, K., Kelly, K., Schneider, R. and Vancini, M. (1967) Clinical inference in nursing: revising judgements, *Nursing Research*, *16*: 38–45.

Hancock, H. and Easen, P. (2006) The decision making processes of nurses when extubating patients following cardiac surgery: an ethnographic study, *International Journal of Nursing Studies*, *43*: 693–705.

Hassani, P., Abdi, A., Jalali, R. and Salari, N. (2016) The perception of intuition in clinical practice by Iranian critical care nurses: a phenomenological study, *Psychology Research and Behaviour Management*, *9*: 31–9.

Hasse, G.L. (2013) Patient-centered care in adult trauma intensive care unit, *Journal of Trauma Nursing*, *20*(3): 163–5.

Health Improvement Scotland (2017) *People at the centre of Health Care. Person-Centred Health and Care*. Available at: https://ihub.scot/media/1036/people-at-the-centre-of-health-and-care.pdf

Heidegger, M. (1962) *Being and Time* (Translated by MacQuarrie, J. and Robinson, E.). New York: Harper & Row.

Henderson, A. (1994) Power and knowledge in nursing practice: the contribution of Foucault, *Journal of Advanced Nursing*, *20*: 935–9.

Herbig, B., Bussing, A. and Ewert, T. (2001) The role of tacit knowledge in the work context of nursing, *Journal of Advanced Nursing*, *34*(5): 687–95.

Hobbs, J.L. (2009) A dimensional analysis of patient-centred care, *Nursing Research*, *58*(1): 52–62.

Hoffman, K., Aitken, L. and Duffield, C. (2009) A comparison of novice and expert nurses' cue collection during clinical decision making: verbal protocol analysis, *International Journal of Nursing Studies*, *46*(10): 1335–44.

Institute of Medicine (2001) *Crossing the Quality Chasm: A New Health Care System for the 21st century*. Available at: https://iom.nationalacademies.org/~/media/Files/Report%20Files/2001/Crossing-the-Quality-Chasm/Quality%20Chasm%202001%20%20report%20brief.pdf

Johnson, R.M. (2015) The changing face of patient care: delivering patient-centered and culturally competent care in an evolving world, *Delaware Medical Journal*, *87*(3): 85–7.

Kelly, J. (2007) Barriers to achieving patient-centred care in Ireland. *Dimensions of Critical Care Nursing*, *26*(1): 29–34.

King, L. and Macleod Clark, J. (2002) The role of intuition and the development of expertise in surgical ward and intensive care nurses, *Journal of Advanced Nursing*, *37*: 322–9.

Kitwood, T. (1997) *Dementia Reconsidered: The Person Comes First*. Buckingham: Open University Press.

Manley, K. (1989) *Primary Nursing In intensive Care*. Harrow: Scutari Press.

Massey, D., Chaboyer, W. and Anderson, V. (2016) What factors influence ward nurses' recognition of and response to patient deterioration: an integrative review of the literature, *Nursing Open*, 1–18.

McCormack, B. and McCance, T. (2010) *Person-Centred Nursing: Theory and Practice*. Oxford: John Wiley and Sons.

McGloin, H., Adam, S. and Singer, M. (1999) Unexpected deaths and referrals to intensive care of patients on general wards. Are some cases potentially avoidable? *Journal of the Royal College of Physicians of London*, *33*: 255–9.

McLean, C., Coombes, M. and Gobi, M. (2016) Talking about persons – thinking about patients: an ethnographic study in critical care, *International Journal of Nursing Studies*, *54*: 122–31.

McQuillan, P., Pilkington, S., Allan, A., Taylor, B., Short, A., Morgan, G., Nielson, M., Barrett, D. and Smith, G. (1998) Confidential inquiry into quality of care before admission to intensive care, *British Medical Journal*, *316*(748): 1853–8.

Mead, N. and Bowers, P. (2000) Patient-centeredness: a conceptual framework and review of empirical literature, *Social Science and Medicine*, *51*: 1087–110.

Meerabeau, L. (1992) Tacit knowledge: an untapped resource or a methodological headache? *Journal of Advanced Nursing*, *17*: 108–12.

Mockford, C., Staniszewska, S., Griffiths, F. and Herron-Marx, S. (2011) The impact of patient and public involvement on UK NHS health care: a systematic review, *International Journal for Quality in Health Care*, November, 28–38.

Morse, J. (2012) *Qualitative Health Research: Creating a New Discipline*. Walnut Creek, CA: Left Coast Press.

NHS Wales (2015) *Health and Care Standards*. Available at: http://www.wales.nhs.uk/sitesplus/documents/1064/24729_Health%20Standards%20Framework_2015_E1.pdf

Nolan, M.., Davies, S. and Grant, G. (2001) *Working with Older People and Their Families: Key Issues in Policy and Practice*. Buckingham. Open University Press.

Nursing and Midwifery Council (NMC) (2015) *The Code. Professional standards of practice for nurses and midwives*. London. NMC.

Odell, M., Victor, C. and Oliver, D. (2009) Nurses' role in detecting deterioration in ward patients: a systematic literature review. *Journal of advanced Nursing*, *65*, 10: 1992–2006.

O'Neill, E., Dluhy, N. and Chun, E. (2005) Modelling novice clinical reasoning for a computerised decision support system, *Journal of Advanced Nursing*, *49*: 68–77.

Owen, M.J. and Holmes, C.A. (1993) Holism in the discourse of nursing, *Journal of Advanced Nursing*, *18*: 1688–95.

Parker, J. and Wiltshire, J. (1995) The handover: three modes of nursing practice knowledge, in Gray, G. and Pratt, R. (eds) *Scholarship in the Discipline of Nursing*. Melbourne: Churchill Livingstone, 151–68.

Radwin, L. (1990) Research on diagnostic reasoning in nursing, *Nursing Diagnosis*, *1*(2): 70–77.

Radwin, L.E., Cabral, H.J. and Wilkes, G. (2009) Relationships between patient-centred cancer nursing intervention and desired health outcomes in the context of the health care system, *Research in Nursing and Health*, *32*(1): 4–17.

Ramezani-Badr, F., Nikbakht, A. and Parsa Yekta, Z. (2009) Strategies and criteria for clinical decision making in critical care nurses: a qualitative study, *Journal of Nursing Scholarship*, *41*(4): 351–8.

Rauta, S., Salantera, S., Nivalainen, J. and Junttila, K. (2012) Validation of the core elements of preoperative nursing, *Journal of Clinical Nursing, 21–22*: 1–9.

Reischman, R. and Yarandi, H. (2002) Critical care cardiovascular nurse expert and novice diagnostic cue utilisation, *Journal of Advanced Nursing, 39*(1): 24–34.

Rew, L. (2000) Acknowledging intuition in clinical decision making, *Journal of Holistic Nursing*, *18*: 94–108.

Rew, L. and Barron, E. (1987) Intuition: a neglected hallmark of nursing knowledge, *Advances in Nursing Science, 10*(1): 49–62.

Ridley, S., Dixon, M., Bodenham, A., O'Riordan, B., Goldhill, D., Bray, K. and Ford, P. (2003) *Evolution of Intensive Care in the UK*. London: Intensive Care Society.

Rogers, C. (1951) *Client Centred Therapy*. London: Constable and Company Ltd.

Rolfe, G., Freshwater, D. and Jasper, M. (2001) *Critical Reflection for Nursing and the Helping Professions: A User's Guide*. London: Palgrave Macmillan.

Royal College of Physicians (2017) *National Early Warning Score (NEWS) 2 Standardising the Assessment of Acute Illness Severity in the NHS*. London: RCP. Available at: https://www.rcplondon.ac.uk/projects/outputs/national-early-warning-score-news-2

Sakalys, J.A. (2006) Bringing bodies back in: embodiment and caring science. *International Journal of Human Caring, 10*(3): 17–21.

Schraeder, B. and Fischer, D. (1987) Using intuitive knowledge in neonatal intensive care nursery, *Holistic Nursing Practice*, 1: 45–51.

Sepsis Trust (2016) *Inpatient Sepsis Screening and Action Tool*. Available at: https://sepsistrust.org/wp-content/uploads/2018/06/Inpatient-adult-NICE-Final-1107-2-1.pdf

Shawver, L. (1998) *Notes on Reading the Birth of the Clinic*. Available at: http://postmoderntherapies.com/foucbc.htm on 26/08/2008.

Slatore, C.G., Hansen, L., Ganzini, L., Press, N., Osborne, M. L. Chesnutt, M.S., & Mularski, R., (2012). Communication by nurses in the intensive care unit: qualitative analysis of domains of patient-centred care. *American Journal of Critical Care, 12*(6): 410–418.

Smith, G., Prytherch, D., Meredith, P., Schmidt, P. and Featherstone, P. (2013) The ability of the national early warning Score (NEWS) to discriminate patients at risk of early cardiac arrest, unanticipated intensive care unit admission and death, *Resuscitation*, *84*: 465–70.

Standing, M. (2005) '*Perceptions of Clinical Decision Making on a Developmental Journey from Student to Staff Nurse*'. PhD Thesis, Canterbury, University of Kent.

Standing, M. (ed.) (2010) *Clinical Judgement and Decision-making in Nursing and Interprofessional Healthcare*. Maidenhead: McGraw- Hill and Open University Press.

Stewart, S. (2001) Towards a global definition of patient-centred care, *British Medical Journal*, *322*: 444–5.

Stiles, K. (2011) Advancing nursing knowledge through complex holism, *Advances in Nursing Science, 34*(1): 39–50.

Tait, D. (2009) '*A Gadamerian Hermeneutic Study of Nurses' Experiences of Recognising and Managing Patients with Clinical Deterioration and Critical Illness in a NHS Trust in Wales.*' Unpublished Doctorate in Nursing Science, Swansea University.

Tanner, C., Patrick, K., Westfall, U. and Putzier, D. (1987) Diagnostic reasoning strategies for nurses and nursing students, *Nursing Research, 36*: 358–63.

Thompson, C. (1999) A conceptual treadmill: the need for 'middle ground' in clinical decision making theory in nursing, *Journal of Advanced Nursing, 30*(5): 1222–9.

Thompson, C. and Dowding, D. (2002) Decision making and judgement in nursing – an introduction, in Thompson, C. and Dowding, D. (eds) *Clinical Decision Making and Judgement in Nursing* (pp. 1–20). Edinburgh: Churchill Livingstone.

Todres, L., Fulbrook, P. and Albarran, J. (2000) On the receiving end: a hermeneutical phenomenology analysis of a patients struggle to cope while going through intensive care, *Nursing in Critical Care, 5*(6): 277–87.

Todres, L., Galvin, K. and Dahlberg, K. (2014) 'Caring for insiderness': phenomenologically informed insights that can guide practice, *International Journal of Qualitative Studies on Health and Well-Being, 9*(1): 1748–2631.

Todres, L., Galvin, K. and Holloway, I. (2009) The humanisation of healthcare: a value framework for qualitative research, *International Journal of Qualitative Studies on Health and Wellbeing, 4*(2): 68–77.

Wolf, D., Lehman, L., Quinlin, R. and Rosenzweig, M. (2008) Can nurses impact patient outcomes using a patient-centered care model? *Journal of Nursing Administration, 38*(12): 532–40.

World Health Organization (WHO) (2015) *Preparing a Health Care Workforce for the 21st Century: The Challenge of Chronic Conditions.* Available at: http://www.who.int/chp/knowledge/publications/workforce_report.pdf?ua=1

Woods, S. (1998) A theory of holism for nursing, *Medicine, Healthcare and Philosophy, 1*: 255–61.

Wu, M., Yang, J., Liu, L. and Ye, B. (2016) An investigation of factors influencing nurses' clinical decision making skills, *Western Journal of Nursing Research*, 1–18.

Zolnierek, C. (2014) An integrative review of knowing the patient, *Journal of Nursing Scholarship, 46*(1): 3–10.

CHAPTER 2

What Triggers Critical Illness?

DESIREE TAIT AND SARA J. WHITE

CHAPTER AIMS

1 To understand what triggers critical illness at a cellular level and how this impacts on cell function.
2 To explore the relationship between changes that occur at cellular level and how this impacts on the person through an examination of the stress and inflammatory response.
3 To explore how personal, cultural and structural factors can trigger and exacerbate critical illness, affect the progression of the patient's condition and impact on their rehabilitation.

INTRODUCTION

This chapter explores the complex and interrelated nature of the triggers that lead to critical illness and it explores the factors that can influence the progression from acute to critical changes in a person's condition. While this chapter introduces and explores these factors from a generic perspective, they have also been applied to a scenario. The chapter begins with an exploration of critical illness from a cellular level and how this relates to the body's stress response and behaviour. We then go on to explore personal, cultural and structural (political) factors that can trigger critical illness as well as influence the morbidity and mortality of the patient concerned.

WHAT ARE THE TRIGGERS THAT CAN LEAD TO CRITICAL ILLNESS AND SUBSEQUENT ADMISSION TO INTENSIVE CARE?

Admission to intensive care occurs when a person is physiologically compromised to the extent that at least one body system is diagnosed as failing, with the potential to lead to further acute deterioration, and that the deterioration has the potential to be reversed (Taskforce of the American College of Critical Care Medicine/Society of Critical Care Medicine, 1999; Intensive Care Society, 2009). Since the 1990s there has been a growing recognition that early detection of physiological change and the use of timely clinical intervention can lead the prevention of further deterioration and the onset of critical illness (Smith and Nielson, 1999; NPSA, 2007). As a consequence policy and clinical guidelines in the last ten years have focused on risk assessment to identify early signs of physiological deterioration and timely intervention (National Institute for Health and Care Excellence (NICE), 2007; Royal College of Physicians, 2012, 2017).

This section begins by exploring the nature of critical illness by examining the triggers for clinical deterioration from the perspective of cell function and cellular injury. Key themes are summarised and applied to a clinical example and links to more detailed cellular physiology and pathophysiology are identified as further reading at the end of the chapter. From a biomedical perspective cell injury occurs when a cell is unable to maintain homeostasis when exposed to injurious stressors. Such stressors include:

- cellular hypoxia
- oxidative stress due to an increase in free radicals
- toxins including infectious agents, medically prescribed drugs, alcohol, social or street drugs
- physical/mechanical stressors such as physical trauma and thermal injury.

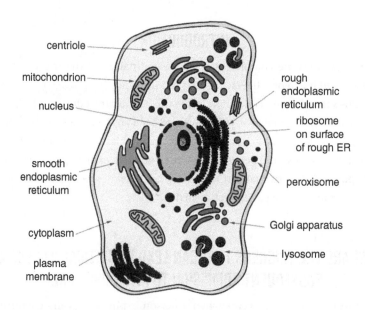

Figure 2.1 Simple anatomy of a cell

Reproduced with permission of © 2016 iatrotec ltd, available at https://www.iatrotec.com/default.asp

According to McCance, Grey and Rodway (2014) the extent of cellular injury depends on a number of specific and modifying factors including:

- cell type
- the level of cell differentiation
- the type of injurious agent
- severity of the injury
- duration of the injury
- nutritional status of the cell
- immunologic and genetic factors.

Figure 2.1 and Bite Size Knowledge 2.1 provide you with a reminder of the structure and key functions of a human cell and organelles.

BITE SIZE KNOWLEDGE 2.1

The function of a generic human cell and its organelles

Table 2.1

Organelle	Function
Nucleus ad nucleolus	Cell division and control of genetic information, replication and repair of DNA
Ribosomes	Provide sites for cellular protein synthesis
Rough endoplasmic reticulum	Is involved with ribosomes in the cells protein synthesis
Smooth endoplasmic reticulum	Involved in the synthesis of steroid hormones
Mitochondria	Contain their own DNA and are involved in the generation of ATP, regulate gene expression in the nucleus, modulate synaptic transmission in brain cells, and trigger systemic inflammatory response
Golgi complex	Process and package proteins from the rough ER into secretory vesicles for transport in and out of the cell
Lysosomes	Contain digestive enzymes that break down bonds in proteins, lipids and carbohydrates. The lysosomal membrane acts as a protective shield protecting the cell from itself
Peroxisomes	Contain oxidative enzymes that produce oxidants that could destroy the cell if not contained within the micro-body. Play a role in alcohol detoxification
Plasma membrane	Control the composition and structure of the space using various methods to facilitate active transport, cell mediated transport, diffusion, cell to cell communication

Regardless of the cell type there are core processes that occur in cell injury and ultimately cell death (McCance et al., 2014). These processes include:

1 Depletion of mitochondrial adenosine triphosphate (ATP) leading to a reduction in the energy capacity of the cell and all cell functions.
2 Early loss of selective membrane permeability leading to cellular swelling.
3 Increase in cellular activated oxygen species (free radicals) leading to destruction of cell membranes and structures as a result of oxidative stress. See Bite Size Knowledge 2.2.
4 Increase in cellular calcium leading to intracellular damage.

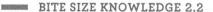 BITE SIZE KNOWLEDGE 2.2

Oxidative stress and reactive oxygen species in critical illness

Oxidative stress occurs when there is an imbalance between the production of reactive oxygen species and nitrogen species (ROS and RNS) and the availability of antioxidants to stabilise the ROS and RNS.

ROS and RNS are free radicals (reactive species) that contain unpaired electrons and are highly reactive with other atoms and molecules in their locality. They include:

• ROS: O_2^- (superoxide anion), OH (hydroxyl radical) and H_2O_2 (hydrogen peroxide)
• RNS: NO (nitric oxide) and $ONOO^-$ (peroxynitrite).

In homeostatic conditions ROS and RNS are constantly produced as a by-product of normal cellular functions such as aerobic respiration using oxidative phosphorylation to produce ATP. Free radicals are also produced as a defence against infection, using radical production to trigger phagocytosis. They also have a role in the regulation of cell reproduction and apoptosis (controlled cell death) (Koekkoek and van Zanten, 2016).

The function of antioxidants is to inactivate and scavenge free radicals in order to maintain a 'reduction-oxidation balance' and prevent oxidative damage. In situations where the production of ROS and RNS exceeds the cell's capacity to retain a balance, oxidative stress occurs. The ROS and RNS react with cell lipids in the plasma membrane, DNA and inactivate enzymes leading to severe cellular damage, cell death, tissue damage and organ dysfunction.

Studies in the last 15 years on the impact of oxidative stress in the critically ill have focused on sepsis and ischaemic reperfusion injury. In sepsis ROS and RNS have been identified as being partially responsible for vascular hypo-reactivity to catecholamine and increased vascular permeability, leading to septic shock and ARDS and paradoxically, where oxygen therapy and inhaled NO have the potential to increase ROS and RNS and can exacerbate further damage (Bernal et al., 2010; Galley, 2011). Extensive studies have also been conducted in the study of ischaemic-reperfusion injury. Reperfusion of ischaemic tissue is essential in order to restore aerobic metabolism and mitochondrial function. However the process of reperfusion can increase the production of ROS and RNS and increase the risk of further damage leading to increased morbidity and mortality (Zweier and Talukder, 2006; Kalogeris et al., 2012).

According to Koekkoek and van Zanten (2016) a number of studies have investigated the use of antioxidant vitamins and trace element supplementation in critically ill patients with some success. However the lack of large randomised control trials limits the validity and generalisability of the findings so far.

The critical factor in relation to cell injury is the absence and or presence of oxygen and cell response to ischaemia and the potential for cell survival is influenced by the:

- severity and duration of the ischaemia
- pathological events initiated by reperfusion of the cells with oxygen.

In order to explore how these processes can impact on a person experiencing an acute deterioration we will examine a case study. Mr Brian Trent, a 62-year-old gentleman underwent the repair of an Abdominal Aortic Aneurysm (AAA) five years ago. Today he has been admitted with acute and severe chest pain which started while walking to the newsagents. He clutched his chest and collapsed on the pavement, a passer-by called for an ambulance and Mr Trent arrived at the cardiac unit within 40 minutes of the onset of his chest pain. He was diagnosed with an inferior myocardial infarction and underwent percutaneous angiography to remove the clots and received two stents, one in his right coronary artery and a second in the right marginal artery. Blood flow was re-established to his heart muscle within 90 minutes of his collapse. In Figure 2.2 the impact of severe ischaemia on Mr Trent's myocardial myocytes, according to the duration of ischaemia, is illustrated.

Timing is critical and in relation to cardiac myocytes, periods of ischaemia lasting less than 5 minutes, followed by reperfusion with oxygen, trigger ischaemic conditioning involving the activation of cell survival programmes that limit the magnitude of injury induced by subsequent exposure to prolonged ischaemia followed by reperfusion (Montecucco et al., 2016). Periods of ischaemia lasting between 5–20 minutess induce myocardial stunning or hibernation and when the cells are reperfused with oxygen contractile function is slow to improve but without progression to infarction and inflammation. Knowledge that cardiac conditioning and cardiac hibernation can occur has led researchers such as Murray et al. (1986) to explore how ischaemic pre-conditioning can reduce the subsequent size of a myocardial infarction (MI) and indeed if ischaemic post-conditioning can be used to reduce the extent of myocardial injury in people presenting with an acute MI. The concept of post-conditioning has however not been tested by rigorous clinical trials and further work is required before clinical interventions can be proposed (Montecucco et al., 2016).

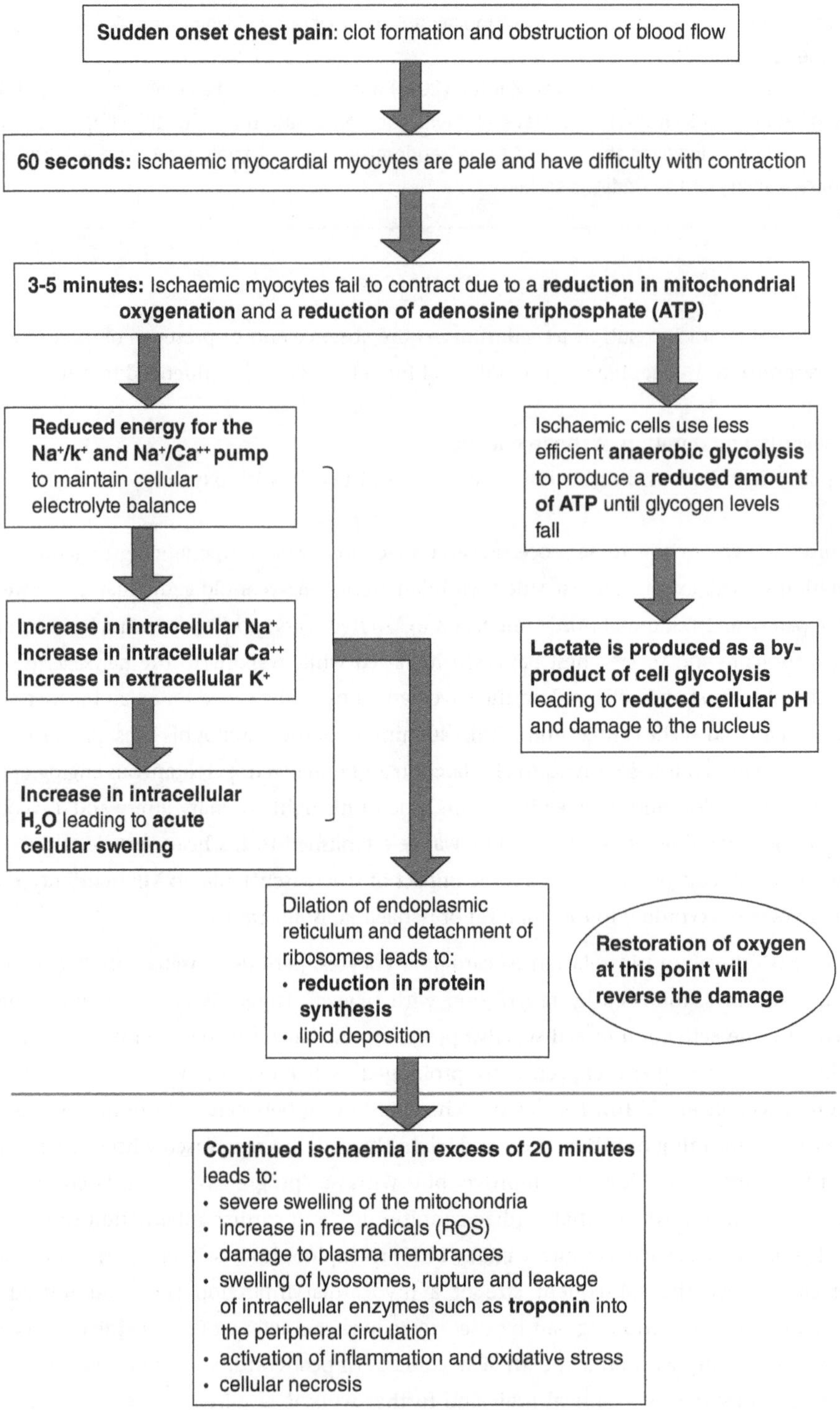

Figure 2.2 The journey of Mr Trent's myocardial cellular ischaemic injury

By the time Mr Trent was admitted to the cardiac unit the four core processes of cellular injury leading to cardiomyocyte death had been initiated. In the heart irreversible cardiomyocyte damage occurs after approximately 20 minutes of ischaemia while in the brain it is less than 20 minutes, and renal cells can survive 30 minutes of ischaemia at normal temperature before cell death is triggered (Kalogeris et al., 2012). Depending on the cell type, once the critical duration of ischaemia has been exceeded cell injury and/or death are inevitable.

Generally the biological events that occur during prolonged ischaemia include:

- anaerobic metabolism
- reduced availability of ATP
- reduced intracellular pH
- loss of the Na^+/K^+ and Na^+/Ca^{++} pumps leading elevated intracellular sodium and calcium
- impaired organelle function
- cellular swelling and swelling of the mitochondria
- damage to plasma membranes
- initiation of the inflammatory response.

These events can be described as the ischaemic components of tissue injury and while re-vascularisation and restoration of blood flow is the primary therapeutic approach, reperfusion *per se* can trigger pathogenic processes that exacerbate the injury primarily caused by ischaemia. Bite Size Knowledge 2.3 summarises the key elements of ischaemia reperfusion injury.

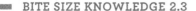 BITE SIZE KNOWLEDGE 2.3

Ischaemia/reperfusion injury

Ischaemia/ reperfusion injury (IRI) refers to the total cellular and tissue injury sustained as a result of (a) prolonged ischaemia (ischaemic component) followed by (b) reperfusion (reperfusion component).

a The onset of prolonged ischaemia triggers the processes of tissue injury (illustrated in Figure 2.2).

b The biochemical changes that occur during prolonged ischaemia contribute to a surge in the generation of ROS and the infiltration of pro-inflammatory neutrophils when oxygen is initially reintroduced into the cells leading to further cell damage.

In a review of the cell biology of ischaemia/ reperfusion (IR) Kalogeris et al. (2012) have summarised four concepts that impact on our understanding of cardiovascular morbidity and mortality. They include:

(Continued)

(Continued)

1 The response to IR is bimodal in that two components of injury exist and the impact of each is dependent on the length of time ischaemia has existed before reperfusion was commenced.
2 Cell injury and dysfunction are triggered by pathological processes involved in (a) ischaemia and second by (b) perfusion.
3 Existing risk factors for IRI are related to factors and events that occur during foetal life (foetal programming) and these can enhance an individual's susceptibility to IRI.
4 The mechanisms that contribute to IRI are complex and multifactorial. They include the following:

    i Ca^{2+} overload leading to mitochondrial and membrane dysfunction
   ii oxidative stress associated with ROS and RNS
  iii endoplasmic and mitochondrial dysfunction
  iv activation of protein kinases
   v inflammatory response
  vi epigenetic changes in gene function
 vii nutritive perfusion deficits
viii protein cleavage products derived from the breakdown of cell proteins.

According to Yellon and Hausenloy (2007) while the biological mechanisms that exist in reperfusion injury are complex, they involve the following processes:

1 generation of ROS fuelled by the introduction of oxygen following reperfusion
2 calcium overload initially triggered by an influx of intracellular calcium during ischaemia is exacerbated by reperfusion
3 opening of the mitochondrial permeability transition pore (MPT) triggered by the increase in calcium that reduces mitochondrial efficiency and ATP production
4 endothelial dysfunction
5 appearance of early triggers for prothrombogenesis
6 pronounced inflammatory response.

In Figure 2.3 these biological processes have been applied to Mr Trent's journey of treatment as the risks of ischaemic/reperfusion injury are managed alongside treatment with percutaneous coronary intervention (PCI) and insertion of stents to facilitate reperfusion. Recent guidelines recommend that fibrinolytic therapy should be initiated for a person presenting with ST elevation MI within 30 minutes of first medical contact when primary PCI cannot be performed within 90 minutes (Huber et al., 2014), with the greatest reduction in mortality and morbidity occurring when reperfusion occurs within 1–2 hours of the onset of symptoms (Kristensen et al., 2014). Mr Trent received PCI within 90 minutes of the onset of this ischaemic event and he was discharged from coronary care four days later. During his time in hospital Mr Trent's haemodynamic status stabilised quickly and he experienced no further chest pain or cardiac arrhythmias. However his history of atherosclerosis means that he remains vulnerable to further episodes of damage to his circulation and haemodynamic integrity (Ramji and Davies, 2015).

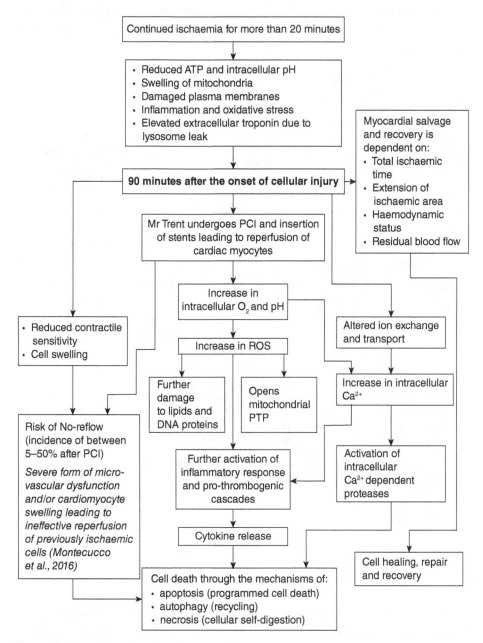

Figure 2.3 Mr Trent's risk of ischaemia/reperfusion injury

WHAT IS THE RELATIONSHIP BETWEEN THE INFLAMMATORY RESPONSE AND CRITICAL ILLNESS?

A key feature of cell injury is acute inflammation, a non-specific, cellular and chemical response that is designed to be the body's second line of defence after physical barriers (the skin) and biochemical barriers on epithelial surfaces have been breached (Rote et al., 2014). You can see a summary of the processes involved in the acute inflammatory response in Figure 2.4.

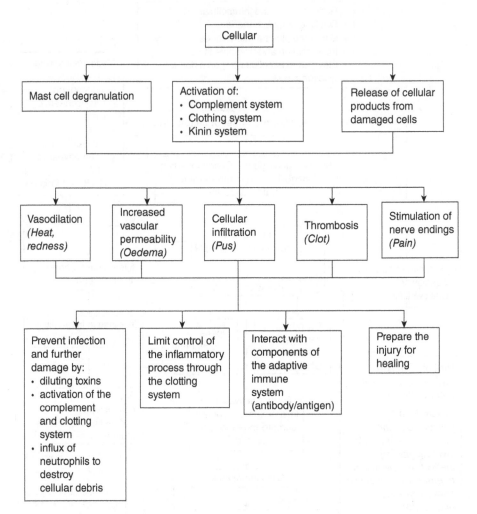

Figure 2.4 The acute inflammatory response

According to Rote et al. (2014) when the inflammatory response is triggered there are three characteristic changes in the micro circulation that occur at the site of injury and these include:

1 vasodilation

2 increased vascular permeability

3 adherence of leucocytes to the inner walls of vessels and their movement through the membrane to the site of injury.

There are also a number of systems and chemicals that contribute to the inflammatory response which are critical to effective defence and recovery. These include the complement, clotting and Kinin systems, all of which are highly interactive and perpetuate the processes required in order to protect cell and tissue function.

The Complement, Clotting and Kinin Systems

The complement system contains plasma proteins that together destroy pathogens and either activate or collaborate with other inflammatory components through three different pathways:

1 chemical pathway (through adaptive immunity – antibody/antigen system)

2 lectin pathway (activated by mannose (sugar) containing bacterial carbohydrates)

3 alternative pathways (activated by gram negative bacterial and fungal cell wall polysaccharides).

These pathways trigger a number of activities designed to perpetuate the inflammatory response including:

a anaphylatoxic activity and degranulation of mast cells

b leucocyte chemotaxis

c opsonisation (flagging) of micro-organisms for destruction

d cell lysis.

The clotting system traps micro-organisms and foreign bodies at the site of inflammation thus preventing the spread of infection to adjacent tissues. It also forms the clot to stop bleeding and support haemostasis as well as providing a fibrin mesh for repair and healing. The Kinin system, in particular bradykinin, triggers some dilation of blood vessels and works with prostaglandins to induce pain, trigger smooth muscle contraction, increase vascular permeability and increase leucocyte chemotaxis (Rote et al., 2014).

The Role of Cytokines

Cytokines are soluble molecules (biochemical messengers) secreted by cells to contribute to the regulation of and response to inflammation. The cytokines involved in the inflammatory response are classified as interleukins (ILs), tumour necrosis factor (TNF-alpha) and interferons (IFNs). Interleukins are produced by cells of the acquired immune system (macrophages and lymphocytes) and are either pro-inflammatory or anti-inflammatory in nature. Figure 2.5 provides a summary of the key cytokines and their role as part of an inflammatory response. Interferons have a protective effect against viral infection and have a role in modulating the inflammatory response. Tumour necrosis factor is another essential cytokine required to support the inflammatory response and has a pro-inflammatory role in the production of inflammatory proteins by the liver (Turner et al., 2014).

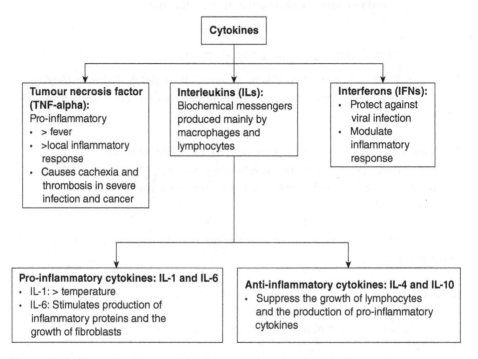

Figure 2.5 The role of some of the key cytokines involved in the acute inflammatory response

Mast Cells

Mast cells are granulated cells (leukocytes) usually located close to blood vessels. These cells are usually found in the endothelial linings of respiratory tract, skin and gastrointestinal tract. They are highly sensitive cells that can be triggered by trauma, chemical agents and by antibodies produced by the adaptive immune system (Urb and Sheppard, 2012; Theoharides and Cochrane, 2004). Once triggered, mast cells are involved in the inflammatory response in two ways: the first response is immediate and is described as degranulation; the second, longer-term response involves the synthesis of inflammatory mediators. During degranulation the mast cells release pro-inflammatory cytokines, histamine which leads to smooth muscle contraction (e.g. bronchospasm) and vasodilation with increased capillary permeability, also neutrophil and eosinophil chemotactic factors are released to attract neutrophils and eosinophils to the site of injury. Chemicals synthesised by the mast cells are involved in perpetuating the inflammatory response and include leukotrienes, which have vascular and smooth muscle effects, prostaglandins which trigger the pain response as well as influencing vasodilation and clotting, pro-inflammatory cytokines and growth factors which trigger proliferation of the endothelial cells, connective tissue and smooth muscle (Rote et al., 2014). Other factors in the inflammatory process involve the relationship between the endothelial lining of blood vessels and platelets. In homeostasis nitric oxide (NO) and prostacyclin (PGI_2) maintain blood flow and pressure through their synergistic action and when in balance inhibit platelet activation. However if cells in the endothelial lining become damaged platelet activation is initiated, the platelets disintegrate and liberate platelet factors which cause a local elevation of the concentration of clotting factors leading to primary haemostasis and simultaneously secondary haemostatic mechanisms associated with the clotting cascade. Further reading related to the relationship between the inflammatory response and atherosclerosis (a chronic inflammatory disorder of the arteries) can be found at the end of this chapter.

WHAT IS THE LINK BETWEEN ACUTE INFLAMMATION AND SYSTEMIC INFLAMMATORY RESPONSE SYNDROME (SIRS)?

We have established that inflammation is essential for the containment of infection and tissue repair. However in situations where there is a severe cellular insult the body produces a non-specific systemic inflammatory response. Proposed by Bone et al. (1992), Systemic Inflammatory Response Syndrome (SIRS) has been identified in a number of situations involving massive cellular trauma. These include:

- burns
- trauma
- pancreatitis
- invasive ventilation
- ischaemia
- bacteraemia, fungaemia, viraemia.

The nonspecific nature of SIRS coupled with the complex interaction between inflammatory mediators means that identifying specific triggers and finding factors to promote resolution of SIRS is difficult and ongoing (Maiden and Chapman, 2014). A summary of the stages of progression from acute inflammation to SIRS is summarised in Figure 2.6.

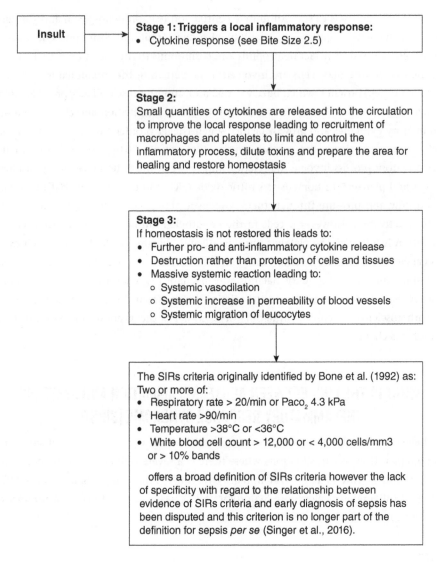

Figure 2.6 The stages of progression from acute inflammation to SIRS

From a pathophysiological perspective the simultaneous triggering of systemic pro-inflammatory cytokines (SIRS) and anti-inflammatory cytokines (Compensatory Anti-inflammatory Response Syndrome (CARS) can lead to one of three general outcomes for the patient:

- uncomplicated rapid recovery
- fulminant multiple organ dysfunction (MOD) and death
- chronic critical illness associated with persistent inflammation, progressive immunosuppression and catabolic syndrome (PICS). (Rosenthal and Moore, 2016)

Studies into the morbidity and mortality of patients diagnosed with SIRS are again difficult to establish because of the wide variety of triggers. However some researchers have identified that the occurrence of SIRS shows an increase on patient mortality at one month and one year. For example Comstedt et al. (2009) found that the presence of SIRS in acutely ill hospitalised medical patients demonstrated an increase in predicted mortality by 7%. Similar findings have emerged in a study of patients presenting with SIRS following trans-catheter aortic valve implantation, where there was a relative increase in mortality of 17% at 30 days and 43% at one year compared to independent predictions (Sinning et al., 2012). The non-specific nature of SIRS and lack of specificity regarding the triggers has also challenged the development of sensitive diagnostic tools and new treatments to improve patient outcome. For example, the current consensus group for defining sepsis (Singer et al., 2016) has identified that due to the lack of specificity when defining the presence of the SIRS criteria (see Figure 2.6) the inclusion of the SIRS criteria described by Bone et al. (1992) is no longer included in the definition of sepsis. Drawing conclusions from this it is clear that physiological processes indicative of a systemic inflammatory response appear to influence the onset of critical illness although not all critically ill patients with sepsis will present with SIRS (Kaukonen et al., 2015). The focus must therefore be on risk assessment and diagnosis of specific features related to clinical deterioration supported by clinical guidance and evidence based practice. So far we have established that the relationship between cellular damage and critical illness is influenced by a number of factors including: the severity of the injury, the length of time cells are exposed to injury, and the body's physiological response to the injury. All types of cellular injury trigger a response and in the next section we discuss the complex relationship between bio-psychosocial triggers as stressors and the development of critical illness.

THE IMPACT OF THE BODY'S STRESS RESPONSE ON HOW A PERSON DEVELOPS AND COPES WITH ILLNESS

Stress can be described as a transactional concept in that it is the body's physiological and behavioural response to an acute stressor with the aim of achieving homeostasis or harmony (Tsigos et al., 2016). In general a person experiences stress when the demand from the stressor exceeds the person's ability to cope or maintain balance. Activation of the acute stress system leads to the triggering of a time limited cluster of behavioural and physiological changes that are adaptive and designed to be stressor specific and to improve a person's chance of survival. However if the stressor becomes chronic the stress response becomes non-specific immunosuppressive and destructive.

Over the years there has been much debate in behavioural sciences and medicine as to whether psychological and social factors which lead to stress can cause diseases and research indicates that the role of chronic stress does contribute to diseases such as cardiovascular disease and cancer. Chronic stress results in long-term, and sometimes permanent, changes to emotional, physiological and behavioural responses (Cohen et al., 2007; McEwen, 2012). Over the last decade much research has been undertaken to explore the effects of stress and many variables explored, for example: cardiovascular disease and stress (Krantz and McCeney, 2002); work and stress (Kivimäki et al., 2012; Health and Safety Executive, 2016) and bio-behavioural factors related to tumour biology (Antoni et al., 2006); stress and prostate cancer (De Sousa et al., 2012); stress and breast cancer (Duiijts et al., 2003); respiratory diseases such as upper respiratory tract infections (Drummond and Hewson-Bower, 1997) asthma (Asthma UK 2016), and autoimmune diseases (Ader, 2008).

Studies tend to agree that whilst humans are very adept at adapting to stress both acute and chronic stress are associated with the development of acute, critical and chronic conditions.

Stressors can be physical and/or psychological and have the potential to lead to a state of disharmony. When disharmony occurs the stress response is triggered and triggers a complex system of interconnected neuroendocrine, cellular and molecular processes leading to physiological and behavioural responses in order to re-establish and maintain homeostasis (Chrousos, 2009; Chrousos and Gold, 1992). These responses are initiated by the secretion of corticotropin-releasing hormone and include:

- increased arousal and alertness
- increased cognition, vigilance and focused attention
- suppression of feeding, gastric motility and reproductive behaviour
- oxygen and nutrients are directed to the central nervous system and stressed body site
- increased respiratory rate and altered cardiovascular tone to increase heart rate and blood pressure
- increased gluconeogenesis and lipolysis
- containment of the stress, inflammatory and immune response.

Hence, as a result of the stress response the individual has enhanced cardiovascular reserve and increased accessibility to fuel for the brain, heart and musculoskeletal system, allowing him/her to take the most appropriate flight or fight action while simultaneously providing a balanced activation of the immune system (Clayton and McCance, 2014). The physiological processes are summarised in Figure 2.7.

How an individual adapts to stress is influenced by a number of factors including genetic, environmental and developmental factors that influence a person's vulnerability to stress and adaptation. A comprehensive assessment and knowing the patient in this context can offer insight into how a person may cope with critical illness, their

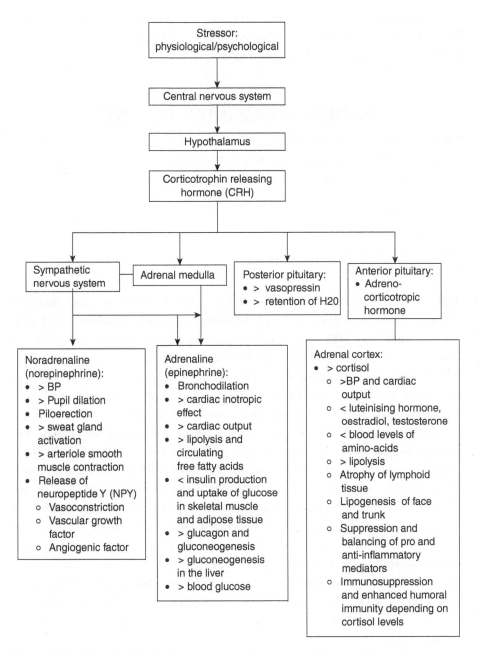

Figure 2.7 The physiological processes and responses triggered by a stressor

rehabilitation and clinical outcome. For example, according to Clayton and McCance (2014) an individual can develop an anticipatory response to stress created by memory and /or conditioning that in some cases can lead to phobias and in others to post-traumatic stress disorder. For some critically ill patients this may be manifested as a post-traumatic stress response to the experience of being critically ill (McGriffin et al., 2016). The factors involved in the triggering of this response however are complex and require further research and are explored in more depth in following chapters.

THE STRESS RESPONSE AND CRITICAL ILLNESS

When a person is exposed to stress a graded response occurs that correlates with the degree of severity of the stress. According to Marik (2009) cortisol and catecholamine levels correlate with:

- the severity of illness/ injury
- the type of surgery
- Glasgow Coma score
- APACHE score.

The acute stress response in critical illness can result in a number of metabolic responses and in particular, stress hyperglycaemia. According to Soeters and Soeters (2012) stress hyperglycaemia and insulin resistance are responses preserved through our evolution to allow the host to survive during periods of severe stress. Not all tissues require insulin to facilitate the uptake of glucose, including the central and peripheral nervous system, bone marrow and red and white blood cells. Subsequently the down regulation of GLUT - 4 receptors due to a reduction in insulin production during the stress response encourages the redistribution of glucose away from skeletal muscle and towards the immune cells and the nervous system (Marik, 2015). The management of stress hyperglycaemia in critical illness has been the subject of considerable debate with several researchers identifying the risks to increased patient morbidity and mortality associated with mild hypoglycaemia and 'tight glycaemic control' (Park et al., 2012; Duning et al., 2010; Vespa et al., 2012). However some studies have found the opposite and according to Badawi et al. (2012) there is a progressive increase in patient mortality associated with blood glucose levels consistently over 6.1 mmols/L. Marik (2015) challenges this finding on the grounds that the study has limited generalisability and so far no other study has been able to replicate the findings. He goes on to argue for conservative glycaemic control involving a detailed assessment of the patient and the factors influencing illness progression and including the presence of existing diabetes.

Stress Hyperlactataemia

A second metabolic response triggered by acute stress is hyperlactataemia. Lactate is a metabolite involved in two processes for adenosine triphosphate production (ATP) including, glycolysis and mitochondrial oxidative phosphorylation.

In stable conditions these two processes steadily metabolise glucose to produce energy:

1 During glycolysis glucose is converted to pyruvate thus generating two molecules of ATP.
2 Pyruvate is then fully oxidised to CO2 and about 36 molecules of ATP through the process of oxidative phosphorylation (Bakker et al., 2013).

Under stressful conditions:

• Glycolysis can increase up to a factor of 1,000 in the presence of glucose in order to meet the increased demand for ATP, producing increased amounts of pyruvate.
• Such a high rate of pyruvate production will saturate mitochondrial functional capacity leading to an accumulation of pyruvate.
• The excess pyruvate is rapidly converted to lactate in order for the second stage of glycolysis to proceed with the assistance of the enzyme lactate dehydrogenase (LDH).
• In this reversible equation lactate is converted to pyruvate during recovery from the stressed state (Bakker et al., 2013).

Thus, lactate production increases under conditions of cellular stress such as sepsis, cardiogenic shock and hyper-metabolic states in order to prevent pyruvate accumulation and to supply the nicotinamide adenine dinucleotide (NAD) needed for phase two of glycolysis. In this way lactate serves as a critical buffer in the acceleration of glycolysis. During this process lactate production inhibits rather than causes metabolic acidosis and while an increase in lactate production coincides with metabolic acidosis, it is an indirect marker rather than a direct cause (Robergs et al., 2004; Gunnerson et al., 2006). This has triggered the proposal that the term 'lactic acidosis' should be replaced by 'hyperlactataemia'.

Lactate can also function as an intermediate fuel that can be exchanged between cells under conditions of acute stress. For example in cardiac muscle during shock and/or beta-adrenergic stimulation, lactate may account for up to 60% of cardiac oxidative substrate (Lopaschuk et al., 2010). Thus according to Barbee et al. (2000) interventions to accelerated lactate clearance during shock could compromise cardiac performance. This finding has been supported by Revelly et al. (2005) where they demonstrated an improvement in cardiac performance following an infusion of sodium lactate in patients with both cardiogenic and septic shock. Similarly in the brain during hypoglycaemia and ischaemia, astrocyte production of lactate has been shown to support neuronal ATP requirements. Similar findings have been shown in liver and kidney cells (Leverve, 1999).

In conclusion, an increase in lactate during critical illness can indicate an acute metabolic stress response that has been triggered by one or more factors and will relate to the severity and type of cellular injury and its impact on tissues and organs. As such, lactate levels can provide an indicator of the severity and duration of the stress response in critical illness and may be used in conjunction with other clinical and diagnostic tools to measure outcome particularly in the early resuscitation of critically ill patients (Bakker et al., 2013).

Maladaptive Coping and the Complexities of Addiction

Some modulators of the stress response are genetic and/or related to physiological mechanisms associated with sex hormone levels. Other modulators include an individual's previous life experiences, exposure to previous stress, educational level and social hierarchy. Some modulators such as nicotine, alcohol and other forms of substance misuse may act to relieve stressors but they can also trigger maladaptive coping which leads to further harm. This can impact directly on the development of critical illness or influence the morbidity and mortality of people who present with maladaptive coping as secondary to the primary cause – such as sepsis. According to Mehta (2016) one in four patients admitted to critical care units will have alcohol related issues that will lead to prolonged length of stay in ICU and increased mortality.

There is no doubt that smoking is an addictive behaviour and causes illnesses and early death from lung cancers, Chronic Obstructive Pulmonary Disease and cardiovascular disease. It is also well known that second-hand smoking has implications for non-smokers. Research undertaken by ASH (2016) (Action on Smoking and Health founded in 1971 by the Royal College of Physicians) indicates that whilst in the UK the numbers of people who have never smoked is increasing there are still approximately 9.6 million smokers, there is still a prevalence amongst men and there is a strong link between cigarette smoking and socio-economic groups (over 30% of manual workers smoke whereas 13% of managerial and professional occupations smoke). There is also an association with the consumption of cigarettes. Here ASH and ONS (2013) report that 55% of smokers who are in the higher social groups are smoking 10 or fewer cigarettes per day compared with 34% in the lower social groups and that the lower social groups smoke more than the higher social groups. Nearly half of unemployed people and the majority of prisoners and homeless people smoke and smoking is twice the national average in people with mental health problems. NICE (2015) suggest that smoking levels in some groups including lesbian, gay, bisexual and transgender (LGBT) people are also high.

Reports from ASH and ONS have resulted in the UK Government issuing a Tobacco Control Plan (Department of Health, 2011a) which set out the Government strategy's to reduce tobacco use over a five-year period within the context of the public health system.

Inhaled cigarette smoke, occupational hazards (such as smoke from biomass fuels or wood burning and associated air pollution) or/and inhalation of noxious particles are major risk factors for the development of Chronic Obstructive Pulmonary Disease (COPD). COPD is a major cause of chronic morbidity and mortality throughout the world; many people suffer from this disease for years, and die prematurely from it or its complications (Global Initiative for Chronic Obstructive Lung Disease, 2017). Indeed Chronic Obstructive Pulmonary Disease (COPD) is the fourth leading cause of death in the world (ibid.). The Global Burden of Disease Study (WHO 2017) 'reports a prevalence of 251 million cases of COPD globally in 2016 and it is estimated that 3.17 million deaths were caused by the disease in 2015'.

Whilst stress and smoking (and second-hand smoking) lead to high levels of respiratory diseases (COPD, upper respiratory tract disease and Asthma), so too can environmental issues such air quality or mould allergies. Here well-known conditions, such as Farmer's lung and Sauna-taker's lung, are caused by mould allergy and people who live in cold damp homes are more likely to have respiratory illness due to the release and inhalation of mould spores (which can also cause symptoms such as rhinitis, itchy eyes, and eczema).

There has been an increase in the range and availability of illicit substances (Opioids, Cocaine, Amphetamines, Ecstasy, Cannabis) (European Monitoring Centre for Drugs and Drug Addiction, 2015). Drug addiction is complex but goes hand in hand with poor health. Physical health is inextricably linked to mental health and vice versa so what is physically good for you is likely to be mentally good for you, and poor physical health leads to negative effects on mental health and wellbeing (Department of Health, 2011b). Thus people who use illicit substances are more prone to mental health problems and people with mental health problems are more prone to using illicit drugs.

The Public Health Institute at Liverpool John Moores University (2018) suggest that there are over 380,000 heroin and crack cocaine users in England. Substance misuse damages both physical and mental health including cardiovascular disease, arthritis, immobility, liver cirrhosis, liver cancer, lung diseases, deep vein thrombosis, Hepatitis B and C, HIV, depression, anxiety, psychosis, delirium and personality disorders (see Chapter 10) . Substance misuse is also associated with homelessness, poor social outcomes including family breakdown, offending and contact with the criminal justice system, poor medication adherence and increased use of community and hospital services.

Obesity and Illness

Obesity is a major public health problem. National Statistics presented by the Health and Social Care Information Centre (2015) show that in 2013 approximately 58–65% of adults were overweight or obese (23–26% of these were obese) in England, Scotland and Wales as are over half of adults in the European Union. The Foresight Report (Butland et al., 2007) project predicted that by 2050 over half of the UK adult population will be obese.

This has implications for society and the economy; and whilst one should recognise that generally obesity tends to be related to changes in society, such as work life, transportation and food production, national statistics presented by the Health and Social Care

Information Centre (UK HSCIC) (2015) highlight that lifestyles of smoking, not eating healthily, not being physically active, hypertension and age were key risk factors for obesity and associated ill health and premature death.

Obesity strongly relates to Thompson '**P**', '**C**' and '**S**' (see Bite Size Knowledge 2.4) levels whereby being overweight or obese is becoming seen as normal and as Butland et al. (2007: 5) state it is 'embedded within a complex societal framework' which will take 'several decades to reverse', because it is associated with health conditions such as type 2 diabetes, hypertension, hyperlipidaemia, cardiovascular diseases, metabolic syndrome, ovarian cancer, cancer of the colon, gall bladder disease, osteoarthritis and stroke (National Audit Office, 2001; Butland et al., 2007). It can lead to reduced quality of life and premature death.

The HSCIC (2015) also highlight that prescription drugs for the treatment of obesity are increasing as are the number of people being admitted to hospital with obesity (primary or secondary diagnosis).

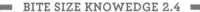 BITE SIZE KNOWEDGE 2.4

Thompson's PCS model

The relationship between inequalities in health and the risk of critical illness can be a major factor in understanding why some people find themselves in a spiral of maladaptive coping and ill health. One way of examining this relationship is through the use of Thompson's (2006) 'P', 'C', 'S' model.

- Whilst the 'P' stands for personal or psychological which includes individual thoughts and feelings, attitudes and actions it also refers to the practice of individual workers and their interactions with individual clients and prejudice which includes the inflexibility of mind that stands in the way of fair and non-judgemental practice. The further away one moves from the personal level the less impact an individual can have and therefore it becomes necessary to move beyond the personal level both in understanding and tackling discrimination and this involves individuals playing their part collectively challenging the dominant discriminatory culture and ideology.
- The 'C' of Thompson's model relates to the shared ways of seeing, thinking and doing and the values and patterns of thought and behaviour and the associated assumed consensus of what is right and what is normal. It therefore produces conformity to social norms.
- The 'S' of Thompson's model relates to the network of social divisions and the power relations that are closely associated with them and also relates to the way in which oppression and discrimination are institutionalised and thus sewn into the fabric of society. It also indicates the wider level of social forces, the socio-political dimensions of interlocking patterns of power and influence. The 'C' is thus embedded within the 'S' level as they owe much to the structure of society and the interlocking matrix of social divisions and the power relations which maintain them.

Nurses cannot be immune regarding issues arising from social structure, and those who focus only on changing an individual's behaviour do not comprehend the complexity of the issues. If holistic nursing care is to be offered nurses need to recognise and understand the root cause of inequalities in health, the social psychology elements and the politico-economic factors (politics, government policies and the economy), which all play a part.

Inequalities in Health

Explanations for inequalities in health can be due to hereditary reasons, behavioural explanations or psycho-social stress (i.e. lifestyle choices) or environmental reasons (i.e. material deprivation/poverty). Annandale and Field (2007) felt that inequalities in health between social groups are inherent in British society. Indeed there are many theories that account for this but social determinants are said to be the foundation. Social determinants of health are the conditions to which people are born, grow, live, work and age in society. Authors (see further reading) argue that deprivation leads to reduced life expectancy, increased child mortality, increased mental illness, obesity, increased use of recreational drugs and alcohol, and increased crime. They argue that people with higher social-economic positions in society have a greater array of life chances and as a consequence have better health (i.e. the lower a person's social position the worse his/her health which is also known as the *deprivation of lower social class* – e.g. individuals with a degree have a longer life expectancy than those without a degree).

Prejudice and Stereotyping

One could argue that an illness is the *tipping point of a crisis*. However using Thompson's **'C'** one could suggest that too often nurses are prejudiced and 'blame' individuals for their illness rather than trying to understand the root cause and help the individual. Prejudice can be any attitude, emotion or behaviour towards a group of individuals and traditionally these have been sexism, racism, ageism or homophobia and a common explanation for this is attributed to upbringing and family circumstances (Brown, 2010). Nowadays it is relatively rare to hear prejudiced views based on these attitudes in public and there is less tolerance of sexist, racist, ageist or homophobic attitudes.

However modern prejudice is thought to be symbolic, aversive, ambivalent racism, subtle prejudice, modern and ambivalent sexism and neo-sexism (see Bite Size Knowledge 2.5: New Forms of Prejudice).

New forms of prejudice

Symbolic prejudice: opposition to social policies seen to favour disadvantaged groups; or social policies which are perceived to be inconsistent with values of freedom of choice or the government, or those who hold power, selecting according to merit, which is perceived to be unfair.

Aversive prejudice: individuals avoiding encounters with members of another group whilst endorsing principles of tolerance – i.e. avoiding interactions with other racial and ethnic groups or racial/ethnic minorities.

Ambivalent racism: when people become aware that they have conflicting beliefs about a group of people who do not belong to their own group and they experience a cognitive dissonance. These feelings are brought about because the individual believes in humanitarian virtues and individualistic virtues (i.e. work hard to improve).

Subtle prejudice: such as ignoring others, or treating others differently or ridiculing others.

Modern and ambivalent sexism (also known as hostile sexism or benevolent sexism): reflects overtly negative evaluations and stereotypes about a gender (e.g. women are inferior to men) or when subjective positive gender equality is demonstrated (e.g. women need protecting by men).

Neo-sexism: a belief that women have achieved equality and women who say otherwise are moaning or trying to gain unfair advantage.

Nonetheless, in the UK evidence suggests that whilst sexist, racist, ageist or homophobic prejudice is decreasing, class prejudice and stereotyping appear to be increasing.

A stereotype is the perception that most members of a group share similar attributes; this stereotyping is a form of categorisation which can originate from the culture people are socialised into, the social structure they are brought up and live in and life experiences.

Stereotyping has generational connotations; for example Brown (2010) explored how in the early 1990s media reports resulted in Germans being known as 'aggressive and ambitious' whereas the British were 'boring and arrogant' and these terms are now embedded into UK culture. Stereotypes generate attributional judgements and negative behaviour of one group of people against another.

Lack of appreciation of stereotypical behaviour can affect judgement and this can lead to acts of prejudice without recognition and as Devine (1989), whose work is widely accepted, stated, 'prejudice is always with us' albeit at an 'unconscious level' and some stereotypical behaviour can enhance motivation and belonging (e.g. belonging to the nursing family).

Social psychologists argue that some stereotyping has elements of truth embedded within it, for example the perception that lower social classes use health services more than higher social classes has an element of true behind it because individuals who are unemployed or live on poor wages and in overcrowded housing have higher levels of illness; or there are perceptions that women are more kind and sensitive than men and this is true when essential biology and social upbringing is understood; or that nurses are known to have similar traits which lead to being caring and compassionate and this is also true when social-psychological and biological traits are explored. Indeed social class stereotypes can influence people's judgement on things like academic level or ability (Darley and Gross, 1983) as do perceptions based on socialisation.

So we will leave prejudice and stereotyping here for you to ponder upon and we will link back to it later in this chapter. Now we will explore how the state of the mind can influence our health and illness; the link between the environment and illness; genetics and illness; Learning Disability and illness; and depression.

Family History/Genetics and Illness

Family histories of high cholesterol, diabetes, or high blood pressure are risk factors for heart disease. Individuals whose parents or siblings develop cancer at an early age are at greater risk of developing cancer themselves. These cancers include:

- Colorectal cancer: Where familial adenomatous polyposis (FAP) almost always leads to colorectal cancer by the time a person is in his or her 40s (Cancer Research UK, 2015).
- Breast cancer: If a woman carries one genetic mutation (in the BRCA1 or BRCA2 genes), her risk of having cancer can be 60%. About 5–10% of breast cancers seem to be caused by currently recognised genetic mutations. If the mother, daughter, or sister has had breast cancer the risk grows two to three times (Cancer Research UK, 2014a).
- Prostate cancer: If a close family member died of prostate cancer before age 50 the chances of a son/sibling/brother having prostate cancer are higher (Cancer Research UK, 2014b).

Learning Disability

A learning disability happens when a person's brain development is affected, either before they are born, during their birth or in early childhood. Learning disabilities such as Down's syndrome are diagnosed at birth whilst others might not be discovered until the child is older. The causes of LD can be due to issues during pregnancy (genetic) or birth (O2 starvation) but sometimes there is no known cause. Conditions such as cerebral palsy and Down's syndrome and autism are associated with having a learning disability; and about 30% of people with epilepsy have a learning disability (NHS, 2016).

Clients with a LD often experience barriers in accessing health care (Garvey et al., 2010), and suffer neglect, abuse and poor quality care often as a result of their needs not being fully understood (Welshman and Walmsley, 2006). Mencap (2007) highlighted that there was poor communication as staff did not respect or listen to family members but often associated challenging behaviour to the LD rather than other issues (pain, confusion, fear) and Garvey et al. (2010) found that there was evidence of discriminatory attitudes.

Depression

Although any illness can trigger depressed feelings, depression is one of most common complications of chronic illness and the level of life disruption it causes. For example people living with diabetes are twice as likely to experience depression as those without diabetes (Lustman and Anderson, 2002); Depression is common among people who have chronic illnesses such as Cancer, Coronary heart disease, Epilepsy, Multiple sclerosis, Stroke (National Institute of Mental Health 2018). Depression can intensify pain and cause fatigue and sluggishness.

Psychological illness may result in physical ill health and physical ill health may result in psychological issues (i.e. post-traumatic stress disorder) and people who develop depression as a result of physical illness have higher morbidity and mortality (see Chapter 11 where psychological illness is explored more).

SO WHAT DOES ALL THIS MEAN FOR HUMANISED NURSING CARE? DO NURSES SHOW PREJUDICE? ARE NURSES JUDGEMENTAL? DO SENIOR NURSES IDENTIFY PREJUDICE OR CHALLENGE BLAME CULTURES?

The NMC clearly state that nurses should not be judgemental or prejudiced, and indeed it is a key element in undergraduate education programmes, but social-psychological research suggest that it is inherent in all, so we would be blinkered if we thought nurses were not in some way, shape or form equal. For example reflect if the following are occurring and how many are challenging to you and your team, and how you are managing these:

- decisions, however small, are being made without patient involvement
- negative attitudes towards obesity, smokers, substance misuse
- poor communication and labelling of people with LD
- lack of knowledge about conditions is leading to indifference, apprehension or fear
- labelling and subtle labelling – i.e. when completing admission forms nurses often put 'retired' in the employment section but this can been seen as labelling, stereotypical as well as dehumanising because it dismisses the whole of the employment history of the client's life
- stereotypical attitudes relating to social class, occupation (or lack of) race and ethnicity
- ambivalent prejudice/favourability of clients with specific causes of illness or cultural/racial characteristics is leading to neglect or discomfort of others
- acts of paternalism or gender differentiation are being employed

- implicit prejudice is happening – i.e. facial muscles give indications of people's likes and dislikes
- a comprehensive health and lifestyle check has not been undertaken in order that planning of humanising nursing care can occur.

TRIGGERS FOR CRITICAL ILLNESS AND HUMANISING DIMENSIONS

Let us return to Mr Trent and his experience of having an MI and summarise in context some of the issues explored in this chapter.

Table 2.1 A summary of Mr Trent's care and how his experience of critical illness can be interpreted using the humanising framework

Humanising dimensions	Critical illness triggers	Managing stressors and coping strategies	Role of expert nurse in support strategies
Insiderness/ objectification	Mr T has a stressful job; he is overweight and tends to eat fast food 4 times per week. His alcohol consumption is 28 units per week Triggers include: • chronic inflammatory response and atherosclerosis • toxic impact of alcohol • psychological stress – elevated blood glucose, increases risk of mitochondrial damage and type 2 diabetes • delayed cellular recovery	Mr T is a director in a company and has long working hours and provides well for his family. He is concerned that the MI may force him to take early retirement and the family's standard of living will be reduced	Enable connectedness by helping staff understand that it is good to take time to listen to Mr T's and his family's fears and anxieties
Agency/ passivity	Mr T is out of his comfort zone and feels unable to decide if it is safe to get up or go to sleep. Mr T does not understand the routine and why it is important • Increased risk of stress hyperglycaemia	Mr T needs a full understanding of - ward routine - roles of staff such as physio - the type of exercise needed - healthy diet - medication - return to work	Ensure staff give Mr T a sound evidence based rationale re why it is important to focus on the present care Discuss recovery time, driving, return to family life
Uniqueness/ homogenisation	Mr T fears that the life he has, which he enjoys, may be lost	The world in which Mr T lives and his fears of what may change in that world due to the MI however small are important to Mr T	Ensure staff are not judgemental about Mr T's lifestyle. Challenge assumptions and examples of modern prejudice being displayed

(Continued)

Table 2.1   (Continued)

Humanising dimensions	Critical illness triggers	Managing stressors and coping strategies	Role of expert nurse in support strategies
	He will be experiencing a sense of grief and loss of role and responsibilities	He has a unique view of that world and this must be recognised if staff are to help him overcome his fears	Enable staff to reflect and learn from any stereotypical behaviour they are showing
Togetherness/ isolation	Mr T does not fully understand the AAA and the reasons why he has now had an MI	He loves his wife and family very much and feels he cannot go on without them. He does fear not being able to provide for them	Involve wife in exploring trigger factors – smoking, diet, exercise and helping to adjust to new lifestyle choices together
Sense making/ loss of meaning	Not understanding what an MI is and the trigger factors He does not know why he is connected to the monitors or why he has a urethral catheter or why staff are concerned about his kidneys when he was admitted for his heart	Staff need to provide Mr T with adequate knowledge of the world he is in at present so he can make sense of the care	Enable staff to recognise that what is 'normal' to them is fear making for Mr T and his family. Help them form questions and answers that are not condescending to Mr T and his family recognising that every situation is potentially new to them
Personal journey/loss of personal journey	Mr T has cardiac pain. He feels weak and helpless. Poor circulation has resulted in Acute Kidney Injury Ischaemic hypo- perfusion and cell damage	Mr T needs a comprehensive understanding of the relationship between body organs – heart, circulation and the kidneys	Enable staff to ensure Mr T has a working knowledge of basic anatomy and physiology and how one has affected the other and the associated care and treatment implications
Sense of place/ dislocation	Mr T is frightened that he may die and leave his wife and children alone Mr T is fearful of being moved to a general ward because of the media stories regarding lack of nursing staff Cultural and structural factors influence a patient's trust in health care systems	Mr T might like to talk through his fears with a counsellor or chaplain or rehabilitation health care professional but he may not know they are available	Ensure staff have a sound evidence base regarding what fears post-MI may bring and can offer coping strategies
Embodiment/ reductionist body	Concerns because he has a friend who has had an MI and the post- medications caused him to be impotent but not wishing to tell nurses of his fears in case he is thought to be weak and unmanly	Mr T may like to talk to a male nurse or to someone from the MI support group or rehabilitation class	Ensure staff are enabling Mr T to make choices. Ensure they have a good working knowledge of support structures that Mr T can access

CHAPTER SUMMARY

There is no distinction or division between bio-psychosocial factors that influence the development of critical illness. A holistic understanding of the person and the consequences of living that led to their critical illness are important factors in understanding their potential for recovery. Chapters 1 and 2 offer insights into how the patient's experience of critical illness can be viewed from a variety of complex integrated and interrelated perspectives. These perspective will continue to be explored in each of the chapters as different patient journeys are explored.

FURTHER READING

Balk, R. (2014) Systemic inflammatory response syndrome (SIRS) where did it come from and is it still relevant today? *Virulence, 5*: 1.

Coulter, A. and Collins, A. (2011) *Making Shared Decision-making a Reality. No Decision about Me, without Me.* London: Kings Fund.

Forsight Report (2008) *Forsight: Mental Capital and Wellbeing: Making the Most of Ourselves in the 21st Century.* Available at: www.gov.uk/government/publications/mental-capital-and-wellbeing-making-the-most-of-ourselves-in-the-21st-century

Marmot, M. (2010) *The Marmot Review. Fair Society, Healthy Lives. Strategic Review of Health Inequalities in England post 2010.* Available at: www.instituteofhealthequity.org/

Picard, M., Wallace, D. and Burelle, Y. (2016) The rise of mitochondria in medicine, *Mitochondrion, 30*: 105–16.

The Acheson Report (1998) Independent Inquiry into Inequalities in Health Report. Available at: www.gov.uk/government/publications/independent-inquiry-into-inequalities-in-health-report

The Wanless Report (2003) *Securing Good Health for the Whole Population.* Available at: http://webarchive.nationalarchives.gov.uk/+/http://www.hm-treasury.gov.uk/media/D/3/Wanless04_summary.pdf

World Health Organisation (2008) *Closing the Gap in a Generation. Health Equity through Action on the Social Determinants of Health.* Geneva, WHO. Available at: http://apps.who.int/iris/bitstream/10665/43943/1/9789241563703_eng.pdf

REFERENCES

Ader, R. (ed.) (2008) *Psychoneuroimmunology* (4th edn). London: Elsevier.

Annandale, E. and Field, D. (2007) Socio-economic inequalities in health, in Taylor, S. and Field, D. (eds) *Sociology of Health and Health Care* (4th edn). Oxford: Blackwell.

Antoni, M.H., Lutgendorf, S.K., Cole, S.K., Dhabhar, F.S., Sephton, S.E., Green, McDonald, P.G., Stefanek, M. and Sood, A.K. (2006) The influence of bio-behavioural factors on tumour biology: pathways and mechanisms, *Nature Reviews: Cancer, 6*(3): 240–8.

ASH (2016) *Action on Smoking and Health*. Available at: www.ash.org.uk

Asthma UK (2016) *Stress and Anxiety*. Available at: www.asthma.org.uk/advice/triggers/stress/

Badawi, O., Waite, M. Fuhrman, S. and Zuckerman, I.H. (2012) Association between intensive care unit-acquired dysglycaemia and in-hospital mortality, *Critical Care Medicine 40*: 3180–8.

Bakker, J., Nijsten, M. and Jansenet, T. (2013) Clinical use of lactate monitoring in critically ill patients, *Annals of Intensive Care, 3*: 12.

Barbee, R., Kline, J. and Watts, J. (2000) Depletion of lactate by dichloroacetate reduces cardiac efficiency after haemorrhagic shock, *Shock, 14*: 208–14.

Bernal, M.E., Varon, J., Acosta, P. and Montagnier, L. (2010) Oxidative stress in critical care medicine, *International Journal of Clinical Practice, 64*(11): 1480–8.

Bone, R.C., Balk, R.A., Cerra, F.B., Dellinger, R.P., Fein, A.M., Knaus, W.A., Schein, R.M. and Sibbald, W.J. (1992) American College of Chest Physicians/Society of Critical Care Medicine consensus conference: definitions for sepsis and organ failure and guidelines for the use of innovative therapies in sepsis, *Critical Care Medicine, 20*(6): 864–74.

Brown, R. (2010) *Prejudice. It's Social Psychology* (2nd edn). Oxford: Wiley-Blackwell.

Butland, B., Jebb, S., Kopelman, P., McPherson, K., Thomas, S., Mardell, J., and Parry, V. (2007) *Foresight. Tackling Obesities: Future Choices. Project Report*. 2nd ed. Government Office for Science. Available at: www.gov.uk/government/uploads/system/uploads/attachment_data/file/287937/07-1184x-tackling-obesities-future-choices-report.pdf

Cancer Research UK (2014a) Available at: https://www.cancerresearchuk.org/about-cancer/breast-cancer

Cancer Research UK (2014b) Available at: www.cancerresearchuk.org/about-cancer/type/prostate-cancer/

Cancer Research UK (2015) Available at: https://www.cancerresearchuk.org/about-cancer/bowel-cancer

Chrousos, G. (2009) Stress and disorders of the stress system, *National Review of Endocrinology, 5*(7): 374–81.

Chrousos, G. and Gold, P. (1992) The concepts of stress and stress system disorders. Overview of physical and behavioural homeostasis, *Journal of the American Medical Association, 267*: 1244–52.

Clayton, M. and McCance, K. (2014) Stress and disease, in McCance, K. and Huether, C. (2014) *Pathophysiology: the Biological Basis for Disease*. St Louis, MO: Elsevier/Mosby.

Cohen, S., Janicki-Deverts, D. and Miller, G.E. (2007) Psychological stress and disease, *Journal of American Medical Association, 298*(14): 1685–7.

Comstedt, P., Storgaard, M. and Lassen, A. (2009) The Systemic Inflammatory Response Syndrome (SIRS) in acutely hospitalised medical patients: a cohort study, *Scandinavian Journal of Trauma, Resuscitation and Emergency Medicine, 17*(67): 1–6.

Darley, J.M. and Gross, P.H. (1983) A hypothesis-confirming bias in labelling effects. *Journal of Personality and Social Psychology, 44*: 20–33.

Department of Health (2011a) *Healthy Lives, Healthy People: a Tobacco Control Plan for England*. HM Government. Available at: www.gov.uk/government/uploads/system/uploads/attachment_data/file/213757/dh_124960.pdf

Department of Health (2011b) *No Health without Mental Health: A Cross-government Mental Health Outcomes Strategy for People of All Ages*. London: Department of Health.

De Sousa, A., Sonavane, S. and Mehta, J. (2012) Psychological aspects of prostate cancer. A clinical review, *Medscape*, *15*(2): 120–7. Available at: www.medscape.com/viewarticle/764044_4

Devine, P.G. (1989) Stereotypes and prejudice: their automatic and controlled components, *Journal of Personality and Social Psychology*, *56*: 5–18.

Drummond, P. and Hewson-Bower, B. (1997) Increased psychosocial stress and decreased mucosal immunity in children with recurrent upper respiratory tract infections, *Journal of Psychosomatic Research*, *43*(3): 271–8.

Duiijts, S.F., Zeegers, M.P. and Bourne, B.V. (2003) The association between stressful life events and breast cancer risk: a meta- analysis, *International Journal of Cancer*, *107*(6): 1023–9.

Duning, T., van den Heuvel, I., Dickmann, A., Volkert, T., Wempe, C., Reinholz, J., Lohmann, H, Freise, H. and Ellger, B. (2010) Hypoglycaemia aggravates critical illness induced neurocognitive dysfunction, *Diabetes Care*, *33*: 634–44.

European Monitoring Centre for Drugs and Drug Addiction (2015) *European Drugs Report: Trends and Developments*. Luxembourg. European Monitoring Centre for Drugs and Drug addiction. Available at: www.emcdda.europa.eu/attachements.cfm/att_239505_EN_TDAT15001ENN.pdf

Galley, H. (2011) Oxidative stress and mitochondrial dysfunction in sepsis, *British Journal of Anaesthesia*, *107*(1): 57–64.

Garvey, F., Wigram, T., Balakumar, T. and Gale, T. (2010) Measuring general hospital staff attitudes towards people with learning disabilities, *Nursing Times*, *106*: 31.

Global Initiative for Chronic Obstructive Lung Disease (GOLD) (2017) *Global Strategy for the Diagnosis, Management and Prevention of Chronic Obstructive Pulmonary Disease*. Available at: https://goldcopd.org/wp-content/uploads/2017/11/GOLD-2018-v6.0-FINAL-revised-20-Nov_WMS.pdf.

Gunnerson, K., Saul, M., He, S. and Kellum, J. (2006) Lactate versus non-lactate metabolic acidosis: a retrospective outcome evaluation of critically ill patients, *Critical Care*, *10*(1): 22.

Health and Social Care Information Centre (2015) *Statistics on Obesity, Physical Activity and Diet*. London: UK Government. Available at: https://digital.nhs.uk/data-and-information/publications/statistical/statistics-on-obesity-physical-activity-and-diet

Health and Safety Executive (2016) *Work Related Stress*. Available at: www.hse.gov.uk/stress/furtheradvice/whatisstress.htm

Huber, K., Gersh, B., Goldstein, P., Granger, C.B. and Armstrong, P.W. (2014) The organisation, functions and outcomes of ST-elevation myocardial infarction networks worldwide: current state, unmet needs and future directions, *European Heart Journal*, *35*: 1526–32.

Intensive Care Society (2009) *Levels of Critical Care for Adult Patients*. London: Intensive Care Society.

Kalogeris, T., Baines, C., Krenz, M. and Korthuis, R. (2012) Cell biology for ischaemia/reperfusion injury, *International Review of Cell Molecular Biology*, *298*: 229–317.

Kaukonen, K-M., Bailey, M., Pilcher, D., Cooper, D.J. and Bellomo, R. (2015) Systemic inflammatory response syndrome criteria in defining severe sepsis, *New England Journal of Medicine*, *372*(17): 1629–38.

Kivimäki, M., Nyberg, S., Batty, G. et al. (2012) Job strain as a risk factor for coronary heart disease: a collaborative meta-analysis of individual participant data, *Lancet, 380*: 1491–7.

Koekkoek, W. and van Zanten, A. (2016) Antioxidant vitamins and trace elements in critical illness *Nutrition in Clinical Practice, 31*(4): 457–74.

Krantz, D.S. and McCeney, M.K. (2002) Effects of psychological and social factors on organic disease: a critical assessment of research on coronary heart disease, *Annual Review of Psychology, 53*: 341–69.

Kristensen, S., Laut, K.G., Fajadet, J. et al. (2014) Reperfusion therapy for ST-elevation acute myocardial infarction 2010/2011: current status in 37 ESC countries, *European Heart Journal, 35*: 1957–70.

Leverve, X. (1999) Energy metabolism in critically ill patients: lactate is a major oxidizable substrate, *Current Opinion Clinical Nutritional Metabolism Care, 2*(2): 165–9.

Lopaschuk, G., Ussher, J. R., Folmes, C.D., Jaswal, J.S. and Stanley, W.C. (2010) Myocardial fatty acid metabolism in health and disease, *Physiology Review, 90*: 207–58.

Lustman, P. and Anderson, R. (2002) Depression in adults with diabetes, *Psychiatric Times, 19*: 1.

Maiden, M. and Chapman, M. (2014) Multiple organ dysfunction syndrome, in Bersten, A. and Soni, I. (2014) *Oh's Intensive Care Manual* (7th edn). Oxford: Butterworth Heinemann/ Elsevier.

Marik, P. (2009) Critical illness corticosteroid insufficiency, *Chest, 135*: 181–93.

Marik, P. (2015) *Evidence Based Critical Care* (3rd edn). Norfolk, VA: Springer.

McCance, K., Grey, T. and Rodway, G. (2014) Altered cellular and tissue biology, in McCance, K. and Huether, C. (2014) *Pathophysiology: The Biological Basis for Disease*. St Louis, MO: Elsevier/Mosby.

McEwen, B.S. (2012) Brain on stress: how the social environment gets under the skin, *Proceedings of the National Academy of Science, 109*(2): 17180–5.

McGriffin, J., Galatzer-Levy, I. and Bonanno, G. (2016) Is the intensive care unit traumatic? What we know and don't know about intensive care and post-traumatic stress responses, *Rehabilitation Psychology, 61*(2): 120–31.

Mehta, A. (2016) Alcoholism and critical illness: a review, *World Journal of Critical Care Medicine, 5*(1) 27–35.

Mencap (2007) *Death by Indifference*. Available at: https://www.mencap.org.uk/sites/default/ files/2016-06/DBIreport.pdf

Montecucco, F., Carbone, F. and Schindler, T. (2016) Pathophysiology of ST-segment elevation myocardial infarction: novel mechanisms and treatments, *European Heart Journal, 37*: 1268–83.

Murray, C., Jennings, R. and Reimer, K. (1986) Preconditioning with ischaemia: a delay of lethal cell injury in ischaemic myocardium, *Circulation, 74*: 1124–36.

National Audit Office (2001) *Tackling Obesity in England*. Available at: www.nao.org.uk/report/ tackling-obesity-in-england/

National Health Service (NHS) (2016). Available at: www.nhs.uk/Livewell/ Childrenwithalearningdisability/Pages/Childrenwithalearningdisabilityhome.aspx

National Institute for Health and Care Excellence (NICE) (2007) *Acutely Ill Patients in Hospital: Recognition of and Response to Acute Illness in Adults in Hospital (NICE Clinical guideline 50)*. London: National Institute of Health and Care Excellence (July).

National Institute for Health and Care Excellence (NICE) (2015) *Smoking: Harm Reduction.* NICE Quality Standard [QS92]. Available at: www.nice.org.uk/guidance/qs92

National Institute of Mental Health (2018) *Chronic Illness and Mental Health.* Available at: https://www.nimh.nih.gov/health/publications/chronic-illness-mental-health/index.shtml#pub2

National Patient Safety Agency (NPSA) (2007) *Safer Care for the Acutely Ill Patient: Learning from Serious incidents.* London: National Patient Safety Agency.

Office for National Statistics (2013) Available at: www.ons.gov.uk/ons/rel/ghs/general-lifestyle-survey/2011/index.html

Park, S., Kim, D., Suh, G., Kang, J.G., Ju, Y.S., Lee, Y.J., Park, J.Y., Lee, S.W. and Jung, K.S. (2012) Mild hypoglycaemia is independently associated with increased risk of mortality in patients with sepsis: a three year retrospective observational study, *Critical Care, 16*: 189.

Public Health Institute. Liverpool John Moores University (2018) *Public Health Reports.* Available at: https://www.ljmu.ac.uk/research/centres-and-institutes/public-health-institute/expertise/drugs

Ramji, D. and Davies, T. (2015) Cytokines in atherosclerosis: key players in all stages of disease and promising therapeutic targets, *Cytokine and Growth Factor Reviews, 26*: 673–85.

Revelly, J.P., Tappy, L., Martinez, A., Bollmann, M., Cayeux, M C., Berger, M.M. and Chioléro, R. L. (2005) Lactate and glucose metabolism in severe sepsis and cardiogenic shock, *Critical Care Medicine, 33*: 2235–40.

Robergs, R., Ghiasvand, F. and Parker, D. (2004) Biochemistry of exercise induced metabolic acidosis, *American Journal of Physiology – Regulatory Integrative and Comparative Physiology, 287*: 502–16

Rosenthal, M. and Moore, F. (2016) Persistent inflammation, immunosuppression, and catabolism: evolution of multiple organ dysfunction, *Surgical Infections, 17*(2): 167–72.

Rote, N., Huether, C. and McCance, K. (2014) Innate immunity: inflammation, in McCance, K. and Huether, C., *Pathophysiology: The Biological Basis for Disease.* St Louis, MO: Elsevier/Mosby.

Royal College of Physicians (2012) National Early Warning Score (NEWS): Standardising the assessment of acute-illness severity in the NHS. London: Royal College of Physicians.

Royal College of Physicians (2017) National Early Warning Score (NEWS)2: Standardising the assessment of acute-illness severity in the NHS. London. Royal College of Physicians.

Singer, M., Deutschman, C.S. and Seymour, C.W. (2016) The third international consensus definitions for sepsis and septic shock (Sepsis-3), *Journal of the American Medical Association, 315*(8): 801–10.

Sinning, J., Scheer, A., Adenauer, V., Ghanem, A., Hammerstingl, C., Schueler, R., Müller, C., Vasa-Nicotera, M., Grube, E., Nickenig, G. and Werner, N. (2012) Systemic inflammatory response syndrome predicts increased mortality in patients after transcatheter aortic valve implantation, *European Heart Journal 33*(12): 1459-68.

Smith, G. and Nielson, M. (1999) ABC of intensive care: criteria for admission, *British Medical Journal, 318*: 1544–5.

Soeters, M. and Soeters, P. (2012) The evolutionary benefit of insulin resistance, *Clinical Nutrition, 31*: 1002–7.

Taskforce of the American College of Critical Care Medicine and Society of Critical Care Medicine. (1999) Guidelines for ICU admission, discharge and triage, *Critical Care Medicine, 27*(3): 633–8.

Theoharides, T. and Cochrane, D. (2004) Critical role of mast cells in inflammatory diseases and the effect of acute stress, *Journal of Neuroimmunology, 146L*: 1–12.

Thompson, N. (2006) *Anti-Discriminatory Practice*. London: Palgrave Macmillan.

Tsigos, C., Kyrou, I., Kassi, E. and Chrousos, G.P. (2016) Stress, endocrine physiology and pathophysiology. www.ncbi.nlm.nih.gov/pubmed/25905226/

Turner, M., Nedjai, B., Hurst, T. and Pennington, D. (2014) Cytokines and chemokines: at the crossroads of cell signalling and inflammatory disease, *Biochimica et Biophysica Acta*, 2563–82.

Urb, M. and Sheppard, D. (2012. The role of mast cells in the defence against pathogens, *PLoS Pathogens, 8*(4):, e1002619.

Vespa, P., McArthur, D., Stein, N., Huang, S., Shao, W., Filippou, M., Etchepare, M., Glenn, T. and Hovda, D.A. (2012) Tight glycaemic control increases metabolic distress in traumatic brain injury: a randomised controlled within-subjects trial. *Critical Care Medicine, 40*: 1923–9.

Welshman, J. and Walmsley, J. (eds) (2006) *Community Care in Perspective: Care, Control and Citizenship*. Basingstoke: Palgrave Macmillan.

World Health Organization (2017) Chronic obstructive pulmonary disease (COPD). Available at: http://www.who.int/news-room/fact-sheets/detail/chronic-obstructive-pulmonary-disease-(copd)

Yellon, D. and Hausenloy, D. (2007) Myocardial reperfusion injury, *New England Journal of Medicine, 357*: 1121–35.

Zweier, J. and Talukder, M. (2006) The role of oxidants and free radicals in reperfusion injury, *Cardiovascular Research, 70*(2): 181–90.

CHAPTER 3

Respiratory Failure

Case Studies: Anna and David

SARA J. WHITE AND FLEUR LOWE

───── CHAPTER AIMS ═══════════════ 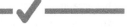 ──────

1 To understand how culture, cultural norms and cultural reasoning may affect critical illness and associated recovery.
2 To discuss the effects of isolation on the critical care patient, family and nurse.

INTRODUCTION

As highlighted in Chapter 1 the knowledge and skills required to provide competent, effective, evidence based care for patients with multiple conditions and the capability to interpret the clinical situation in order that the care offered is the best, is vital for critical care nurses. As such, the ability to have clinical decision making skills needed in respiratory care requires a sound knowledge base of respiratory anatomy, physiology, pathophysiology and pharmacology and it is assumed that those reading this chapter have that knowledge. Consequently the authors of this chapter appreciate the expertise of nurses who independently evaluate a patient's condition and make decisions about how to plan, implement and evaluate care. Therefore for this chapter we have chosen two case studies to focus upon and link the humanising health care dimensions to, and you may wish to refresh your memory regarding this by revisiting Chapter 1. The first case is of Anna; a 76-year-old lady with a history of chronic respiratory problems where we shall speak of culture, sepsis and delirium. The second is of David; a 45-year-old gentleman with a short history of acute respiratory failure (see Bite Size Knowledge 1: Type I & Type II Respiratory Failure) and here we shall focus upon perceptions of critical illness and isolation. Whilst, as you read the case studies, other co-morbidities will be evident (such as Acute Kidney Injury which will be explored in subsequent chapters) the focus of this chapter is culture, sepsis, delirium and isolation and throughout we offer ideas for discussion and staff development.

BITE SIZE KNOWLEDGE 3.1

Type I & Type II Respiratory Failure

Respiratory failure is a syndrome in which the pulmonary system fails in one or both of its gas exchange functions. In practice, it is classified as either hypoxaemic (type I) or hypercapnic (type II).

Type I hypoxaemic respiratory failure is characterised by an arterial oxygen tension (PaO_2) lower than 60 mm Hg with a normal or low arterial carbon dioxide tension ($PaCO_2$). Common aetiologies include cardiogenic or non-cardiogenic pulmonary oedema, pneumonia, and pulmonary haemorrhage. It is the most common form of respiratory failure. However, the distinction between acute and chronic hypoxaemic respiratory failure cannot be readily made on the basis of arterial blood gases, whereas the clinical markers of chronic hypoxemia, such as polycythaemia or cor-pulmonale, suggest a longstanding disorder.

Type II hypercapnic respiratory failure is characterised by a high $PaCO_2$ and hypoxemia. The pH level depends on the bicarbonate level, which, in turn, is dependent on the duration of hypercapnia. Common aetiologies include severe airway disorders such as asthma, chronic obstructive pulmonary disease and neuromuscular disease. Acute hypercapnic respiratory failure develops over a very short period (minutes to hours) and tends to have a pH of less than 7.3. Chronic respiratory failure develops over a longer period such as several days which allows time for renal compensation and an increase in bicarbonate concentration resulting in a slightly decreased pH level.

Hypoxemia is the major immediate threat to organ function and needs correcting immediately together with stabilising haemodynamic status. The underlying pathophysiology and causes of the respiratory failure need exploring and the specific treatment tailored accordingly (McChance and Huether, 2010).

CASE STUDY 3.1: ANNA

This case study is about Anna and whilst the co-morbidities of Anna are acknowledged the focus of this case study is on culture, communication, stereotyping and barriers to care delivery. Anna is a 76-year-old lady who moved to England from Eastern Europe in late February. In her culture Anna was the matriarch. Her family told how normally her English was broken but understandable. She lives with her grandson and two lodgers. Normally she is independent. However, because of a fractured humerus a package of care was developed to help her with washing, dressing, breakfast and lunch while her family members are working. Her past medical history (PMH) and medications are shown in Box 3.1 below.

In March Anna was found on the floor at home by her son. She was admitted to hospital with acute confusion. Her son stated that she was not normally confused. The initial diagnosis was sepsis from a Chest Infection and a Urinary Tract Infection (see Tables 3.1 and 3.2) and therefore she was commenced on the Sepsis pathway (see Bite Size Knowledge 3.2: Sepsis) and given analgesia, IV fluids, oxygen, and antibiotics.

BOX 3.1

Anna's Past Medical History and Medications

Past medical history
- asthma
- agoraphobia
- paranoid schizophrenia
- essential hypertension
- type 2 diabetes mellitus
- retinopathy
- breast cancer
- stage 3 cardiovascular disease
- hiatus hernia
- recent fracture of humerus.

Medications
- omeprazole
- ramipril
- metformin
- chlorpromazine
- procyclidine
- ramitidine
- quinine
- seretide
- salbutamol.

Table 3.1 Anna's blood results

	Day 1	Day 3
Na (Sodium)	127	130 mmol/L
K+ (Potassium)	4.5	3.5 mmol/L
Urea	10.2	14.4 mmol/L
Creatinine	196	174 mmol/L
eGFR (Estimated glomerular filtration rate)	22	26
CRP (C-reactive protein)	317	297 mg/L
Lactate	1 mmol/L	
WBC (White blood count)	14.7	11.2 10^9/L

(Continued)

Table 3.1 (Continued)

	Day 1	Day 3
Neutrophils	12.9 10⁹/L	9.3 10⁹/L
Hb (Haemoglobin)	9.2 g/dL	8.8 g/dL
CK (Creatine kinase)	456 U/L	456 U/L
INR (International normalised ratio)	1.2	
APTT (Activated partial thromboplastin time)	1 secs	
Glucose	13.8	

Table 3.2 Anna's observations

	Day 1	Day 1	Day 1	Day 1	Day 1	Day 1	Day 2	Day 3	Days 4&5
Time	09:35	09:56	10:21	13:14	18:35	23:30	08:00	06:00	08:30
BP	174/140	167/90	163/83	166/83	126/63	150/60	150/76	152/99	160/92
Pulse	122 (r)	120	119	113	114	89	105	106	88
Temp	39.2	40.1	-	36.9	37	36.9	36.8	36.5	36.4
Resp	36	44	34	36	40	32	27	30	34
O₂ sats	93%	97%	94%	92%	96%	96%	100%	92%	94%
GCS	15	14							
BG	16.9	13.2		20.9	25.1	25	22.9		
O₂	air	15L Venturi	15L Venturi	15L Venturi	15L Venturi	60% Humidi	60% Humidi	60% Humidi	60% Humidi
Pain	3/10								

 BITE SIZE KNOWLEDGE 3.2

Sepsis

Sepsis, also referred to as blood poisoning or septicaemia, is a potentially life-threatening condition triggered by an infection or injury. Sepsis Six is the name given to a bundle of medical therapies designed to reduce the mortality of patients with sepsis. It consists of three diagnostic and three therapeutic steps, all to be delivered within one hour of the initial diagnosis of sepsis.

1 titrate oxygen to a saturation target of 94%
2 take blood cultures

3 administer empiric intravenous antibiotics
4 measure serum lactate and send full blood count
5 start intravenous fluid resuscitation
6 commence accurate urine output measurement.

(See the NICE guidelines 2016: www.nice.org.uk/guidance/NG51/chapter/recommendations)

Anna was admitted to a side room on an oncology ward because there were no medical beds available. Here she was reassessed by the medical Foundation doctor (F1) at 10.21, the medical registrar at 10.40 and by the consultant at 13.57. The assessments concurred with the initial diagnosis and due to her PMH a poor recovery was expected.

On **Day 2** Anna remained unstable and confused. Her chest X-Ray (CXR) showed worsening consolidation. During the night she pulled out her urethral catheter and persistently tried to get out of bed. Anna's Metformin, used to manage her diabetes, was stopped on admission because her Glomerular Filtration Rate (GFR) was 22; however, her glycated haemoglobin (Hba1c) was 56 so blood sugar control was managed with 10 iu of Lantus. Anna's resuscitation status was discussed with her son, and because he felt that normally Anna was healthy and independent, he wanted full treatment. Anna was more receptive of immediate care being offered by her son and grandson.

During **Days 3, 4 and 5** Anna was regularly seen by the Critical Care Outreach Team (CCOT). They noted that she had pulled another catheter out; that she had crackles throughout her chest and that air entry to her right base was reduced; as this indicated Pulmonary Oedema she was given Frusemide. Oxygen was required to maintain adequate saturation levels but as Anna was very unsettled and confused she was non-compliant with it. Tirelessly she tried to climb out of bed. CCOT noted that she had not had her bowels open for at least four days.

On **Day 6** Anna's consultant felt that because of her continuing low oxygen saturations (88%), left apex expiratory wheeze, quiet lung bases, weak intermittent cough and irregular blood sugars, she had clinically deteriorated. Anna's confusion continued and she had pulled out the third urethral catheter. Consequently questions were raised regarding withdrawing active treatment. However on **Day 7,** whilst the CXR still showed left sided consolidation and a right pleural effusion possibly due to fluid overload, Anna was alert and talking in full sentences. She had her bowels open in the night and her third urethral catheter was draining well (it was removed on **Day 9**). Her son and grandson conversed with her to note that she had been trying to get out of bed because she needed the toilet and did not want to soil the bed.

Between **Days 8 and 14,** with physiotherapist input, Anna mobilised well. Her grandson assisted her with a shower on **Day 13**. Whilst she remained hypertensive, Acute Kidney

Injury was evident (Urea averaged at 16.3 and Creatinine at 206) and her air entry remained reduced in the right base, she was using her inhalers well and her fluid balance and blood sugars remained stable.

Anna continued to make progress despite oral Candida being diagnosed and on **Day 18** she was moved to a medical ward and discharged home on **Day 20.**

DISCUSSION OF ANNA'S CASE STUDY

Anna's case study contains several physical and psychological issues; she had pneumonia, a urinary tract infection and constipation and was being managed as a 'medical outlier' in a side room on an oncology ward. So linking back to Chapters 1 and 2, consider patient-centred care, the humanising framework and what triggers may have led to her critical illness and consider what her needs and issues are.

We would suggest that her psychological needs were not met because her confusion and agitation were deemed to be due to her septic state and worsening condition rather than the fact that she was in a foreign country with a different culture, that English was not her first language and no one conversed with her to determine what her needs were. The family dynamics were alien to the ward staff and the fact that intimate immediate care was being given by male family members made the female ward staff uncomfortable.

So let us first address Anna's asthma which was exacerbated by a chest infection. Patients with asthma experience exacerbations during the natural course of their disease, requiring a visit to the primary care physician, emergency department or/and hospital admission. The standard of care for acute exacerbation management includes provision of supplemental oxygen, mechanical ventilation, short-acting inhaled bronchodilators, systemic corticosteroids and antibiotics. The overlap of asthma and Chronic Obstructive Airways Disease (COPD) in older patients is an important clinical consideration and multiple exacerbations tend to lead to patients being classified as COPD (Kim and Rhee, 2010; Irwin and Rippe, 2012; Schive et al., 2013; Pierson, 2013; Dixit et al., 2015). Anna's full medical history was not in the UK so information was obtained from her family. The medical staff explored whether Anna should be resuscitated if the need arose and whether treatment should continue. Williams (1989), who reviewed psychosocial literature on COPD, highlighted that many of the quality of life instruments and disability measures used by medical staff were inadequate. Accordingly the involvement of family members who knew Anna the best was of paramount importance and consequently full medical treatment and interventions as guided by British Thoracic Society (2016) were upheld.

So let us now address the issue of Anna's psychosocial care and culture. Anna had removed several urethral catheters, was trying to get out of bed to go to the toilet and was not complying with treatments such as oxygen. Staff appeared to consider that the confusion was due to her complicated past medical history and her present sepsis and we are sure that some of this is true because as we know sepsis can cause acute confusion, delirium (see Bite Size Knowledge 3: Delirium) and agitation (Nervenarzt, 2011; Tsuruta and Oda, 2016). But Anna's situation was more complicated, because she was new to living in the UK, was not conversant with the language or culture of the organisation and, when her family members tried to help her with intimate care, the ward staff were unhappy. Consequently let us explore the apparent lack of conversing with Anna.

BITE SIZE KNOWLEDGE 3.3

Acute Delirium

Delirium, from the Latin *delirare* meaning 'to swerve off the path', is a common, complex clinical syndrome characterised by disturbed consciousness and cognitive function or perception. It has an acute onset and fluctuating course and is associated with poor outcomes if not diagnosed and treated early.

The pathophysiology of delirium is not completely understood. Research suggests it is due to a neurotransmitter abnormality with cholinergic deficiency that affects multiple spheres of the central nervous system (Hsieh et al., 2013; Elie et al., 2001; Meagher et al., 2000). There are multiple causes and predisposing factors and it is the most common mental health issue found in the general hospital setting with reports of up to 80% in critically ill patients. Mortality ranges between 22% and 76%, with the elderly more prone (Miller, 2008).

Delirium can be misdiagnosed as dementia or depression, as some symptoms can overlap and all three syndromes can coexist. Successful management relies on daily assessment using a validated screening tool and a combination of prevention techniques and early treatment.

(See: NICE guideline 2010: https://www.nice.org.uk/guidance/cg103)

As highlighted Anna pulled out several urethral catheters and was persistently trying to get out of bed. Whilst her confusion could have been due to a pathophysiological issue (such as a low sodium level) Anna's behaviour was associated with her being acutely confused due to her underlying diagnosis, but in fact she was trying to go to the toilet and save the embarrassment of soiling the bed. There was a mismatch of communication here. Staff had made assumptions that her behaviour was because she was confused, informed the family accordingly and adopted a parent-like state (see Bite Size Knowledge 3.4: Transactional analysis). However, Anna needed to pass urine and have her bowels open but due to her illness could not recall the English words to ask for assistance to go to the toilet, so she attempted to go alone as one would expect an adult to do normally and not revert to the childlike behaviour of asking permission. Indeed lack of communication in health care creates situations where errors can occur, and errors caused by a failure to communicate and/or misinterpretation of needs are a persistent problem in today's healthcare organisations. One could suggest that staff had not been respectful in ensuring a positive adult to adult relationship with Anna where she understood the necessity of having a staff member present when she went out to the toilet. Unfortunately complaints about poor communication are one of the top three reasons for hospital complaints investigated by the Ombudsman Service. Another common reason is staff attitude (Parliamentary and Health Service Ombudsman, 2014) and there is also a history regarding how the nursing profession, which has claimed that they offer holistic care in fact fails to do so as gaps in holistic patient care are evident because staff focus on physical illness and treatment only (Drury and Hunter, 2016). There is a wealth of research that clearly indicates there are strong positive relationships between a healthcare team member's communication skills and a patient's capacity to follow through with medical recommendations. The Institute for Health Care Communication (2011) discuss how the core elements of good communication lead to patient satisfaction and highlight the need for person- and family-centred care (see Chapter 1). Partnerships between healthcare practitioners and patients where the preferences of the individual are honoured are key to person- and family-centred care. Putting the patient, and the family, at the heart of every decision and the building of a therapeutic relationship (O'Connell, 2008) by empowering them to be genuine partners in their care are vital in offering empathetic and compassionate care, and this could have been offered to Anna, yet one could suggest that this did not always occur and consequently suboptimal care (McQuillan et al., 1998) due to a lack of cultural understanding occurred.

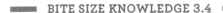 **BITE SIZE KNOWLEDGE 3.4**

Transactional analysis

The psychiatrist Eric Berne developed transactional analysis (TA) on the principle that individuals communicate from one of three parts (or ego-states) of our personality, these being based on work by Sigmund Freud, and are:

- 'Taught' ego-states (parent state), which are a set of thoughts, feelings and behaviours we have learnt from our parents or other significant people and which have two stages: nurturing and controlling.
- 'Thought' ego-states (adult state) tend to be the most rational part of our personality and relate to the here and now.
- 'Felt' ego-states (child state) which are learnt from childhood and have three stages: the spontaneous and playful 'natural child'; the curious and exploring child and the adaptive or fitting in or rebelling child.

Freud suggested that adults choose which state to communicate from and a transaction will succeed when we respond to others from the state expected, e.g. from the same level or from critical parent to adaptive child (Stewart and Joines, 2012).

Transactional analysis has a supportive base which is non-judgemental, secure and respectful and is a powerful tool which healthcare providers can use to give themselves more options when conversing and responding to patient needs and ensuring that a positive relationship is forged.

CULTURE, CULTURAL NORMS AND CULTURAL REASONING

Let us now discuss the apparent lack of understanding of culture, cultural norms and cultural reasoning, and how this may have led to Anna being labelled 'confused', which in turn may have hindered her recovery (see Bite Size Knowledge 3.5: Culture).

BITE SIZE KNOWLEDGE 3.5

Culture

The origins of the word 'culture' derive from the Latin 'colere', which means to tend to the earth and grow, or cultivation and nurture.

Culture is the characteristics and knowledge of a particular group of people. It is defined by the shared patterns of behaviours and interactions and group identity which are fostered by learned socialisation and social patterns unique to the group; experience, beliefs, values, attitudes, meanings, hierarchies, religion, notions of time, roles, spatial relations, concepts of the universe, and material objects, arts, music, cuisine and possessions acquired by a group of people. This occurs over the course of generations through individual and group striving and a cumulative deposit of knowledge.

No doubt you have heard of terms such as Western culture, Eastern culture, Latin culture, Middle Eastern culture, African culture etc., but many countries in the interconnected world of the twenty-first century have multiple cultures, which are in themselves constantly changing and developing. However the history of specific cultures should not be forgotten, as they are riddled with conflicts of religion, ethnicity, ethical beliefs etc. Consequently the fluidity of culture makes it difficult to define in any one way.

There are many dimensions of culture and cultural variations that are associated with disease and illness. These include socioeconomic, environmental, dietary, behavioural and genetic variations such as sickle-cell anaemia, occurrences of diseases such as coronary artery disease, chronic rheumatic disease, hypertension, obesity, cancers, liver cirrhosis.

In simple terms culture is a word for people's genetic history and their way of life. Different cultural groups think, feel, and act differently and the position that the ideas, meanings, beliefs and values people learn as members of society determines human nature. This uniqueness of a human and their complex whole is what nurses need to recognise as they practice. They should not be ethnocentric and believe that their own culture is superior to that of others.

We know that healthcare providers are socialised into the culture of their profession and that this professional socialisation occurs as they enter into the work environment. For many this is as a non-qualified healthcare provider, such as a healthcare support worker or apprentice, and for others it is as they enter studentship for their chosen profession. Dinmohammadi et al. (2013) feel that professional socialisation teaches a set of beliefs and practices, norms, habits, rituals and each has its own language, which is quickly adopted by those new to the profession. Moving from the complexities of understanding oneself to understanding others is also part of education. Naturally we try to simplify things by looking for similarities and ignoring differences and as such we oversimplify people, which links back to previous discussions on stereotyping. Cultural identity (Higgs and Jones, 2000) is often underpinned by physical appearance, dress and distinctive customs. Yet when an ill person enters a hospital they are often stripped of this identity as the professionals work to cure the illness. In this inherent desire to help a person regain their health, professionals are caught up in the pressures of their work, the need to make quick decisions and clinical judgements and, as a result, the cultural identity of the individual is often forgotten.

Cultural shock can be applied to Anna's situation. Cultural shock was a term first used by Oberg in 1960. He spoke about people's attempts to adapt to a new culture and whilst there has been much debate over his work (e.g. see Ward et al., 2001, who use the term cultural distance), the term cultural shock is a useful one to help us consider how Anna might have been feeling and how the staff may have felt. Cultural shock means that when an individual (i.e. Anna) enters another's culture (i.e. the hospital ward) a different understanding and interpretation of situations happen and thus confusion and frustration transpire. Different reactions to the ones expected by those native to the situation also occur. For the native to the culture (i.e. the nursing staff) they may not understand why the one encountering the new culture (Anna) is responding, or not responding, in such a way. Fundamental to the care of Anna there was a lack of understanding of her as a person and an associated breakdown in communication between Anna, her family and the nurses. Communication difficulties and their impact on care have been readily explored (see above) by authors such as Helman, 2007 and MacLachlan, 2006 who have shown that cultural differences in intercultural interactions have the potential to cause confusion and dissatisfaction both for the patient and the healthcare provider.

It is not uncommon for nurses to interpret the 'medical language', treatments and associated care for patients and families, but an appreciation of the cultural construct from Anna's perspective was important. Nurses are the ones whose presence with the patient is most constant. However, the provision of patient and family attentiveness can be challenging and psychologically and emotionally demanding. As such, many nurses cope by distancing themselves from the patient and family and just perform that which is necessary for safe patient care, as they involve themselves in the flurry of activity on the rest of the ward. If staff appreciated that some of Anna's confusion was not because of her illness but related to a lack of understanding of the English language being used, and that routine and rituals are used by all to establish a sense of comfort, they might have foreseen that the strange environment of the noisy, brightly lit hospital environment disrupted Anna's normal circadian rhythms and that her comfort was breached. Whilst comfort measures may seem ordinary, when compared to life saving treatments, for humans comfort is vital to wellbeing as is establishing trust, rapport and reassurance (O'Connell, 2008).

Strategies could have been put in place to minimise the confusion (see Table 3.3: Humanising health care for Anna). Cultural awareness, knowledge acquisition and knowledge about her culture which are critical elements of effective clinical reasoning might have enabled staff to take the time to recognise Anna as the family matriarch. As such, her son and grandson offering intimate care was deemed an honour for them and an expectation by Anna. Barriers between staff and Anna as a person may not have occurred.

Therefore now let us consider another important element of care delivery. It is important to recognise the impact of the advances in medicine, pharmacology and technology that have led to a greater chance of recovery from critical illness. Undoubtedly 30 years ago Anna's PMH and admission presentation would have led to her death; however with early detection and advances in treatments the prospect of recovery is greatly improved. It was recognised that Anna had sepsis and she was appropriately commenced on treatments as outlined in the Sepsis pathway (National Institute for Health and Care Excellence [NICE] 2016).

Early recognition and treatments were key to the development of Intensive Care units in the early 1960s, albeit that development of critical services and prioritisation started with Florence Nightingale (1850s) and the use of St. Jorgens Hospital in Copenhagen in 1952 to care for acutely unwell individuals with leprosy who were dying of respiratory failure. In the UK recognising and responding to deterioration was prominent in the 1990s, and the Department of Health commissioned a review of critical care services which led to the Comprehensive Critical Care (2000) document. This detailed the creation of 'Outreach teams' to provide and support the care of sick patients on the ward, i.e. 'critical care without walls' (Hillman, 2002), which was a concept whereby intensive care staff (intensivists and nurses) offered their help and expertise to those who were acutely unwell on the general wards, which in turn led to the development of CCOT. The expert CCOT nurses are not only skilled regarding knowing how and what to do and 'knowing how and when to respond' (Benner et al., 1999: 498), but have practical wisdom and the ability to recognise ever-changing conditions and interpret and forecast them. They work closely with members of the multi-disciplinary team to pool together clinical perspectives to enhance patient care.

Table 3.3 Humanising health care for Anna

Humanising dimensions	Bio-psychosocial triggers	Managing stressors and coping strategies	Role of expert nurse in support strategies
Insiderness/ objectification	Anna is new to the UK. She is a matriarch in her culture. She has a complex PMH and associated medications. Recently a package of care has been initiated. During the acute stage of her ill health she is dependent on staff.	Anna's son and grandson are helping her adjust to UK living. They help with intimate care needs and when not present staff need to help Anna.	Enable connectedness by helping staff to understand that it is therapeutic for Anna's son and grandson to undertake ALD's with/for Anna. Encourage staff to question their own understanding of culture. Enable staff to reflect on social norms and roles and treating patients as an individual.
Agency/passivity	Anna is confused at present and she has reverted to her native tongue and view of the world.	Anna needs help, in her native tongue, to understand what is occurring and what is expected and to make choices if she is to overcome this ill health.	Ensure staff have an evidence based rationale for care. Ask family to write down key words and phrases in Anna's native tongue and English to enable communications Use a picture point.
Uniqueness/ homogenisation	Due to her present view of the world Anna is unsure of her surroundings, what staff are saying and what is expected of her.	Anna wants to go to the toilet. She does not understand the urethral catheter and the need to call the nurse before mobilising. She needs intimate care.	Ensure staff do not belittle Anna by assuming confusion rather than lack of understanding. Enable staff to understand Anna's uniqueness and what is occurring. Involve Anna's family as much as possible. Encourage reflection on cross-cultural practitioner–client communications.
Togetherness/ isolation	Family are important to Anna and her grandson and son help her. She is adjusting to living in the UK and culture.	Anna is an outlier on an oncology ward and therefore viewed as a problem. Anna's son and grandson help her with personal needs and staff feel this is inappropriate. When Anna's family are not present she is isolated.	Support staff to recognise that spending time with Anna and using comprehensive communication strategies will enhance recovery. Encourage staff and family to help Anna maintain contact with the outside world and everyday occurrences.
Sense making/ loss of meaning	Anna is confused as people are speaking to her in her second language and explanations are not making sense.	Explanations should regularly be given in her native tongue.	Enable staff to appreciate what is causing fear and anxiety for Anna.

Humanising dimensions	Bio-psychosocial triggers	Managing stressors and coping strategies	Role of expert nurse in support strategies
			Ensure staff have a rationale for the care and use multiple strategies to empower Anna's understanding and being active in her recovery; for example - optimise position to aid lung function - work with physio and OT - strict fluid balance - set goals for oral fluid and nutrition - set goals in relation to her regaining control of her activities of daily living.
Personal journey/ loss of personal journey	Normally independent, having a package of care was intrusive for Anna. She is unsure of time and place due to her present ill-health. She is concerned about soiling herself but understanding how complex going out to the toilet is challenging.	Anna needs a thorough regular explanation of what is occurring to her and how she can help have a safe and quick recovery. She needs help to understand what is occurring and what will occur tomorrow, next week and in the future.	Enable staff to ensure Anna understands: - necessary anatomy and physiology - sepsis - monitoring of fluid status, hypoxia etc. - health care and treatment.
Sense of place/ dislocation	The strangeness of the location is upsetting Anna. She does not know the ward routine or what is occurring to her.	Anna needs explanations given in her native tongue so she can feel safe and secure.	Involve Anna's family in creating an environment that reminds her of home, with essential words and phrases written in her native language and English. Ensure staff have a sound evidence base regarding recovery from sepsis to enable short- and long-term goal setting.
Embodiment/ reductionist body	Anna is anxious because staff do not understand what she wants and who she is.	Anna needs staff to understand her needs and wants and associated culture.	Ensure staff allow Anna to make choices. Ensure staff have a good working knowledge of support structures that Anna uses and can access. Assist staff to understand culture and enable them to gain cultural awareness. Challenge ethnocentricity.

Anna was seen by CCOT nurses many times during her stay and appropriate treatments were offered although they were not caring for her as attentively as ward nurses. Yet there were issues with Anna being in a side room on an oncology ward rather than a specialist medical ward. Although many patients have co-morbidity and, as such, nurses should have knowledge about conditions other than their own speciality, there is no doubt the perception that, as an 'outlier', Anna did not belong on the ward and consequently she may have received suboptimal care delivery. McQuillan et al. (1998) highlighted that suboptimal care implied a lack of knowledge and this tended to relate to the significance of clinical findings involving dysfunction of airway, breathing and circulation. Quirke et al. (2011: 183) also explored the concept of suboptimal care and showed that those who were acutely ill on wards deteriorated because the 'abnormal vital signs are either not recognised or are treated inappropriately; that there are delays in diagnosis, treatment or referral, poor assessment and inadequate or inappropriate patient management'. It appears the nurses were attributing Anna's confusion and anxiety to her chest infection and UTI rather than other physiological conditions or her lack of understanding of what was occurring. Possibly they did not appreciate the effects that issues such as low sodium and constipation were having. Maybe they had negative perceptions of ageing based on their own societal upbringing, whereas the son and grandson had different perceptions of ageing and had a better understanding of her physical and mental integrity and health status. Maybe the medical staff had 'sown do not resuscitate seeds' and this in turn had led to suboptimal care delivery. Who knows? However, what we do know is that Anna's care was not humanised. Clinical decision making skills when caring for Anna involved thinking wider than the diagnosis, as she had complex health needs. Anna was vulnerable and the trust in the healthcare provision was diminished because of the language barrier. But healthcare providers have obligations of beneficence as the fiduciary relationship (based on a trust) between nurse, patient and family, which is based on dependence, reliance and trust, is established. Good clinical judgement is based on clear communication between healthcare providers and this requires willingness to listen, trust and have mutual respect, but one questions if this occurred. The power of this case study points to the multiple skills needed to care for this complex lady and the extended skills of the expert nurse who can view her holistically with significant attention being paid to her cultural needs and dynamics and connected wellbeing.

SUMMARY OF ANNA'S CASE STUDY

This case study has shown how the power of language and cultural understanding can have significant effects on the patient journey and recovery. It has highlighted how Anna's care was not always humanised and how staff needed to recognise the benefits of working with Anna and the family.

FACILITATING LEARNING

1 The Institute for Health Care Communication (2011) discuss how the core elements of good communication lead to patient satisfaction. Do you know what core elements are?

   Exercise: Use 'The Communication Quiz' (www.mindtools.com/pages/article/ newCS_99.htm) to assess.

2 Communication in health care is still a persistent problem. Facilitate a discussion regarding why this might be and how it can be prevented. Use transactional analysis to explore examples from practice.

3 What strategies could be used to enable communication with non-English-speaking patients?

4 What is your understanding of culture? What is ethnocentricity?

5 How is chest assessment undertaken?

6 What wheezes may occur for those with Pulmonary Oedema; those with Bronchospasm; those with sputum?

7 What is the difference between Acute Kidney Injury and Chronic Kidney Disease and what does the GFR rate tell us?

CASE STUDY 3.2: DAVID

This case study is about David, a 45-year-old man. David has no past medical history, does not normally take any medications, has never smoked or taken illicit drugs, drinks no more than 10 units of alcohol per week, weighs 100kg, is 1.829 metres tall and normally enjoys excellent fitness. He has not travelled abroad recently. His wife and two children, whom he dotes on, are also fit and well. David successfully built up his own business, which he recently sold and he was planning a new venture.

David was admitted to the Acute Medical Unit (AMU) via the Emergency Department (ED) during the evening. He presented with a 2-week history of progressive shortness of breath (SOB) following flu-like illness with myalgia, coryzal symptoms and night sweats. His shortness of breath led to him visiting his GP who commenced him on a Salbutamol inhaler. Four days prior to admission he saw his GP again who commenced him on a course of Amoxicillin. However there was no improvement and he had SOB upon minimal exertion and climbing stairs; consequently he attended the local walk in clinic who advised him to attend the ED.

On admission he was examined by a Foundation year 2 doctor who used the ABCDE assessment process (see Table 3.4: ABCDE Assessment of David and Table 3.5: David's Blood results).

Table 3.4   ABCDE Assessment of David

Airway:

- patent.

Breathing:

- respiratory rate 20
- talking in full sentences
- SpO_2 85% on air
- peak expiratory flow 260 L/min
- dull percussion note both lower lobes
- coarse crackles and reduced air entry to left mid and lower lung zones and right base
- producing green sputum
- SpO_2 increased to 93% on 15 litres O_2 via non-rebreath mask.

Cardiovascular:

- pale, sweaty and clammy. T-shirt soaked
- heart rate 102/min, regular and strong
- blood pressure 139/98
- temperature 37.1
- moist oral mucosa
- urine output >0.5ml/kg/hr (Urea and Creatinine levels normal)
- arterial blood gas (ABG) on 15L O_2 shows: pH 7.42, pCO_2 4.9 kPa, pO_2 10.2 kPa, HCO_3 24.6 mmol/L, lactate 0.7 mmol/L.

Disability:

- Glasgow Coma Score 15/15
- retrosternal chest pain on coughing only
- blood sugar 6.3 mmol/L
- pupils equal and reactive to light.

Exposure:

- no peripheral oedema
- no calf swelling
- no rashes
- abdomen soft, non-tender, no organomegaly.

Electrocardiogram: sinus tachycardia.

Chest x-ray: patchy consolidation in the left lower zone.

Blood results **(Table 3.5)** showed raised inflammatory markers, reduced platelets and deranged liver function tests. Blood cultures and sputum culture taken.

Atypical antigen screen including H1N1 flu swabs, hepatitis B & C and HIV screen – NAD.

Table 3.5 David's Blood results

	Day 1	Day 3	Day 4
Na	137	136	138 mmol/L
K+	4.3	4.4	4.5 mmol/L
Urea	6.3	5.1	6.3 mmol/L
Creatinine	90	69	87 mmol/L
eGFR	87	>120	90
CRP	67	31	20 mg/L
Lactate	1.1	1.4	0.7 mmol/L
WBC	12.5	9.8	10.7 10⁹/L
Neutrophils	9.4	7.7	8.1
Hb (Haemoglobin)	140	139	143 10⁹/L
Plt (Platelets)	427	407	412
GGT (Gamma-glutamyltransferase)	272 IU/L		
ALT (Alanine aminotransferase)	145 IU/L		
ALP (Alkaline phosphatase)	135 IU/L		
Billirubin	11 mmol/L		

David was given a provisional diagnosis of community acquired pneumonia (CAP). The sepsis screening tool identified that he had a moderate to high risk of sepsis and he was commenced on the Sepsis 6 pathway (see: Bite Size Knowledge 3.2: Sepsis). He was prescribed and given co-amoxiclav and clarithromycin antibiotics as per hospital policy for CAP. Intravenous 0.9% saline administration began and he was encouraged to drink plenty.

Following initial treatment he was transferred to the AMU into a bay with five other patients. The CCOT were alerted. Later that night David was reviewed by the Intensive Care Unit (ICU) Specialist Registrar who prescribed Tamiflu (an antiviral medicine for treatment of flu). David was moved to a side room.

Early afternoon on **Day 2** a repeat ABG showed worsening type 1 respiratory failure with a PaO$_2$ of 8.22 kPa, although it is noted that David briefly removed his oxygen to eat just prior to the sampling. The ICU consultant reviewed him and decided that he did not require high flow nasal oxygen at this stage. However if he deteriorated further this therapy would be appropriate. He was encouraged to keep the oxygen mask on and he had a relatively settled night.

Midday on **Day 3** a repeat ABG showed a PaO$_2$ of 9.9 kPa which CCOT discussed with the medical consultant, as a pulmonary embolus could not be ruled out. A repeat chest x-ray showed no further change. The medical consultant reviewed him and for patient safety prescribed Dalteparin (a low molecular weight heparin/anti-coagulant). A subsequent Computed Tomographic Pulmonary Angiography (CTPA) showed extensive left sided consolidation but no visible clot.

On **Day 4** David told CCOT that he had had a restless night and admitted to feeling very anxious about his illness and the lack of improvement. He continued to need high flow oxygen via a non-rebreath mask, although he was coping with having saline nebulisers driven with 6L oxygen for short periods (oxygen saturations dropping to 91%). Later that day he weaned to 98% oxygen via a humidified system.

Over the **next 5 days** he gradually improved, enabling the oxygen to be weaned. No causative organism was identified and he was moved out of the side room. He was eventually discharged home with a two-week course of clarithromycin to cover mycoplasma pneumoniae. He was asked to have a CXR and follow up appointment in outpatients in two weeks.

DISCUSSION OF DAVID'S CASE STUDY

There are discussion points here relating to community acquired pneumonia and causes of mycoplasma pneumoniae and associated treatment such as NIV, and high flow nasal oxygen. You may also like to link David's case study to the humanising dimensions explored in Chapter 1. The discussion here however focuses on perceptions of critical illness and isolation.

At 45 David considered himself to be young and healthy. He believed that pneumonia was an illness that affected older people and did not understand how he could have contracted it, especially the possibility of H1N1. Although he feared that he might die from this illness, he took comfort from knowing that he had provided financial security for his family. Whilst it is often not possible to remove the cause of a patient's fear and anxiety, in David's case the life threatening pneumonia, the nurse must support patients and offer help to modify the anxiety and enable them to make any necessary behaviour adaptations. However David was isolated and this impacted on channels of support.

The stress of critical illness threatened David's sense of wholeness, security and control, and the possibility of dying was a very real fear. The ICU doctor warned him of the possibility of High Flow Nasal Oxygen (HFNO2) (Gotera et al., 2013), Non Invasive Ventilation (NIV) (see Kinnear, 2002), intubation and ventilation if he deteriorated further. The Patients Association (2018) talk about how people want to be kept informed about events that affect their health but unfortunately they often feel they are not kept adequately informed. David was given the news about ventilation in the middle of the night when he was tired, exhausted and unable to make sense of it all and one could suggest that clinical forethought and judgement here was lacking here (see Chapter 1).

Shortly after this conversation David was isolated in a side room, where he had no-one to ask to explain the technical terms, or to comfort and reassure him. He felt a loss of control as he did not know how to take his mind off the situation because he needed a coherent explanation of the situation communicated at his level of understanding (see Bite Size Knowledge 3.6: Isolation).

BITE SIZE KNOWLEDGE 3.6

Isolation

The practice of isolating a patient, also termed barrier nursing, is instigated in response to a suspected or confirmed infective pathogen, whose mode of spread cannot be eliminated through hand washing alone, and therefore poses a risk to others.

Reverse barrier nursing enables an immunosuppressed patient to be protected from potentially infective pathogens carried and transmitted by those caring for them. This process is enhanced by reversing the airflow current to enable potentially contaminated air to be replaced with clean air. Isolation can have negative and positive effects on patients and staff caring for them (further explored later in the chapter).

Hospital staff who ignore the presence of a patient, regardless of how alert the patient is, contribute to the patient's sense of isolation. The term presencing is a blend of presence and sensing. Hersel (2009) defines it as the therapeutic use of self, adopting a caring attitude and paying attention to an individual's needs. It is not merely a physical presence, but requires the giving of one's full attention to the person, and the ability to actively listen.

Further insecurities emerged a few days later. These related to issues such as length of hospitalisation, financial implications, wellbeing of family and permanent physical limitations. Again David felt a loss of control whereas normally he is capable and strong. He could not even do the simplest of tasks without getting short of breath and feeling exhausted. This left him feeling frustrated and frightened. Although a nurse checked his observations every hour (see Table 3.6: David's observations), he knew they were busy and he did not feel that he could detain them too long from attending to the needs of other patients. The daily medical ward round also felt rushed and the doctors did not have time to listen and help him make sense of his situation. The wearing of a Personal Protective Equipment (PPE) mask also hampered communication. When talking to each other we rely to an extent on reading and interpreting facial expressions. However, the mask hides these visual clues and voice clarity is distorted, making those with strong regional or foreign accents even harder to understand.

In this situation, presencing can be a meaningful strategy for alleviating distress and anxiety in the critically ill patient. According to Bizek (2012) when a nurse uses

Table 3.6 David's observations

	Day 1	Day 1	Day 2	Day 2	Day 3	Day 4	Day 5	Day 6	Day 7
Time	**19:42**	**21:20**	**05:00**	**09:35**	**06:30**	**10:00**	**16:00**	**10:30**	**10:00**
BP	139/98	145/100	131/50	135/90	133/83	120/70	100/60	107/83	111/87
Pulse	91	76	77	80	77	72	69	82	94
Temp	37.1	37	36.6	37.2	36.7	37.1	36.7	36.6	37.1
Resp	20	24	26	22	24	20	16	16	17
Sat's	85%	94%	89%	94%	93%	97%	96%	94%	94%
AVPU	A	A	A	A	A	A	A	A	A
BS	6.3		6.4		5.9				
O$_2$	15L RM	15L RM	15LRM	15L RM	15L RM	15L RM	80%Hum	80%Hum	40%Hum
Pain	0/10	0	0	0	0	0	0	0	0

presence, the focus is not on tasks or on what else he or she has yet to do. Energy and attention are directed at the patient and his or her needs and feelings. Presencing can provide reassurance. It is not merely a verbal skill, in the form of realistic encouragement and clarifying misconceptions, but goes further than that. It means making a conscious effort to use all of one's capacity in a more intentionally healing way (Quin, 2000).

David's needs must be sensitively considered and he needed to be given time to unburden himself and be helped to make sense of things that were causing him fear and anxiety. The reassuring cliché 'you'll be all right', which is often said to comfort, only reinforces a sense of distance by denying the patient's feelings as being real, and it discourages further expression of fears and questions and this in turn heightens stress.

Unfortunately, whilst isolation is often necessary for the protection of the patient and others, it can increase the risk of patient deterioration going unnoticed, as the patient in a side room is not a priority for the caregiver. Studies have shown that healthcare workers spent half as much time in direct patient care with isolated patients as they did with non-isolated patients (Kirkland and Weinstein, 1999; Saint et al., 2003). Another potential detrimental effect of isolation is loneliness and boredom (Barratt et al., 2010). However, David found the experience of privacy and the relative quiet of a single room positive as, during the first three days, he was too tired to feel bored. He slept for long periods during the day and when he started to recover, his family and friends were encouraged to visit; he also had his iPad and mobile phone to break up the monotony of the day.

There are other positive aspects to being nursed in isolation. Physical assessments and discussions regarding David's illness and symptoms were done in private, thus maintaining confidentiality which is not easily achieved behind closed curtains. He was also able to have private time with his wife to discuss concerns regarding their immediate future. He could also make private phone calls to her, day or night, without disturbing other patients. David's dignity with bodily functions was also maintained, as the room had en-suite shower and toilet and because these were close to his bed he was able to maintain a degree of independence and control. However, he was at risk of worsening hypoxia and breathlessness when he removed his oxygen mask to use the toilet, and the nurse asked him to use a urinary bottle by his bed. However this did not address his needs around showering and defecation, though subsequently another nurse attached a length of oxygen tubing to his non-rebreath mask, which was long enough to enable him to reach the en suite.

Isolation would ordinarily provide a more peaceful and quiet environment where David would be able to rest and benefit from improved sleep quality. However, because of the increased need for monitoring and vigilance, with one to two hourly clinical observations for the first 36 hours, this was not achieved until **Day 3**. The impact was lessened with the use of a monitor that provided continuous readings of oxygen saturations, heart rate and respiratory rate and the blood pressure cuff was left in situ at night and set to record automatically at set intervals, which David said did not disturb his sleep.

Isolation can have a negative impact on the nurse delivering care. This may take the form of frustration, when they do not have the necessary equipment in the room and there is no-one around to locate it for them. Nursing a patient in isolation increases workload, is time consuming and can be uncomfortable when donning PPE, such as tight fitting masks and gowns that trap body heat. There may also be a fear of contracting infection due to lack of knowledge about infectious diseases and mode of spread.

The nurse can also experience increased stress because the support structure that a team gives when on an open ward is limited when caring for a patient who is in isolation. Consequently fear of coping alone and not knowing what to do if something untoward occurs, can manifest itself in the nurse's clinical decision making. An example of this was when David's oxygen saturations fell below the recommended target level. Instead of assessing why this might be, looking for contributing factors such as anxiety, recent exertion or recent removal of the face mask, the immediate response was to call a junior doctor, who took an ABG which merely confirmed what was already known, but no answer as to why. Literature emphasises the need for critical thinking to improve clinical judgement and decision making (Mishoe, 2003; Tanner, 2006; Banning, 2008) and this requires the gathering of appropriate data and sufficient information to interpret, analyse, evaluate, infer and explain the situation, before a judgement about the best course of action is made.

AMU nurses deal with a variety of critically ill patients and they frequently have to make astute clinical decisions about the priority and delivery of care. In addition, patients often have a short length of stay due to the constant need for acute beds. A core skill AMU nurses therefore have to develop is adaptability in managing complexities of patient care and a constant state of flux (Griffiths, 2010). Time is a critical factor in decision making. Time constraints in an AMU pose difficulty in making astute decisions, often leading to increased intuitive information handling with less seeking of additional information to support decision making (Thompson et al., 2004). In addition, a novice uses strict rules to make a decision, in David's case the nurse performing hourly observations and telling a doctor they feel comfortable communicating with, and in turn the junior doctor taking an ABG and subsequent referral to the CCO nurse. Here the CCO nurse evaluated the observations within the wider context of David's situation and elicited further information. By observing David directly, asking him questions and listening to his concerns the following cues were gathered:

- David had recently removed his oxygen mask to have a drink
- he had mobilised to the toilet and back
- his increased breathlessness increased his anxiety
- he had noted the abnormal observations, because the machine was alarming
- he perceived that the nurse and the junior doctor were anxious about his condition.

After the CCO nurse sat with David and explained the physiological effects of his illness and encouraging relaxing, therapeutic breathing techniques, he was able to see his O2 saturations improving. Knowing he had contributed to this improvement empowered him and gave him a much needed sense of control, reassuring and reducing his anxiety. Thus it is important to listen to the patient and enable them to gain knowledge, so that they can contribute to their care and develop strategies to manage their fears.

Caring for critically ill patients in isolation can be a positive experience for nurses. Repeated exposure within the context of a supportive team with access to clinical experts will improve knowledge, develop skills in problem solving, organisation and time management, critical thinking and decision making and team working. It can be empowering as the nurse can fully concentrate on their needs while in the room with them. There is opportunity to have time with the patient's family to share and understand their hopes and fears and build therapeutic relationships with them. The wider team can provide support by ensuring that they meet other patients' needs while the nurse caring for the needs of the patient in isolation are met.

The expert nurse needs to have and show the skills of confidence, competence, active listening, presencing, knowledge and experience, effective communication, critical thinking, analytical, evidence based reflective and intuitive practice which is persistent and empowering.

For David the expert nurse needs to acknowledge David's fears and explain and explore the impact of illness, the pathophysiology and disease progression, knowledge of infectious disease and potential outcome in language he understands but without frightening him, thus giving him sufficient knowledge to help him process the information in the context of his situation and symptoms. The expert nurse can then explore what he can do to help himself and why it is important, giving him back some control and responsibility; this includes keeping the oxygen on, deep breathing exercises, expectorate sputum, good oral fluid intake, rest in between activities and 'listening to his body'. For family the explanation of the disease and the impact is similar but the nurse can also explain what they can do to help him; for example short frequent visits with a limited number of visitors; help David keep in contact with the outside world by talking about his children, parents, friends, everyday occurrences, headline news and bring him some comforts from home.

The expert nurse can also help develop the fearful junior nurse with regard to their knowledge of critical illness and understanding of the monitoring and therapeutic interventions. They can also help junior nurses develop skills in managing the emotional labour of the work, by building resilience strategies, emotional intelligence, mutual respect and reciprocity, and understanding the humanising care needs of David (see Table 3.7: Humanising health care for David).

SUMMARY OF DAVID'S CASE STUDY

This case study has shown how a lack of patient understanding of a respiratory condition and how inappropriate delivery of news can cause significant patient stress. It has shown how, had a humanising care philosophy been used, nursing care could have been enhanced.

━━━ REFLECTIVE EXERCISE 3.1 ━━━━━━━━━━ ━━━━━

1 How might a critical illness impact on a young previously fit and healthy alpha male?
2 How does pneumonia affect the respiratory system and how does it evolve?
3 What is H1N1 and how does it spread?
4 How would you explain HFNO2 and NIV to David?
5 How would you break bad news and how would you support the patient afterwards?
6 How might you create a healing environment?
7 How do you foster trust?
8 How would you foster hope?
9 What are the physiological effects of anxiety?
10 How would you enable David to regain some control?

Table 3.7 Humanising health care for David

Humanising dimensions	Bio-psychosocial triggers	Managing stressors and coping strategies	Role of expert nurse in support strategies
Insiderness/objectification	David has recently sold his business. He considers himself to be fit and well with an active lifestyle.	David is relieved that he sold his business two weeks ago, as his wife and children will be financially secure if he doesn't recover from this illness.	Enable connectedness by helping staff to understand that it is therapeutic to take time to listen to David's fears and anxieties and what specifically makes him think he is going to die.
Agency/passivity	David doesn't understand why, given his healthy lifestyle, he has become so ill. David doesn't comprehend why he feels so weak and breathless and is afraid to mobilise because he is attached to continuous oxygen. He also fears falling asleep, in case he doesn't wake up again.	David needs a thorough explanation of the physiological effects of: - pneumonia - oxygen therapy - nebulisers - breathing exercises - adequate rest - the role of the physio.	Ensure staff are able to give David a sound evidence based rationale for focusing on the current care and how he can contribute to this.
Uniqueness/homogenisation	David fears he will not recover from this critical illness. He believes he might die and leave his wife to cope alone and that he will not see his children grow up.	David has a perception of his situation that has been influenced by the media and this is reinforced by his isolation in a side room. David is relieved he sold his business and takes comfort from knowing that his wife and children will be financially secure if he dies.	Ensure staff do not belittle David for his way of thinking about his illness. Enable staff to help David re-emphasise his uniqueness and that he doesn't have to accept the media hype. Involve wife in helping David to continue to be part of any discussions and decision making relating to his family.
Togetherness/isolation	David doesn't understand why he has been moved to a side room, when previously he was in a 6-bedded bay and nurses didn't need to wear protective clothing. He is worried his wife and children won't be allowed to visit him.	David is isolated and feels that no-one has the time to talk to him and explain to him what is happening.	Enable staff to recognise that spending time with David will enhance his recovery process. Involve wife and children in maintaining David's contact with the outside world and everyday events in his family's life.

Humanising dimensions	Bio-psychosocial triggers	Managing stressors and coping strategies	Role of expert nurse in support strategies
Sense making/loss of meaning	David thought that pneumonia was something older or infirm people get. He doesn't understand why his observations are measured hourly, why his urine output and how much he drinks are being measured and why he has to have so many blood tests. He is frightened when the monitor he is connected to alarms.	David needs a thorough explanation of the rationale for monitoring his: - vital signs - fluid balance - oxygenation - blood results. David needs to understand and be empowered.	Enable staff to appreciate that what is normal for them is fear inducing for David. Ensure staff are able to explain the rationale for their care and empower David in taking an active part, for example: - optimising his position to aid lung function - documenting his intake on the fluid chart - setting goals for his oral intake and frequency of breathing exercises.
Personal journey/ loss of personal journey	David feels weak and helpless.	David needs a thorough explanation of the effects of oxygen depletion and infection on his body organs.	Enable staff to ensure David has a working knowledge of basic anatomy and physiology, the effects of sepsis and hypoxia and the associated care and treatment implications.
Sense of place/ dislocation	He is not used to being on his own in a hospital environment.	David is able to use his laptop computer and mobile phone to keep in touch and to help him manage his stress.	Involve wife to help create an environment in the side room that has reminders of home, for example photos, own clothes, iPad. Ensure staff have a sound evidence base regarding the recovery phase post pneumonia and encourage and enable David to set short and long-term goals.
Embodiment/ reductionist body	Isolation is causing David to be preoccupied with his body's changes and focus on what he can't do instead of what he can do.	David would like to talk to a doctor but thinks they are too busy to speak to him. David may like to talk to a clinical psychologist or chaplain or rehabilitation health care professional, but he may not know they are available or what they can offer.	Ensure staff are enabling David to make choices. Ensure they have a good working knowledge of support structures that David can access.

CHAPTER SUMMARY

These case studies seemingly portray both sides of the same coin and yet are very diverse in their complexity. They are linked, in a broad sense, through the experience of critical illness, the fight to breathe and to survive. However, the profound impact on the individuals, how they cope and travel along the road to eventual recovery could not be more different. Along the way they encounter many obstacles and setbacks. Professionals from novice to expert attempt to understand and help them navigate this path. These unique experiences provide opportunities for learning and growth in our understanding of what it means to humanise the care we give critically ill patients. One illness or problem/need is different from one person to another and in one culture to another. Staff need to develop skills to see cultural differences and work with patients and family to develop a good working relationship, which helps the client and does not hinder recovery. Pre-understandings that inform the way we view people are based on socialisation etc., and are inherent in all and these can produce stereotypical behaviour and prejudice. However, exposure and understanding of different cultures should be recognised as a key skill and one that needs to be developed in all. The knowledge base and reflexivity of staff at all levels needs to be developed and using case studies which explore the professional gaze and humanising dimensions can help with this.

FURTHER READING

Abad, C., Fearday, A. and Safdar, N. (2010) Adverse effects of isolation in hospitalised patients: a systematic review, *Journal of Hospital Infection*, 76: 97–102.

Atkinson, D. (2013) 'Nursing observation and assessment of patients in the acute medical unit', Thesis. University of Salford, UK. http://usir.salford.ac.uk/29466/

Benner, P. (1994) *Interpretive Phenomenology: Embodiment, Caring and Ethics in Health and Illness*. Thousand Oaks, CA: Sage.

Benner, P. and Tanner, C. (1987) Clinical judgement: how expert nurses use intuition, *American Journal of Nursing*, 87(1): 23–31.

Benner, P. and Wrubel, J. (1982) Clinical knowledge development. The value of perceptual awareness, *Nurse Educator*, 7: 11–17.

Benner, P. and Wrubel, J. (1989) *The Primacy of Caring: Stress and Coping in Health and Illness*. Palo Alto, CA: Addison-Wesley.

Coulter, M.A. (1989). The needs of family members of patients in intensive care units, *Intensive care Nursing*, 5: 4–10.

Hammond, F. (1995) Involving family in care within the intensive care environment. A descriptive study, *Intensive and Critical Care Nursing*, 1: 256–64.

Holden, C. (2013) *Transactional Analysis in Bite Sized Chunks. Book 1: The Ego States; Book 2: Strokes and Hungers; Book 3: People Play Games*. Whole Deen Publishing, UK.

Madeo, M. (2003) The psychological impact of isolation, *Nursing Times*, *99*(7): 54.

Murdoch, I. (1991) *The Sovereignty of the Good*. London: Routledge.

National Institute for Health and Care Excellence (NICE) (2007) *NICE Guidelines [CG50] Acutely Ill Adults in Hospital: Recognising and Responding to Deterioration*. www.nice.org.uk/guidance/cg50

Schon, D. (1987) *The Reflective Practitioner: How Professionals Think in Action*. New York: Basic.

Spector, R.E. (2010) *Cultural Diversity in Health and Illness* (7th edn). London: Pearson.

White, S. and Stancombe, J. (2003) *Clinical Judgement in the Health and Welfare Professions. Extending the Evidence Base*. Maidenhead: Open University Press.

REFERENCES

Banning, M. (2008) A review of clinical decision making: models and current research, *Journal of Clinical Nursing*, *17*(2): 87–95.

Barratt, R., Shaban, R. and Moyle, W. (2010) Behind barriers: patients' perceptions of source isolation for MRSA, *Australian Journal of Advanced Nursing*, *28*(2): 53–9.

Benner, P.M., Hooper-Kyriakidis, P. and Stannard, D. (1999) *Clinical Wisdom and Interventions in Critical Care. A Thinking-in-action Approach*. London: Saunders.

Bizek, K. (2012) *The Patient's Experience with Critical Illness*. Available at: http://ferronfred.eu/onewebmedia/ThePatient'sExperienceWithCriticalIllness.pdf

British Thoracic Society (2016) *Guidelines and Quality Standards*. Available at: www.brit-thoracic.org.uk/guidelines-and-quality-standards/

Department of Health (2000) *Comprehensive Critical Care: A Review of Adult Critical Care Services*. Available at: http://webarchive.nationalarchives.gov.uk/20130107105354/http:/www.dh.gov.uk/prod_consum_dh/groups/dh_digitalassets/@dh/@en/documents/digitalasset/dh_4082872.pdf

Dinmohammadi, M., Peyrovi, H. and Mehrdad, N. (2013) Concept analysis of professional socialization in nursing, *Nursing Forum*, *48*(1): 26–34.

Dixit, D., Bridgeman, M.D., Andrews, L.B., Narayanan, N., Radbel, J., Parikh, A. and Sunderram, J. (2015) Acute exacerbations of Chronic Obstructive Pulmonary Disease: diagnosis, management, and prevention in critically ill patients, *Pharmacotherapy*, *35*(6): 631–48.

Drury, C. and Hunter, J. (2016) The hole in holistic patient care, *Open Journal of Nursing*, *6*: 776–92.

Elie, M., Cole, M.G., Primeau, F. J., Bellavance, F. (2001) Delirium risk factors in elderly hospitalized patients. *Journal of General Internal Medicine*. https://doi.org/10.1046/j.1525-1497.1998.00047.x

Gotera, C., Díaz Lobato, S., Pinto, T. and Winck, J.C. (2013) Clinical evidence on high flow oxygen therapy and active humidification in adults. *Portuguese Journal of Pulmonology*, *19*(5): 217–227.

Griffiths, P. (2010) A community of practice: the nurses' role on a medical assessment unit, *Journal of Clinical Nursing*, *20*: 247–54.

Helman, C.G. (2007) *Culture, Health and Illness* (5th edn). London: Hodder Arnold.

Hersel, J.A. (2009) Presence in nursing practice: a concept analysis, *Holistic Nursing Practice*, *23*(5): 276–81.

Higgs, J. and Jones, M. (2000) *Clinical Reasoning in the Health Professions* (2nd edn). Oxford: Butterworth Heinemann.

Hillman, K. (2002) Critical care without walls, *Current Opinion in Critical Care*. *8*(6): 594–9.

Hsieh, S.J., Ely, E.W., & Gong, M.N., (2013) Can intensive care unit delirium be prevented and reduced? Lessons learned and future directions, *Annals of the American Thoracic Society*, *10*(6). https://doi.org/10.1513/AnnalsATS.201307-232FR

Institute for Healthcare Communication. (2011). *Impact of Communication in Healthcare*. Available at: http://healthcarecomm.org/about-us/impact-of-communication-in-healthcare/

Irwin, R.S. and Rippe, J.M. (2012) *Intensive Care Medicine* (7th edn). Philadelphia: Lippincott Williams and Wilkins.

Kim, S.R. and Rhee, Y.K. (2010) Overlap between Asthma and COPD: where the two diseases converge, *Allergy Asthma Immunology Research*, *2*(4): 209–14.

Kinnear, W. for British Thoracic Society Standards of Care Committee (2002) BTS guideline: non-invasive ventilation in acute respiratory failure, *Thorax*, *57*: 192–211.

Kirkland, K.B. and Weinstein, J.M. (1999) Adverse effects of contact isolation, *Lancet*. *354*: 1177–8.

MacLachlan, M. (2006) *Culture and Health: A Critical Perspective Towards Global Health* (2nd edn). Chichester: John Wiley & Sons Ltd.

McChance, K.L and Huether, S.E. (2010) *Pathophysiology. The Biologic Basis for Disease in Adults and Children* (7th edn). Canada: Elsevier Mosby.

McQuillan, P., Pilkington, S., Allan, A., Taylor, B., Short, A. and Morgan, G. (1998) Confidential inquiry into quality of care before admission to intensive care, *British Medical Journal*, *316*(7148): 1853–8.

Meagher, D. J., O'Hanlon, D., O'Mahony, E., Casey, P.R. and Trzepacz, P.T. (2000) Relationship between symptoms and motoric subtype of delirium. *Journal of Neuropsychiatry and Clinical Neurosciences*. https://doi.org/10.1176/jnp.12.51

Miller, M.O. (2008) Evaluation and management of delirium in hospitalized older patients. *American Family Physician*. 78 11; 1265-70.

Mishoe, S. (2003) Critical thinking in respiratory care practice: a qualitative research study, *Respiratory Care*, *48*(5): 500–16.

National Institute for Health and Care Excellence (NICE) (2010) Delirium: diagnosis, prevention and management (Clinical guideline 103). Available at: https://www.nice.org.uk/guidance/cg103 [accessed 3 May 2011].

National Institute for Health and Care Excellence (NICE) (2016) *NICE Guidelines NG51 Sepsis: Recognition, Diagnosis and Early Management*. Available at: www.nice.org.uk/guidance/indevelopment/ng51/documents

Nervenarzt, D. (2011) Summary of clinical neurological diagnosis of sepsis-associated delirium, *Biotech, Healthcare and Medical Resources*, *82*(12): 1578–83.

Oberg, K. (1960) Cultural shock: adjustment to new cultural environments, *Practical Anthropology*, *7*: 177–88.

O'Connell, E. (2008) Therapeutic relationships in critical care nursing: a reflection on practice, *Nursing in Critical Care*, 13(3): 138–43.

Parliamentary and Health Service Ombudsman (2014) *Complaints about Acute Trusts 2013–2014*. Available at: www.ombudsman.org.uk/organisations-we-investigate/what-our-data-tells-us/quarterly-reports-complaints-about-nhs-trusts/complaints-about-acute-trusts-2013-14-and-april-september-2014-15

The Patients Association (2018) Available at: https://www.patients-association.org.uk/

Pierson, D.J. (2013) Oxygen in respiratory care. A personal perspective from 40 years in the field, *Respiratory Care*, 58(1): 196–204.

Quin, J.F. (2000) The self as healer: reflections from a nurse's journey, *American Association of Critical Care Nurses Clinical Issues*, 11(1): 68–76.

Quirke, S., Coombs, M., and McEldowney, R. (2011) Suboptimal care of the acutely unwell ward patient: a concept analysis, *Journal of Advanced Nursing*, 67(8): 1834–45.

Saint, S., Higgins, L.A., Nallamothu, B.K. and Chenoweth, C. (2003) Do physicians examine patients in contact isolation less frequently? A brief report, *American Journal for Infection Control*, 31: 354–6.

Schive, M., Phan, C., Louie, S. and Harper, R. (2013) Critical Asthma Syndrome in the ICU. Clinical Review, *Allergic Immunology*, 48: 31–44.

Stewart, I. and Joines, V. (2012) *TA Today: A New Introduction to Transactional Analysis*. (2nd edn). Chapel Hill, NC: Lifespace Publishing.

Tanner, C. (2006) Thinking like a nurse: a research based model of clinical judgement in nursing, *Journal of Nursing Education*, 45(6): 204–11.

Thompson, C., Cullum, N. and McCaughey, D. (2004) Nurses' information use and clinical decision making – the real world potential for evidence based decisions in nursing, *Evidence Based Nursing*, 7: 66–72.

Tsuruta, R. and Oda, Y. (2016) A clinical perspective of sepsis-associated delirium. *Journal of Intensive Care* 4(18). Available at: http://jintensivecare.biomedcentral.com/articles/10.1186/s40560-016-0145-4 [accessed 1 August 2016].

Ward, C., Bochner, S. and Furnham, A. (2001) *The Psychology of Culture Shock* (2nd edn). London: Routledge.

Williams, S.J. (1989) Chronic respiratory illness and disability: a critical review of the psychosocial literature, *Social Science and Medicine*, 28(8): 791–803.

CHAPTER 4

Haemodynamic Instability

Case Study: Joseph Knight

JONATHAN BRANNEY AND DEBBIE BRANNEY

━━━ CHAPTER AIMS ━━━━━━━━━━━━━━━━━ ━━━

1 To analyse the challenges of delivering humanised care to people who are critically ill in a highly technical and busy clinical environment.
2 To evaluate a generalised approach to the promotion of humanised care towards a person critically unwell with acute myeloid leukaemia and neutropenia, using the Humanising Care Framework.
3 To evaluate the support required by inexperienced nursing staff towards delivering safe and effective humanised care to people who are critically ill.

INTRODUCTION

This chapter explores the issues highlighted in a complex critical care scenario; it aims to encourage critical reflection on the practical and ethical challenges of providing safe and effective humanised nursing care in the contemporary critical care environment.

Haemodynamic instability/failure is frequently a feature of critical illness (Vincent and de Backer, 2013). Haemodynamic instability is a term which at one extreme might be used to describe the condition of a patient whereby one or more measurements of cardiovascular function are not in the normal range, but not clearly pathological, through to the other extreme, circulatory failure or shock leading to organ hypoperfusion and, ultimately, death. In a large multicentre prospective cohort study, some degree of haemodynamic failure was evident on admission in around one third of patients (Vincent et al., 1998). A similar proportion of patients had evidence of haemodynamic instability in a more recent study involving 198 intensive care units (ICUs) across 24 countries in Europe (Vincent et al., 2006). Critical care nurses therefore are regularly delivering care to haemodynamically unstable patients, which can require a high level of knowledge, skill and experience. While the nurse's technical expertise is no doubt vital in achieving successful outcomes for patients, the delivery of that care ought to be optimal when done within the context of humanised, person-centred care (see Chapter 1).

In the following case study, a senior nurse supports a staff nurse in the care of a patient, whom we will call Mr Joseph Knight, who was haemodynamically unstable. You are invited to consider that you were that senior nurse, and intermittently questions will be posed where you might pause to consider the issues raised. Think about the clinical decisions that were made, the support offered to the junior nurse, and what you would have done. The case study is likely to feature instances from clinical practice similar to your own experience, providing an ideal opportunity to reflect on your own practice, to reflect on decisions you made in the past, and what you might do differently tomorrow.

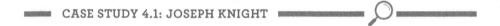

CASE STUDY 4.1: JOSEPH KNIGHT

Support of Junior Staff by the Expert Nurse

Shortly after handover, the nurse in charge of the critical care unit for the day shift has asked you, as a senior critical care nurse, to supervise a junior staff nurse in the administration of intravenous (IV) drugs. The staff nurse in question has been allocated to care for Mr Joseph Knight, a 75-year-old gentleman recently diagnosed with acute myeloid leukaemia and admitted to hospital for further investigations and treatment in the oncology ward. The treatment there included transfusion of blood products, but this, alongside mild heart failure (see Chapter 5), had resulted in circulatory overload and pulmonary oedema, a recognised albeit less common transfusion reaction (see Table 4.1: Transfusion reactions – six most common in order of prevalence).

Mr Knight's condition had deteriorated and he had been admitted to critical care for non-invasive ventilatory support (see Chapter 3) and continuous haemodynamic monitoring. An added complication was neutropenia induced by chemotherapy, with the risk of neutropenic sepsis meaning Mr Knight had to be nursed in a side room.

Mr Knight, who liked to be called Joe, was a retired joiner and widower, had two children and three grandchildren who lived nearby, all of whom he loved dearly, and he described himself as grumpy (confirmed by his sons). His past medical history included asthma, mild heart failure, paroxysmal atrial fibrillation and anxiety; he was rather fed up with his list of ailments. We will learn more about Joe's healthcare journey as the case unfolds. Let us first consider the scenario from the perspective of the staff nurse caring for him.

The staff nurse, whom we she call Angela, was in her first post since graduating from university and had been accepted onto the NMC register only a few months previously.

Table 4.1 Transfusion reactions – six most common in order of prevalence

Transfusion reaction	Prevalence (per 100,000 units transferred)	Symptoms	Timing of symptoms	Interventions
Febrile non-haemolytic	1,000 – 3,000	Incremental increase > 1°C above baseline and no other new symptoms	During	Close observation, frequent vital signs. If stable continue with transfusion.
Allergic	112.2	Hives, rash, itching of skin, throat, eye, tongue swelling	During	Stop transfusion and assess patient. If severe reaction check patient ID and unit ID and compatibility. Administer antihistamines. Only restart transfusion if mild reaction which responds to antihistamines.
Delayed serological or haemolytic	Serological: 48.9–75.7 Haemolytic: 40	Haemolytic: Dark urine or jaundice (45–50%), fever; chest, abdominal or back pain; dyspnoea; chills; hypertension	24h to 28 days after	Most patients do not require treatment other than additional transfusions to maintain desired haemoglobin.
Transfusion-associated circulatory overload	10.9	Bronchospasm, dyspnoea, tachypnoea and hypoxaemia, copious frothy pink-tinged fluid, chills, rigors, hypotension, nausea or vomiting, feeling of impending doom, back or chest pain, intravenous sitepain, cough	Within 4–6 hrs	Stop transfusion, keep intravenous line open, assess patient, check patient ID and unit ID and patient compatibility. Treat symptoms as indicated (adrenaline, antihistamines, steroids; oxygen and respiratory support, diuretics; fluid, blood pressure, and renal support). Chest radiograph for presence of bilateral interstitial infiltrate, if suggestive of transfusion-related acute lung injury. Blood cultures (patient and product), if high clinical suspicion of sepsis. Do not resume transfusion. Notify blood transfusion laboratory; return unit with administration set, plus post-transfusion patient sample. Associated products can be quarantined.
Anaphylactic	8		During	As for transfusion-associated circulatory overload.
Acute haemolytic	2.5-7.9	Sudden onset fever or chills, pain, hypotension, dyspnoea, haemoglobinuria	During	Stop the transfusion and assess patient.

From her experiences as a student Angela had become convinced that critical care was the area that she wanted to work in and her first few months in post had confirmed this. She was aware of being on a steep learning curve from the first day and had been closely supervised and supported with access to post-registration education. Angela was now delighted to have finally been given the chance to prove that she could work more independently as afforded by the geography of nursing Mr Knight in a side room. She was used to always having an experienced nurse close by her on the unit, and while that was reassuring, the extra autonomy felt like acknowledgment that she was ready to progress in her career. Equally, she was frustrated at not yet being able to administer IV drugs and needing to be helped with this.

Reflection

Does the allocation of a junior staff nurse to Mr Knight give you any cause for concern? As a senior critical care nurse, what support do you think Angela would need in caring for a critically ill person like Joe, and in a side room?

It happened to be the case that on this shift the patient caseload in the critical care unit was particularly challenging with complex and time-consuming medical and nursing care required by all patients. The more experienced nurses had been allocated to those patients with particularly complex needs while, relatively speaking, Mr Knight was considered to have less complex needs. There were fewer dependent patients in the high dependency unit and on another occasion Angela would have been allocated there. However, there was another junior nurse there already being supported in her leadership and management skills by senior staff. It might be considered that the allocation of a junior nurse to Mr Knight indicated that the skill mix was suboptimal. On the other hand, it could also be considered that the skill mix available was used optimally while affording development opportunities to junior staff, important for the future development of the service. A skill mix that is adaptable and that remains optimal for every possible case-mix is not realistic. Therefore the approach outlined here could well be considered as commensurate with recommended standards for nurse staffing in critical care (Bray et al., 2010). While the situation of an inexperienced nurse being faced with caring for a highly dependent patient presents a challenge, it also presents a great opportunity for the expert nurse to facilitate the learning of the junior nurse while ensuring the patient receives the appropriate care.

After receiving handover from the nightshift staff nurse, Angela knew that one of the first things she had to do was to organise the giving of fluids and drugs prescribed for Mr Knight and she got to that immediately. It was around that time that you were asked to check and administer the IV drugs with Angela. Let us now consider the scenario from your point of view, as the senior critical care nurse.

When you entered the side room Angela immediately indicated both verbally and non-verbally that she would like assistance with checking the IV drugs. She wanted to get these done as they were holding her back from attending to Mr Knight's basic or essential care needs. However, after acknowledging Angela you instinctively scanned to assess the situation first (see Figure 1.2, Chapter 1). You looked first of all at Mr Knight and you rapidly noted that he appeared pale and sleepy but apparently reasonably comfortable in a semi-recumbent position in bed. His breath sounds were suggestive of a moist chest but his respiratory effort was not excessively laboured. You glanced at the monitoring equipment as you approached to introduce yourself to Joe and explain to him why you were in the room, and you noted that he had a PICC (peripherally inserted central catheter) line which was in situ for chemotherapy with one extra lumen available for drugs. You then returned to check the drugs with Angela.

Angela wished first to administer IV paracetamol but you noticed that there had already been obtained a unit of packed red cells requested from the blood bank by the night staff nurse. With only one IV lumen available, giving the blood first would delay administering the IV drugs which could not be given concurrently. However, it was not clear exactly how long the blood had been out of refrigeration and you knew that the transfusion should be completed within four hours of leaving temperature-controlled storage according to guidelines (Harris et al., 2009) otherwise a precious resource would be wasted. You pointed out to Angela that since some of Mr Knight's drugs were prescribed orally there was no compelling reason why the paracetamol might not be given orally instead of IV. Indeed, when a patient is capable of taking medication orally, according to a recent systematic review the balancing of risks and benefits favours oral over IV administration of paracetamol (Jibril et al., 2015). You balanced delaying the other IV drugs against spoiling the blood and decided to administer the blood first.

Reflection

What issues are raised during the decision making needed in relation to drug administration here? Do you endorse the actions based on the experienced nurse's critical thinking as outlined above? What would you have done?

Complicating the situation above, a nurse from the oncology ward arrived soon after to administer Mr Knight's chemotherapy, and she was not best pleased to find this had to be delayed and she started discussing how and when the chemotherapy might be started. You were conscious of the risk of Mr Knight feeling objectified (see Table 4.2: Humanising health care for Mr Joseph Knight) so you purposefully included him, and Angela, in the conversation by explaining what the discussion was about. This hopefully will have reduced any anxiety that may have been provoked by discussing Joe's care in front of him, but not involving him.

Table 4.2 Humanising health care for Mr Joseph Knight

Humanising dimensions	Bio-psychosocial triggers	Managing stressors and coping strategies	Role of expert nurse in support strategies
Insiderness/Objectification	Recently diagnosed with acute myeloid leukaemia and promptly admitted to hospital for treatment. This presents a challenge to Joseph's personal and subjective view of his world with little time for mental processing.	Coping with new diagnosis of cancer might provoke a great deal of fear about the future, and an unwelcome reminder of his wife's death from cancer. Happening in a short time-frame this could feel overwhelming.	Joseph should be facilitated to feel like a person, not simply a recipient of care. Care ought not to be 'done to the leukaemia patient' but 'delivered for and with Joseph Knight, a person with cancer'. He should be encouraged and given time to express his concerns and feelings while the nurse actively listens. This will help to reduce Joseph's stress and help him to feel valued.
Agency/passivity	The pathophysiology of leukaemia and the side-effects of chemotherapy, combined with breathlessness, all contribute to exhaustion and subsequent loss of independence.	While Joseph is a proud man who believes in hard work (he was a self-employed joiner all his working life), his family report that he has readily adopted the 'sick role'. Equally he finds it very uncomfortable being in an unfamiliar environment over which he feels little control.	Exhaustion allowing, Joseph should be involved as a partner in the planning of his care. Plan care carefully to avoid interruptions to rest. Informed consent and choice whenever possible should be regular features of care and self-care should be encouraged when possible to reduce passivity. TV/radio/music that Joseph can select himself should be offered.
Uniqueness/homogenisation	Critical illness and admission to hospital are preventing Joseph from taking part in the roles and activities that contribute to his sense of self.	Joseph is unable to fully participate in his roles as grandfather, father and active member of the local football team supporters' club.	Promote the use of Joseph's preferred name by all staff when communicating with him. Arrange for viewing of football matches when possible. Start a diary and complete with Joseph's likes/dislikes and things that are important to him.
Togetherness/isolation	Joseph's ability to communicate is hampered by breathlessness, exhaustion and non-invasive ventilation. He is required to be physically isolated due to the heightened risk of infection due to neutropenia, and his family are currently restricted from visiting due to coughs/colds.	Being isolated from his family, who are particularly close since his wife's death, will be particularly stressful for Joseph.	Promote family communication by facilitating phone calls, use of a mobile phone, video-calling if possible. Encourage family and members of his football supporter's club to send cards, letters, photos to keep Joseph up-to-date and feeling in touch with the world outside his room. Family and friends should be encouraged to contribute to the diary, and the nurse should read this to Joseph if he does not feel like reading it. The nurse can also use humour and self-disclosure where appropriate to help Joseph feel like a fellow person, not merely a recipient of care.

Humanising dimensions	Bio-psychosocial triggers	Managing stressors and coping strategies	Role of expert nurse in support strategies
Sense making/loss of meaning	The new diagnosis alongside the investigations, treatments and new terminology could contribute to a feeling of bewilderment.	Joseph had not long been moved from the oncology ward to critical care and he may not have had time to make sense of what was going on. Moving from one area to a noticeably more technically complex area of care could be most unsettling.	Throughout the shift the nurse should explain the structure of the day and what to expect. Information which is provided from monitors, tests and various staff members should be pieced together and explained in terms that Joseph can readily understand.
Personal journey/loss of personal journey	The new diagnosis and change to his health status may hinder the achievement of any of Joseph's life goals.	It may feel to Joseph like his chances of achieving life goals have been stripped away from him.	The nurse should find out Joseph's goals and aspirations. Provide encouragement as to how these might still be achieved or modified.
Sense of place/ dislocation	As for any critically ill person, being in an unfamiliar critical care environment can be unpredictable and frightening.	Being in a critical care unit can provide an assault on the senses. Sights such as wires, monitors and staff in uniform might appear alien; smells may be unfamiliar and unpleasant; sounds may be disturbing and unsettling.	With Joseph's permission put his letters/photos etc. on the wall to make the room feel more like 'home'. Compassionate communication with appropriate humour will build rapport and help make Joseph feel 'safe'. Rest, especially at night, should be facilitated with eye mask/ear plugs. Facilitate normal activities where possible, e.g. Joseph may want to place a bet on a football game or order his favourite takeaway meal.
Embodiment/ reductionist body	Critical illness has rendered Joseph relatively immobile and unable to fully participate in his usual life activities.	Physiological monitoring, invasive investigations and administration of treatments may contribute to Joseph feeling detached from his body.	The expert nurse will be able to role model to junior staff the mastery associated with the delivery of care that is both highly technical at times but at all times humanised. Effectively explain the reasons for monitoring, other aspects of care and the roles of the different healthcare professionals involved.

The dilemma described above was indicative of Angela's inexperience for how best to manage the drug and fluid administration, and liaise with oncology staff. In fact, this early situation allowed you to further establish after discussion with Angela that she did not have a clear plan for how to best organise the shift to maximise the timely delivery of care for Joe. The drugs were viewed as a task to be done that was getting in the way of what she really wanted to do, deliver 'care' to Joe. We will return to consider this potential tension between what might be described as basic nursing care, such as personal washing, which arguably has a more obvious humanising dimension, and highly technical care such as IV drug administration, as characterised by the technologised critical care environment.

While the blood infusion was underway, the electrocardiogram (ECG) monitor alarmed and the monitor displayed fast (> 130 beats/minute) atrial fibrillation (AF). Angela looked to you for guidance. You promptly reassessed Mr Knight who appeared concerned at the alarm and you calmly explained to him what was happening and that you were working to resolve the situation. There were no typical signs or symptoms of immediate transfusion reaction such as rigors, lumbar pain, dyspnoea, hypotension or haemoglobinuria as associated with an acute haemolytic transfusion reaction nor of an anaphylactic reaction. However, you recognise it is prudent to stop the infusion until more information is obtained (Delaney et al., 2016). It was logical to then consider electrolyte imbalance particularly since Mr Knight was receiving diuretics. You instructed Angela that a sample should be drawn from Joe's arterial line for arterial blood gas (ABG) analysis to check his serum potassium level in particular and to check when the last venous sample was analysed for urea and electrolytes (U+Es). Once she had drawn the arterial sample you reminded Angela to take it to the analyser immediately to reduce the risk of a haemolysed sample giving a falsely high potassium reading. His serum potassium level was 3.4 mmol/L, probably due to polyuria due to frusemide to offload fluid. Blood results also revealed a low magnesium (0.84 mmol/L). [There is some contention as to the efficacy of magnesium for cardioversion in AF (Kotecha, 2016). However, serum magnesium < 0.9 mmol/L is generally considered low (Romani, 2018) therefore warrants correction.] Administration of IV potassium and magnesium was now the priority and with electrolyte correction, sinus rhythm was restored and the transfusion was recommended without further event.

Throughout the period of care outlined above, regular communication was important with the anaesthetist to agree the management plan and prescribe the required fluids. However, during this particularly busy shift with a complex caseload of patients the siting of an intravenous cannula which would assist in the delivery of medication was deemed low priority. Ordinarily you would have sited the cannula yourself, but you recognised that due to poor venous access there was a risk of causing discomfort to Joe without successful cannulation. Thus, it was deemed best to wait for the expertise of the anaesthetist, albeit a source of frustration for you, and Angela when trying hard to deliver timely and effective person-centred care (see Chapter 1).

DISCUSSION: TECHNOLOGY VERSUS HUMANISATION

The modern ICU is a highly technical environment where patients are typically attached to a variety of physiological monitoring and organ-support systems, both invasive and non-invasive, with one of the main roles of the critical care nurse being to record and respond to the outputs from this technology. While these systems will be crucial for preserving the lives of patients, concern has been raised that too great a focus by the nurse on the equipment, and the physiological readings they produce, might present an impediment to humanised care, with the person being forgotten behind the screen (Almerud-Österberg, 2010). This is an understandable concern due to the risk of the objectification of the patient, with the potential for the loss of meaning by the person as they might be considered, from this standpoint, only as a 'body' with little or no 'uniqueness' beyond their physiology (see Table 4.2: Humanising health care for Mr Joseph Knight). As legitimate a concern as this might be, Barnard and Sandelowski (2001) argue that technology versus humanisation ('humane nursing care') is a false dichotomy. Rather than leading to a negating of the self, technology might be viewed as assisting the person to be the 'self' they desire – 'well'. The example we described earlier, of fast AF being identified on the ECG which allowed for timely treatment and a good outcome for Mr Knight, is a clear case for the benefits of technology. It was key though that the nurses caring for him explained what was happening, what the plan of action was, invited and responded to his concerns, and explained what to expect next to show Mr Knight that he was valued and would therefore feel valued as a fellow human being.

To emphasise the importance of social or emotional intelligence in nursing, it is reassuring to note than in our increasingly technologised world nurses are one of the least likely occupational groups to be replaced by computerisation owing to the high degree of social intelligence required which machines are not even close to replicating (Frey and Osborne, 2013). Monitoring in ICU is best done by computers which are not susceptible to lapses of concentration or need for rest breaks (Clifford and Clifton, 2012), but they will never 'know' the patient and be able to integrate that technical knowledge with the thoughts, hopes and wishes of the person and make them feel valued and safe.

Rather than technology *per se* presenting a risk to humanised care, the real risk comes from what Barnard and Sandelowski (2001: 372) describe as 'technique':

> Technique refers to the formation of a system comprised of human, organisational, political, and economic structures, which are aimed towards the absolute efficiency of methods and means in every field of human endeavour.

Therefore, it is the organisation and running of the healthcare systems in which nurses work, where patients are to be 'processed' as efficiently as possible by increasingly specialised staff whose remit is but one facet of the person, for example, the person's reason for admission rather than their overall wellbeing, that are the real threats to person-centred care. This dovetails with the challenges of delivering person-centred care in ICU. In considering whether it is myth or reality that such care is delivered in ICU, Rattray and McKenna (2012) highlight that while it is 'likely' that much of the care in ICUs is generally person-centred, the softer skills of care, compassion and communication, essential for person-centred care, are more difficult to evidence than safety and effectiveness (ibid.). And since 'organisation of care tends to be driven by policy, targets, resources and external drivers' (Rattray and McKenna, 2012: 225) it is not always easy for nurses to deliver the care they wish to. However, with a staff nurse to patient ratio of 1:1 in the UK, the ICU arguably presents the greatest opportunity for regular person-centred care during the in-hospital patient journey.

Reflection

What risks to person-centred care do you see from technology? From the organisation of the health system in which you work?

PERSON-CENTRED CARE – FAMILY AND HUMOUR

When a patient is in hospital away from their family, friends and all that is familiar, there is a strong risk of loneliness. Added to that needing to be nursed alone in a side room, as was the case for Mr Knight, assisting patients with feelings of isolation (see Table 4.2: Humanising health care for Mr Joseph Knight) is an important part of the care plan. For Mr Knight, family was very important and regular visits from his sons and family were both encouraged and facilitated. Photos and cards for the room were encouraged to promote a sense of place while Mr Knight was in relative isolation. While visitors can bring physical and psychological benefits to patients and be an important source of advocacy and information, nurses have not always regarded visiting positively, in contrast to patients and visitors (Gibson et al., 2012). In a study that sought the views of ICU nurses in the UK (20 ICU nurses via focus groups) and Australia (51 ICU nurses via questionnaires) the importance of families was universally acknowledged; however the UK-based nurses were generally less favourable towards visiting and more likely to view visiting family as a burden (Kean and Mitchell, 2013). Study limitations need to be factored into interpreting this finding, notably the UK study was in one ICU only; the Australian study, in two ICUs, had only a 26% response rate (51 of 197 surveys returned). However, the findings are instructive in that, despite having a more restrictive policy in terms of the hours visitors could attend, in the Australian ICUs there appeared to be a stronger culture of involving the family in the patient's care (ibid.). This could explain why family were less likely to be viewed as a hindrance to the nurses getting on with their work, as they were involved in the work. Detail was not given as to the care family members were specifically involved in, nor which family members tended to do this. Nevertheless, properly managed, the involvement of family can be a real asset to patient recovery, and potentially to some aspects of the workload of the critical care nurse.

The importance of family access, both for the patient and the family member, has been poignantly underscored by a recent campaign in England called John's Campaign, started by Nicci Gerrard and named after her father who had dementia and quickly deteriorated while in hospital (Jones-Berry, 2016). Ms Gerrard believed his marked deterioration was in large part due to being isolated from his loved ones and while her campaign seeks to improve family access to patients with dementia, the plight of this group of vulnerable patients highlights the importance of family, friends and familiarity to recovery. Nurses are the cornerstones in making sure that patients receive the family access they need during their period of illness. The importance of family to Mr Knight was evident in his level of animation when his sons visited. His mood lifted, he began eating more when his family brought food he wanted to eat rather than hospital meals and began to regain his independence. While his sons recognised the importance of this and visited dutifully, they disclosed to nurses that they felt their father liked to 'play the sick role' (see Bite Size Knowledge 4.1: Functionalism and the sick role) especially since the death of their mother.

═══ BITE SIZE KNOWLEDGE 4.1 ═══════════════ ══════════

Functionalism and the sick role

Functionalism can be seen as an analogy between society and a biological organism (Barry and Yuill, 2016). Just as the various organs of a living thing work together in order to maintain the whole, society, from a functionalist perspective, is made up of a number of systems and institutions that work together to produce social order. Functionalists hold that society usually operates in a smooth and consensual manner (Giddens and Sutton, 2017). Illness is therefore seen as a dysfunction, which can disrupt the flow of the normal functioning of society. Talcott Parsons argued that sickness was a social and not a purely biochemical condition (White, 2016). Crucially, he also felt that individuals could make choices about their illnesses, based upon the idea that the sick role was learned behaviour via socialisation (Giddens and Sutton, 2017). For functionalists, an essential element in ensuring that society is well maintained is the need for individual motivations to be in line with the values of the societal system (Barry and Yuill, 2016). Without this central value system it is held that

(Continued)

(Continued)

society would cease to function, because its cohesiveness could not be ensured. Thus, Parsons felt that people must be prevented from choosing to abdicate from society whenever they wanted, hence his conception of the sick role (White, 2016).

The sick role is characterised by Parsons as a temporary, medically sanctioned form of deviant behaviour, a niche provided for the individual to recuperate from illness free from the stresses of everyday life (Annandale, 2014). The rights of the sick person are that they are not held personally responsible for being sick and are entitled to certain rights and privileges, including a withdrawal from normal responsibilities. However, these rights are founded on the responsibilities to endeavour to get well and to consult a medical expert and agree to be a patient. Adherence to these conditions allows those surrounding the sick person to accept the validity of his/her claims (Giddens and Sutton, 2017).

Reflection

What would you say to Mr Knight's sons in response to them believing he 'plays the sick role'?

Your response might include explaining that you understand why they might feel that way, thus helping to legitimise their view and assist in reducing any guilty feelings. It can be mentally and physically exhausting juggling work and family as well as visiting and worrying about a family member who is seriously unwell. You might also explain however that Mr Knight's behaviour is also perfectly rational. When anyone is unwell it is common to seek secondary gain (Fishbain et al., 1995) by perhaps emphasising symptoms in front of those whose sympathy we seek. You might even take the opportunity to point out that there were bound to have been times when they sought secondary gains from their dad!

While this last comment might sound flippant, and could be interpreted as such if not delivered in the appropriate context, humour can be an effective way of building rapport and, in fact, there is evidence that humour can contribute to a humanised experience for patients and their families, as well as staff. From two ethnographic studies conducted in critical and palliative care settings, Kinsman Dean and Major (2008) concluded that respect for the personhood of individuals was evident in the humour shared with patients. A comment from one patient's wife was particularly notable in that she felt that when staff took time to laugh and joke with her and her husband, they were seeing them as persons and not merely recipients of care (Kinsman Dean and Major, 2008). Humour thus is commensurate with achieving person-centred care. Further to that, the rapport that may be achieved through humour creates trust such that information might be more readily shared by patients and their caregivers which might prove vital in promoting patient recovery. In the critical care environment there were a number of instances of humour being used to relieve tension and facilitate team cohesion (ibid.), important not just for effective team work but job satisfaction in an otherwise stressful critical care environment. After a period of critical illness around 20% of patients are psychologically traumatised in the year after discharge from a critical care unit (Bienvenu and Gernstenblith, 2017). It is speculative that humour while in critical care might prevent such psychological trauma, but at the very least might provide the patient with some happier memories from a difficult time.

Over a few days, Mr Knight was weaned off the non-invasive ventilation, and improvement occurred slowly with the support of effective physiotherapy and nursing care. He transferred back to the oncology ward for continuation of chemotherapy before being discharged home after around a week, to the care of primary care healthcare staff, and his family.

CHAPTER SUMMARY

In this chapter we have, through the case study of Mr Joseph Knight, described how an expert nurse might facilitate the development of a junior nurse to deliver safe and effective humanised care to a critically ill person. While technical critical care can be delivered in a humanised, person-centred way, nurses are trying to achieve this against the obstacles provided by the organisation of healthcare systems such as bed turn-around and staffing levels. We have considered how this might be achieved in what is a highly technical and often stressful environment, for staff and patients and their families. Safe and effective nursing care needs to include knowledge and skills pertaining to pathophysiology, such as the management of haemodynamic instability. But it will only be person-centred if we remain vigilant about caring for the whole person, and not the monitor.

REFLECTIVE EXERCISE 4.1

1 Review Table 4.2: Humanising health care for Mr Joseph Knight and see where it can be added to or amended.
2 Consider what communication strategies you could employ when facilitating junior staff to develop their knowledge and limit their need to prioritise technology over offering person-centred humanised care.
3 Consider how the expert nurse may demoralise junior staff and propose strategies to prevent this.
4 Consider how your staff may have negative views related to perceptions of functionalism and how you may develop their learning.

REFERENCES

Almerud-Österberg, S. (2010) Visualism and technification – the patient behind the screen, *International Journal of Qualitative Studies in Health and Wellbeing 5*: 5223. Available online: DOI: 10.3402/qhw.v5i2.5223.

Annandale, E. (2014) *The Sociology of Health and Medicine: A Critical Introduction*, (2nd edn). Cambridge: Polity Press.

Barnard A. and Sandelowski, M. (2001) Technology and humane nursing care: (ir)reconcilable or invented difference? *Journal of Advanced Nursing, 34*(3): 367–75.

Barry, A. and Yuill, C. (2016) *Understanding Health: A Sociological Introduction* (4th edn). London: Sage Publications.

Bienvenu, O.J. and Gernstenblith, T.A. (2017) Posttraumatic stress disorder phenomena after critical illness, *Critical Care Clinics, 33*(3): 649–58.

Bray, K., Wren, I., Baldwin, A., St-Ledger, U., Gibson, V., Goodman, S. and Walsh, D. (2010) *British Association of Critical Care Nurses (BACCN) Standards for Nurse Staffing in Critical Care*. London: BACCN, Critical Care Network Nurse Leads, Royal College of Nursing Critical Care and In-Flight Forum.

Clifford, G.D. and Clifton, D. (2012) Wireless technology in disease management and medicine, *Annual Review of Medicine, 63*: 479–92.

Delaney, M., Wendel, S., Bercovitz, R.S., Cid, J., Cohn, C., Dunbar, N.M., Apelseth, T.O., Popovsky, M., Stanworth, S.J., Tinmouth, A., Van De Watering, L., Waters, J.H., Yazer, M. and Ziman, A. (2016) Transfusion reactions: prevention, diagnosis, and treatment, *The Lancet, 388*(10061): 2825–36.

Fishbain, D.A., Rosomoff, H.L., Cutler, R.B. and Rosomoff, R.S. (1995) Secondary gain concept: a review of the scientific evidence, *Clinical Journal of Pain, 11*(1): 6–21.

Frey, C.B. and Osborne, M.A. (2013) *The Future of Employment: How Susceptible Are Jobs to Computerisation?* University of Oxford. Available at: www.oxfordmartin.ox.ac.uk/downloads/academic/The_Future_of_Employment.pdf

Gibson, V., Plowright, C., Collins, T., Dawson, D., Evans, S., Gibb, P., Lynch, F., Mitchell, K., Page, P. and Sturmey, G. (2012) Position statement on visiting in adult critical care units in the UK, *Nursing in Critical Care, 17*(4): 213–18.

Giddens, A. and Sutton, P.W. (2017) *Sociology* (8th edn). Cambridge: Polity Press.

Harris, A.M., Atterbury, C.L.J., Chaffe, B., Elliot, C., Hawkins, T., Hennem, S.J., Howell, C., Jones, J., Murray, S., New, H.V., Norfolk, D., Pirie, L., Russell, J. and Taylor, C. (2009) *Guideline on the Administration of Blood Components*. London: British Committee for Standards in Haematology.

Jibril, F., Sharaby, S., Mohamed, A. and Wilby, K.J. (2015) Intravenous versus oral acetaminophen for pain: systematic review of current evidence to support clinical decision-making, *Canadian Journal of Hospital Pharmacy, 68*(3): 238–47.

Jones-Berry, S. (2016) Campaign fights for family access to dementia patients, *Nursing Older People, 28*(10): 6.

Kean, S. and Mitchell, M. (2013) How do intensive care nurses perceive families in intensive care? Insights from the United Kingdom and Australia, *Journal of Clinical Nursing, 23*: 663–72.

Kinsman Dean, R.A. and Major, J.E. (2008) From critical care to comfort care: the sustaining value of humour, *Journal of Clinical Nursing*, 1088–95.

Kotecha, D. (2016) Magnesium for atrial fibrillation, myth or magic? *Circulation: Arrhythmia and Electrophysiology*, *9*:e004521. Available online: www.ahajournals.org/doi/pdf/10.1161/circep.116.004521?hits=10&FIRSTINDEX=130&searchid=1&resourcetype=HWFIG&RESULTFORMAT=&maxtoshow=&

Rattray, J. and McKenna, E. (2012) Person-centred care in intensive care: a myth or reality? *Nursing in Critical Care*, *17*(5): 225–6.

Romani, A. (2018) Assessment of magnesium deficiency, *British Medical Journal Best Practice*. Available at: http://bestpractice.bmj.com/topics/en-gb/1137

Vincent, J.L., and de Backer, D. (2013) Circulatory shock, *New England Journal of Medicine, 369*: 1726–34.

Vincent, J.L., de Mendonca, A., Cantraine, F., Moreno, R., Takala, J., Suter, P.M., Sprung, C.L., Colardyn, F. and Blecher, S. (1998) Use of the SOFA score to assess the incidence of organ dysfunction/failure in intensive care units: results of a multicenter, prospective study. Working group on 'sepsis-related problems' of the European Society of Intensive Care Medicine, *Critical Care Medicine, 26*: 1793–800.

Vincent, J.L., Sakr, Y., Sprung, C.L., Ranieri, V.M., Reinhart, K., Gerlach, H., Moreno, R., Carlet, J., Le Gall, J.R. and Payen, D. (2006) Sepsis in European intensive care units: results of the SOAP study, *Critical Care Medicine, 34*: 344–53.

White, K. (2016) *An Introduction to the Sociology of Health and Illness London* (3rd edn). London: Sage Publications.

CHAPTER 5

Cardiac Failure

Case Study: Michael

SARA J. WHITE AND FLEUR LOWE

CHAPTER AIMS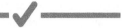

1 To understand the complexity of sustaining a large anterior ST elevation myocardial infarction (STEMI).
2 To appreciate the complexity of an intra-aortic balloon pump and Non-Invasive Ventilation (High Flow Nasal Oxygen and CPAP) used in cardiac failure.
3 To explore the role of the senior nurse in relation to humanising the care of a client in a complex situation and associated leadership and management of staff.

INTRODUCTION

This chapter explores Michael's journey through a complex myocardial infarction, the predicaments experienced by his wife Jean, who stayed with him throughout his stay, and those of the Coronary Care Unit (CCU) staff and the Critical Care Outreach Team (CCOT).

Before we introduce you to Michael remind yourself about Myocardial Infarction (MI), Cardiogenic Shock (CS) and Ventilation/Perfusion mismatch – see Bite Size Knowledge 5.1: Myocardial Infarction and Cardiogenic Shock and Bite Size Knowledge 5.2: Ventilation/ Perfusion (VQ) mismatch.

Throughout the case study we need to remember that whilst these symptoms are occurring Michael and Jean will probably have high levels of anxiety and emotional reactions.

BITE SIZE KNOWLEDGE 5.1

Myocardial Infarction (MI) and Cardiogenic Shock (CS)

MI occurs when the coronary blood supply is insufficient to meet the myocardium's oxygen and nutrient demand. This leads to ischaemia and progresses to myocardial damage and death (Copstead and Banasik, 2007). There are a number of conditions that cause an imbalance between demand and supply such as hypertrophy, vascular disease and atherosclerosis (McCance and Huether, 2014).

MI is subdivided into sub-endocardial or non-ST-elevation MI (NSTEMI) and transmural or ST-elevation MI (STEMI). NSTEMI presents with ST depression and T-wave inversion. STEMI presents with ST elevations. Although both types of MI need interventions, patients with STEMI have a higher risk of serious complications.

MI can cause significant structural and functional changes to cardiac tissues, leading to cardiogenic shock. This is a life-threatening condition involving insufficient blood flow to the body's tissues and organs. The impaired heart function is unable to pump blood effectively around the body causing persistent hypotension and tissue hypo-perfusion, despite adequate intravascular volume and left ventricular filling pressure.

Other pathogenic conditions that can cause CS include sepsis, cardiomyopathy, aneurysm, myocarditis, dysrhythmias, pulmonary embolism and valvular disorders (Grossman and Porth, 2013).

Cardiogenic shock is rare, but often fatal if not treated immediately. Mortality is estimated at 50%. Early mechanical revascularisation is a therapeutic strategy that reduces mortality (Drakos et al., 2009).

BITE SIZE KNOWLEDGE 5.2

Ventilation/Perfusion (VQ) mismatch

The V/Q ratio is used to assess the efficiency and adequacy of the matching of two variables. Ventilation is the air that reaches the alveoli, while perfusion (denoted as Q) is the blood that reaches the alveoli via the capillaries. The V/Q ratio is defined as the amount of air reaching the alveoli per minute to the amount of blood reaching the alveoli per minute. These two variables constitute the main determinants of the blood oxygen and carbon dioxide concentration. In a typical adult, 1 litre of blood holds approximately 200ml of oxygen. The typical V/Q ratio in the lung as a whole is 0.8, though actual values differ between the lung apices and bases and lung positioning i.e. gravity.

V/Q mismatch is a general term for both shunt and dead space. Shunt is perfusion without ventilation, for example pulmonary oedema or pneumonia. Dead space is ventilation without perfusion and is the volume of a breath that does not participate in gas exchange; anatomic dead space is determined by airways anatomy and physiologic dead space is a functional measurement based on the ability of the lungs to eliminate carbon dioxide. Pulmonary embolus is an example where severe respiratory dysfunction leads to a higher percentage of dead space and ventilation-perfusion mismatch as the ventilation and perfusion of gaseous exchanging unit are not matched (Copstead and Banasik, 2007). A V/Q mismatch can cause a type I respiratory failure (see Chapter 3: Bite Size Knowledge 3.1: Type I & Type II Respiratory Failure).

CASE STUDY 5.1: MICHAEL

This case study is about Michael, a 67-year-old recently retired bricklayer, who lives with his wife Jean. He presented as an emergency admission following a sudden onset of central crushing radiating chest pain which extended into both arms and was associated with nausea, sweating and clamminess. He had experienced angina-type pain for two weeks. His past medical history included hypercholesterolaemia and trans-urethral resection of a bladder tumour. He stopped smoking 35 years ago, drinks alcohol occasionally and takes no medication.

Following diagnosis of a large anterior ST elevation myocardial infarction (STEMI) and cardiogenic shock Michael was taken for Primary Percutaneous Cardiac Intervention (Weitsman and Meerkin, 2013; NICE, 2013) with 1 drug-eluting stent to his left main and left anterior descending arteries and intra-aortic balloon pump (IABP) insertion (Fajadet and Chieffo (2012) and Bite Size Knowledge 5.3: Intra-Aortic Balloon Pump).

On admission to the CCU he continued with IABP 1:1, slow intravenous fluids, anti-platelets and boluses of loop diuretics. His nausea, bouts of vomiting and epigastric pain continued until Day 6.

BITE SIZE KNOWLEDGE 5.3

Intra-Aortic Balloon Pump

The intra-aortic balloon pump (IABP) is a circulatory assist device used to support the left ventricle when a disorder causes a low cardiac output; these include haemodynamic support during and after Percutaneous Coronary Intervention, unstable angina, cardiogenic shock, pre-operatively in high risk patients, mechanical complications post myocardial infarction.

The IABP is inserted percutaneously through the femoral artery and positioned in the descending thoracic aorta. The catheter tip lies distal to the left subclavian artery and proximal to the renal thoracic aorta. The tip should be visible on chest X-Ray (CXR) between the 2nd and 3rd intercostal space.

(Continued)

(Continued)

The size of the IABP is dependent on patient's height thus preventing occlusion of the renal and subclavian arteries. Inflation and deflation of the balloon catheter is timed to the cardiac cycle. The balloon is connected to a console that regulates the inflation and deflation with the passage of helium, which easily dissolves in blood and prevents the risk of air emboli if the catheter ruptures.

Inflation occurs just after the closure of the aortic valve, causing an increase in diastolic arterial pressure and an increase in cardiac output. Deflation occurs in systole causing a decrease in aortic end diastolic pressure, ventricle wall tension and an increase in stroke volume. These increase blood pressure, coronary artery perfusion and myocardial oxygen supply, and decrease pulmonary artery pressure, myocardial oxygen demand and myocardial work by reducing afterload.

The central lumen of the catheter allows monitoring of the arterial pressure in the descending aorta during the cardiac cycle. The IABP is able to identify the beginning of the cardiac cycle through a variety of triggers. The choice of trigger varies depending on the patient's clinical situation (Krishna and Zacharowski, 2009; Fajadet and Chieffo, 2012).

On **Day 2** Michael's Oxygen (O2) requirement increased. An echocardiogram showed severe left ventricular impairment with an ejection fraction of 25–34% (normal = 50–75%). He was prescribed anti-platelet, Aldosterone antagonist, Angiotensin-converting enzyme inhibitor and Beta blocker medications and the IABP was weaned to 1:2. However on **Day 3** Michael's blood pressure and O2 saturation dropped and the IABP reverted to 1:1. His CXR showed pulmonary oedema which was treated with loop diuretic and non-invasive ventilation (NIV) with continuous positive airway pressure (CPAP) of 5cm – 7.5 H2O. That night he developed supraventricular tachycardia with further chest pain which was treated with diamorphine, potassium supplements and a class III anti-ar-rhythmic. His cardiac rhythm changed to atrial fibrillation (AF) occasionally reverting to sinus rhythm (SR). AF is the most common sustained arrhythmia in the elderly. It is associated with an increased risk of stroke and those with a history of MI have a higher risk of AF (Krijthe et al., 2013).

On **Day 4** there was no improvement. An arterial blood gas showed type I respiratory failure (see Chapter 3) and a fully compensated moderate metabolic acidosis. Metabolic acidosis occurs when the body either produces excessive quantities of acid or when the kidneys fail to remove enough acid. This leads to acidaemia with blood pH <7.35 caused by an increased production of hydrogen ions or the inability of the kidney to form bicarbonate. Symptoms include chest pain, palpitations, headache, altered mental status, nausea, vomiting, abdominal pain, altered appetite and weight gain, muscle weakness, bone and joint pain. Signs include Kussmaul respirations, stupor, seizures, cardiac arrhythmias and hypotension.

Consequently Michael was commenced on a loop diuretic infusion and 10cm H2O of CPAP and later, when his temperature, C-reactive protein and White Cell Count elevated and he developed haemoptysis, he was screened for sepsis and prescribed antibiotics for a suspected hospital acquired pneumonia (see Chapter 3: Bite Size Knowledge 3.2: Sepsis).

On **Day 5**, when not receiving NIV Michael was hypoxic. He was finding the CPAP mask uncomfortable and not tolerating it by **Day 6**. Later that evening, he was escalated to and reviewed by CCOT and intensive care unit (ICU) specialist registrar (SpR) and consultant; his NIV was changed to high flow nasal oxygen (HFNO2) with 60L/min and 75% O2 with good effect and tolerated well (see Bite Size Knowledge 5.4: High Flow Nasal Oxygen (HFNO2); Continuous Positive Airway Pressure (CPAP); Biphasic Positive Airway Pressure (BiPAP). He remained in CCU overnight in view of transfer risk with ongoing PEEP and IABP. Later that night he developed Fast AF and hypokalaemia which was effectively treated with potassium and Magnesium Sulphate supplements.

Potassium is an abundant electrolyte with 98% found inside the cell and 2% in blood serum. Normal value is 3.5 - 5.5 mmol/l. Homeostasis is maintained through balancing oral intake with renal excretion and by shifting potassium between intracellular and extracellular compartments. Hypokalaemia (<3.5 mmol/l) is associated with a higher risk of atrial fibrillation (Wahr et al., 1999).

Magnesium is an essential constituent of many enzyme systems, particularly those involved in energy generation and maintenance of the intracellular environment. The largest stores are in the skeleton. Magnesium is excreted mainly by the kidneys and is therefore retained in renal failure. Since Magnesium is secreted in large amounts in the gastrointestinal fluid, excessive losses in diarrhoea, stoma or fistula are the most common causes of low levels. Deficiency may also occur in alcoholism or as a result of treatment with certain drugs. Magnesium sulphate is recommended for the emergency treatment of serious arrhythmias, especially in the presence of hypokalaemia (Sica et al., 2002).

BITE SIZE KNOWLEDGE 5.4

High Flow Nasal Oxygen (HFNO2); Continuous Positive Airway Pressure (CPAP); Biphasic Positive Airway Pressure (BiPAP)

Acute hypoxaemic respiratory failure and the need for mechanical ventilation is associated with high mortality (Esteban et al., 2013). There is evidence to suggest that non-invasive positive pressure ventilation (NIV) reduces the need for endotracheal intubation and mortality among patients with severe cardiogenic pulmonary oedema (Patel et al., 2016; Vital et al., 2013; Ferrer et al., 2003; Delclaux et al., 2000; Martin et al., 2000). NIV decreases the work

(Continued)

(Continued)

of breathing (WoB) and improves gas exchange. CPAP is an effective NIV when treating pulmonary oedema associated with left ventricular failure and fluid overload. BiPAP is indicated where, due to hypoventilation, there is inability to maintain adequate gas exchange. This NIV mode increases tidal volumes to a set inspiratory pressure as well as ensuring CPAP.

HFNO2 therapy delivers optimally heated, humidified oxygen via nasal cannula at high flow rates (up to 60L/min). This generates low levels of positive pressure in the upper airways and results in improved oxygenation and may also decrease physiological dead space by flushing expired carbon dioxide from the upper airway, a process that potentially explains the observed decrease in the WoB (Nishimura, 2015; Lee et al., 2013, Corley et al., 2011). It is increasingly used because of its ease of implementation, tolerance and clinical effectiveness.

During the early hours of **Day 7** Michael bled from the femoral artery IABP insertion site. Pressure was applied and the medical and ICU SpRs and on-call cardiology consultant offered advice throughout. He was transferred to the ICU where diuretics were carefully regulated as his cardiac rhythm was very sensitive to hypokalaemia. Low weight molecular heparin was also given. Meanwhile his HFNO2 was reduced to 35% and IABP reduced to 1:3 ratio and removed on **Day 9**. However on he had FAF and was given a cardiac glycoside. His ECG showed ST elevation in leads V2-4. He also needed HFNO2 of 60%; however this was gradually reduced and discontinued on **Day 11** where he received 4L of O2 via nasal cannula. Unfortunately on **Day 12** his O2 requirement and infection markers increased and his CXR showed further pulmonary oedema needing further diuretics and HFNO2 was recommenced (**Day 13**).

During the evening of **Days 14 and 15** he had increased breathlessness and an ECG confirmed further myocardial infarction (12 hour troponin was 887ng/mL - normal = 0.01 ng/mL); he was bradycardic and a vasoconstrictor sympathomimetic administered; a CXR still showed pulmonary oedema and left mid-zone consolidation, consequently he was commenced on 100% O2 via BiPAP NIV and further antibacterial and loop diuretics given.

On **Day 16** Michael had a short episode of asystole requiring chest compressions and an antimuscarinic drug; his intermittent bradycardia persisted and he was dependent on NIV and inotrope. Transfer to a specialist hospital was sought but there was no bed available and consequently active treatment continued until **Day 24** when he was transferred.

During his stay Michael developed pressure sores over bridge of nose and philtrum (Grade 2), and tips of ears (Grade 1) from NIV devices and colloid dressings were applied; Grade 3 on his sacrum. He developed multiple mouth ulcers and on **Day 19** a nasogastric (NG) tube was inserted for administering medication. NG nutritional supplements commenced on **Day 22**.

DISCUSSION OF MICHAEL'S CASE STUDY

So far we are conversant about the clinical aspects of Michael's journey namely myocardial infarction, cardiogenic shock and the Ventilation/Perfusion (VQ) mismatch. We have also explored IABP and HFNO2. It should be noted that considerable developments have occurred during the last 10 years including the widespread application of emergency primary PCI for treatment of patients with STEMI. In addition, the new drugs such as platelet inhibitors and thrombin-inhibitors are increasingly being used and may lead to increased bleeding risks with IABP. As technology continues to develop rapidly, it is essential that centres undertaking PCI and IABP are appropriately equipped and that staff are competent in caring for these patients. This requires a robust training and development programme and an agreed escalation protocol if the patient requires additional organ support. Because of its complexity and potentially life-threatening complications, patients with an IABP should be cared for in a level 2 facility as defined by the Department of Health (DoH) (2000) who define level 2 as: 'Patients requiring more detailed observation or intervention, including support for a single failing organ system or post-operative care and those stepping down from higher levels of care'. As highlighted the first three days of Michael's stay his needs could be met in CCU, a level 2 facility. However, by **Day 4** it was clear that as well as cardiac and respiratory failure he had also developed sepsis, thus his care needs required transfer to a level 3 facility i.e. ICU; 'Patients requiring advanced respiratory support alone or basic respiratory support, together with support of at least two organ systems. This level includes all complex patients requiring support for multi-organ failure' (DoH, 2000).

So this leads us to question why CCOT and ICU staff were not involved with Michael's care until **Day 6** and why was Michael not transferred to a level 3 facility until **Day 7**, despite a clear escalation protocol.

The CCU nurses caring for Michael were competent in the management of IABP and CPAP in relation to its use in acute LVF; however recognition of ventilatory complications associated with ongoing LVF, pneumonia and sepsis required a more expert level of knowledge. The patient was compliant and uncomplaining, which may have masked the critical nature of his condition and early recognition of worsening. However Jean and the nurses became increasingly concerned by his deterioration which resulted in Jean staying by his bedside. This is an example of togetherness as Jean sought to make sense of the situation. The nurses were also concerned and recognised that they needed help and referred Michael to CCOT for help with his ongoing hypoxaemia and dependency on CPAP.

Capability and Competency

Capability describes ability to perform a specified task and over time and practice capabilities can develop into competence. According to the Health and Safety Executive (2017) competence is defined as the combination of training, skills, experience and knowledge that a person has and their ability to apply them in order to perform a task safely. The NMC (2015) states that nurses must be able to safely use invasive and non-invasive procedures, medical devices, and current technological and pharmacological interventions, and, where relevant, provide information that takes account of individual needs and preferences **(NB: from 2019 New NMC standards become applicable).** However is this capability or competence? To be competent the nurse requires in-depth understanding of, and the aptitude to respond to, adults' full range of health and dependency needs. Being able to deliver care to meet essential and complex physical and mental health needs, nurses must be able to provide leadership in managing nursing care, understanding and coordination of inter-professional care and liaison with specialist teams.

Bradshaw and Merriman (2008) argued that when Bradshaw first spoke about competency in 1998 there was no agreed consensus to determine nurses' competence and despite major changes in nurse education and preparation to prepare the 'knowledgeable doer', rather than one who is competent, there is still confusion, albeit that Benner (1984) placed competence in the middle of her novice to expert continuum. Benner (1984) stated that competent practitioners are consciously able to plan their actions but tend to lack flexibility and speed.

Competency includes having the insight to be aware of one's own expertise or limitations and Coles and Fish (1997) feel that in order to practise effectively and intelligently practitioners require a combination of underlying knowledge, critical thinking capacity and attributes that are transferable to different situations and the ability to explain the situation to non-health-care professionals so they can understand what is occurring (sense making).

In 2002 Watson explored clinical competence and stated that it was easier to value and measure scientific and technical aspects of care but the artistic and humanistic aspects of nursing, such as empathy and attentive listening skills, are more difficult to measure. Yanhua and Watson (2011) evaluated clinical competence in nursing and found that whilst competence-based education is evident, the issues related to competence definition have yet to be resolved.

Using Banner's benchmark in Michael's situation, we can see that the complexity of his care needs could not realistically be met by a capable or indeed a competent nurse but needed an expert nurse. Linking this to the humanising dimensions, could capable nurses truthfully enable Michael and Jean make sense of the situation? Also we have to ask ourselves how a practitioner maintains competence and confidence when they are not regularly exposed to caring for patients needing IABP and CPAP.

As nurses undertake more specialist roles, strategies need to be in place to ensure competencies are maintained. This highlights one of the difficulties facing nurses working in specialist roles. Maintaining competencies and meeting the demands of continuing professional development can pose problems. Understanding the realities of these roles and considering how nurses can be supported in practice is therefore a priority. A competency framework should reflect the continuum of development evident among specialities, recognising that some staff may enter specialist roles at a developmental level, progressing to become proficient and then expert practitioners. In level 2 and 3 facilities the staff on duty should at all times reflect this skill mix, so that when a patient's condition deteriorates an expert is on hand to assess, intervene and escalate promptly.

NIV Delivery Devices, Pressure Ulcers and Nutrition

As highlighted Michael sustained several pressure ulcers and as such could not tolerate the NIV delivery devices. Rathore et al. (2016) report that there are many complications of NIV facial masks including pressure-related skin and tissue necrosis and Michael developed pressure ulcers. Thompson (2005) indicates that a pressure of >/= 35 mmHg, which is above the normal capillary filling pressure of the skin, for more than two hours will cause tissue damage and ischaemia. Michael certainly had a facial mask and HFNO2 for prolonged periods and his nursing records indicate that the mask was regularly removed to relieve pressure (although the documentation does not evidence this occured every two hours). A good point of contact for assistance in the trust Michael was being cared for, is from the Respiratory Nurse Specialist (RNS). The RNS has a multitude of pressure-relieving devices, such as a full face mask, and is the trust point of contact should escalation be needed; principles of safeguarding and trust policy state that Grade 3 pressure ulcers need escalating; however, documentation does not indicate whether or not assistance or escalation occurred. There were, however, many contributing factors to Michael's skin breakdown, such as periods of poor skin hydration due to the necessary high doses of diuretics (needed for his cardiac and pulmonary issues and which resulted in hypotension) and lack of nutritional intake.

Reflection

Consider what knowledge you and your team have about what is understood by adequate nutritional intake?

Nutritional Intake

At the end of the case study you will note that it states that Michael did not receive nutritional supplements until **Day 22**. During HFNO2 use there is no nostril for a naso-gastric tube and Michael's notes indicate that he was managing some nutrition and he was prescribed nutritional drinks when in ICU; however his skin breaking down indicates that he possibly had inadequate nutrition. Yalcin et al. (2013) identified that the most common cause for insufficient nutritional practice is lack of nutritional knowledge in nurses.

Generally nurses are taught that adequate amounts of fats, carbohydrates, proteins, vitamins and minerals are essential for normal cellular function as they convert to adenosine triphosphate (ATP) which is the major source of energy for all body cells. Nurses are also taught that the recommendations for a healthy cardiac diet include having regular meals, eating five portions of fruit and vegetables a day, reducing saturated fat, salt, sugar, red meat and alcohol (BHF, 2016; WHO, 2003); and that a poor diet may cause health problems such as blindness, anaemia, obesity, metabolic syndrome, cardiovascular disease, diabetes, osteoporosis etc. but are nurses aware that when an individual is critically ill and nutritional intake is low, catabolism occurs?

Catabolism is a set of metabolic pathways that breaks down molecules into smaller ones that are oxidised to release energy, or used in other anabolic reactions. Large molecules (such as polysaccharides, lipids, nucleic acids and proteins) are broken down into smaller molecules (such as monosaccharides, fatty acids, nucleotides, and amino acids, respectively). This reduces muscles mass as the body searches for sources of energy to keep vital organs functioning therefore turns to muscle mass for those energy foods; this in turn causes excess cellular wastes including lactic acid, acetic acid, carbon dioxide, ammonia, and urea (McCance and Huether, 2014). Consequently providing enteral nutrition early to people with critical illness, such as Michael, may prevent catabolism and reduce their infection risk (Desai et al., 2014).

Indeed NICE (2006) highlight that screening for malnutrition and the risk of malnutrition should be carried out on all hospital inpatients on admission and this should be regularly reassessed, and that nutrition support should be considered in people at risk of malnutrition who 'have eaten little or nothing for more than 5 days and/or are likely to eat little or nothing for the next 5 days or longer' (NICE, 2006: section: 1.3.2). However, they stress that caution should be taken for seriously ill people and that it should be commenced at 'no more than 50% of the estimated target energy and protein needs' to prevent refeeding problems. The amount can increase to meet 'full needs over the first 24–48 hours according to metabolic and gastrointestinal tolerance'. Consequently had early feeding commenced for Michael it may have also helped to prevent weight loss, overcome weakness and fatigue and assist with cardiac repair. One questions if staff needed more education regarding essential nutrition and the benefits because early escalation to the dietician should have occurred.

Leadership and Educational Needs of Staff

We will now further explore the leadership and educational needs of the staff. As highlighted throughout Michael's stay there were safety issues related to the use of HFNO2 and IABP. It appears that CCU staff needed more knowledge regarding HFNO2 and ITU staff and CCOT needed more knowledge regarding IABP. This section will concentrate on leadership and education and what lessons can be learnt for future patient care needs.

Leadership should be demonstrated by all levels of staff as they focus on the needs and preferences of the patient and next of kin. Staff should take personal responsibility for meeting needs whilst adhering to government strategies and policies, legislation, professional codes of practice and guidelines, research and the NHS Constitution (DoH, 2015). In critical care the nurses are the functional heart of this as they give patient and family care a distinct perspective of the outcome of inter-professional practice decisions being made. However, lack of knowledge leads to stress, a feeling of disempowerment and fear (Kendall-Gallagher et al., 2016). In this case study there appeared to be the fear of challenging a decision made by a senior staff. In the care of Michael staff who may have lacked knowledge appeared to be unable to either voice their concerns and/or highlight their knowledge limitations. We recognise that fear and apprehension sometimes limit critical and creative thinking, decision making and problem solving. Subsequently it seemed that ward leaders did not notice staff trepidation and left inexperienced staff in charge of Michael's care; and although once CCOT were involved, and voiced concerns, and highlighted the importance of both knowledge and patient location they were not managing Michael continually and thus the situation did not alter. The Care Quality Commission (CQC) produced 'Fundamental Standards' (CQC 2014) for health and social care staff to measure safety and quality and several of the standards related to the safety and suitability of equipment; staff being properly qualified and trained; adequate numbers of staff; and the development and education of staff which are all key to this case study.

Contino (2004) stresses that critical care nurse leaders need to have divergent, dynamic and inspiring leadership skills as they collaborate with colleagues and peers in the everyday multifaceted challenges. At the heart of leadership strategies and styles is motivation, which is the energy behind performance as research shows that motivated people are more productive than unmotivated people; Bite Size Knowledge 5.5: motivational theories, management theories and leadership styles offers some of the theories and the origins and the facilitated learning explores the way forward with these.

REFLECTIVE EXERCISE 5.1

- Which management and leadership style was adopted by those caring for Michael?
- Which management and leadership style would you adopt and why?
- How would these help to motivate staff?
- Look at the CQC (2012), 'Essential Standards' nos 11–14. What knowledge do your staff need?

━━━ BITE SIZE KNOWLEDGE 5.5 ━━━━━━━━━━━━

Motivational theories, management theories and leadership styles

Motivational theories

1 **Content Theory:** based on why people behave in a particular manner, and divided into:

   Instinct: Flight or Fight.

   Need: Psychological; safety; belongingness; esteem; self-actualisation. (Alderfer, 1972; Maslow, 1943).

2 **Process Theory:** based on how processes work to direct an individual's effort into performance:

   Reinforcement Theory – based on reward and punishment (Skinner, 1953).

   Expectancy Theory – based on how rewards shape the decisions and actions people make, i.e. desire to make effort worthwhile (Vroom, 1995).

   Equity Theory – based on perception of work and perceived fairness (Adams, 1963).

   Goal-setting Theory – Suggests that the expected goal is the motivation, i.e. goal leads to higher performance, or praise or incentives (Locke, 1968).

Management theories

1 **Classical / Scientific / Bureaucratic / Administrative / Management Approach** based on rules and procedures, formal structures and hierarchy, and information flow (Gopee and Galloway, 2014).
2 **Human Relations / Behavioural / Informal Approach** takes account of psychological and social needs of employees (Maslow, 1943, 1987; Herzberg et al., 1959).
3 **Systems Approach** – belief that the organisation can be closed or open with open being one which interacts with its environment by way of inputs, throughputs, and outputs (Miner, 2005).
4 **Contingency Approach / Situational** – effective management is dependent upon the interplay between the application of effective management behaviours (Miner, 2005).
5 **Postmodern Approach** – suggests that all situations need to consider alternative approaches to situation resolution (Patersen and Bunton, 1997).

Leadership Styles include: **Traditional / Formal / Informal / Attempted / Effective / Charismatic / Political / Shared / Elected / Imposed** (see Gopee and Galloway, 2014).

You may have highlighted that possibly staff adopted a classical style whereby they were waiting for instruction from another more dominant professional (Radcliff, 2000), or that there was a breakdown in understanding the complexity of the situation. You may also have highlighted that a traditional leadership style was used when a more informal one may have been appropriate. What you should also have highlighted was that there was a need to educate staff in management of HFNO2, IABP, pressure-relieving strategies and nutrition.

Whilst peer-learning is a rich source of learning it is only appropriate when there are knowledgeable expert practitioners on duty and this was not always so in Michael's case study. Indeed lifesaving equipment cannot be learnt by 'trial and error' when in use and adequate training should have occurred before the need to use them. One could question whether if staff had more knowledge about the equipment it may have been used more appropriately and in a more timely way, and this may in turn have enabled Michael to overcome his illness quicker and prevented transfer to a centre of excellence. Had he had good nutrition, pressure ulcers and pain may have been prevented.

You may have established a lack of knowledge regarding essential standards and made a plan to motivate your staff to enhance their knowledge. Undeniably motivated individuals are more open to change and transition (Sullivan and Garland, 2013) and had this been recognised they might have adopted a self-education approach or as Paulo Freire (an educator and philosopher , a lead advocate of critical pedagogy) stated, 'Knowledge emerges only through . . . the restless, impatient, continuing, hopeful inquiry human beings pursue in the world, with the world, and with each other', but when oppressed there is a fear of freedom to develop and seek alternative approaches to situation resolution.

Let us now further consider humanising health care for Michael. Refer back to Chapters 1 and 2 to remind yourself about the philosophy underpinning humanising health care.

▬▬ REFLECTIVE EXERCISE 5.2 ▬▬▬▬▬▬▬▬▬▬ ▬▬▬

Consider the following:

- Was Michael's care humanised? Did staff enable connectedness, recognising his uniqueness and enabling his need for togetherness with Jean?
- Did staff fully support and enable Michael and Jean to have a broader view of Michael's symptoms and treatment and aid sense making?
- How could staff have enabled them to have a broader view of his symptoms and treatment?

Now have a look at Table 5.1: Humanising health care for Michael and see what we thought. What have you highlighted that we have not and vice versa. Understanding and knowledge are key to the care of Michael and inability to offer this may be seen as dehumanising. Galvin and Todres (2013) speak of capacity to care and how

Table 5.1 Humanising health care for michael

Humanising dimensions	Bio-psychosocial triggers	Managing stressors and coping strategies	Role of expert nurse in support strategies
Insiderness/ Objectification	Michael recently retired and being normally fit and active he was looking forward to spending quality time with Jean and their family. Having sustained a major heart attack he finds it difficult to come to terms with it and the ramifications. During the acute stage of ill health he is dependent on staff.	Michael is given 1:1 care, because his illness needs continuous close monitoring. Michael's family need regular contact and health status information. During deterioration Michael needs continual reassurance and Jean's presence.	Enable connectedness by helping staff understand that it is therapeutic for Michael to voice his disappointment and frustration with his illness.
Agency/passivity	Michael needs bedrest. The IABP limits movement and lying position. Frequent nausea and vomiting, contributing to him developing back pain. Without the NIV mask Michael struggles to breathe and maintain adequate oxygen levels. The pressure from the mask and head straps is uncomfortable. As he deteriorates he becomes increasingly passive and dependant. He allows Jean to communicate his needs.	Michael needs frequent assistance to relieve pressure on his back and sacrum. He needs regular analgesia and anti-emetics. He needs regular breaks from the NIV mask and oral fluid for comfort.	Encourage staff to explore alternative equipment (i.e. profile bed and mattresses), to optimise positioning and comfort. Encourage staff to seek advice from experts (i.e. respiratory nurse, CCOT, ICU doctor) who can advise on alternative NIV methods and more ergonomic masks providing more comfort and suitability for long-term use. Facilitate staff to recognise passive dependence and encourage facilitation of patient participation.
Uniqueness/ homogenisation	Michael complies with all his treatment; despite feeling very ill and uncomfortable from the NIV equipment he does not complain.	Michael needs referral for expert advice and intervention regarding the management of ongoing hypoxia.	Facilitate staff to appreciate that an uncomplaining, compliant patient can be a subtle sign of clinical deterioration.
Togetherness/isolation	As Michael deteriorates, he wants Jean to be constantly with him; he feels most anxious at night.	Jean is very attentive and acts as a spokesperson for Michael.	Assist staff to consider the impact of critical illness for the patient and their family's emotional and psychological wellbeing.

Humanising dimensions	Bio-psychosocial triggers	Managing stressors and coping strategies	Role of expert nurse in support strategies
	This constant vigilance is affecting Jean; she's struggling to cope with Michael's deteriorating health. She becomes increasingly anxious, exhausted and angry when staff suggest she upholds visiting hours and goes home to rest.	They need to be together. Jean's interventions and conversation help to ease Michael's discomfort and anxiety.	Ensure staff are aware of other support (i.e. chaplain and psychologist). Encourage staff to explore alternatives with Jean, (i.e. resting during the day and being with Michael at night).
Sense making/loss of meaning	Michael has been referred to a specialist hospital for ongoing management. Michael and Jean are told of a possible heart transplant. Deterioration and waiting for a bed causes increasing anxiety.	Michael is offered diazepam to ease his fear and anxiety; this he sometimes accepts. His life threatening illness leads to his family wishing to stay.	Enable staff to make sense of: a) the impact on family members when a loved one is deteriorating b) feelings of desperation and powerlessness in coping with finite resources.
Personal journey/loss of personal journey	Michael's optimism and hope of making a meaningful recovery recedes as condition deteriorates. His world has been turned upside down.	Michael needs continuous technical intervention and monitoring. The activities and interaction are repetitive.	Enable humanised care by getting to know who Michael is as a person. Enable staff to ensure Michael has knowledge of his illness, associated care and treatment implications.
Sense of place/ dislocation	CCU and ICU are strange and frightening environments. The IABP and monitors frequently alarm. Michael is disturbed hourly as nurses record vital signs and check invasive arterial catheters.	Michael needs staff attending to his needs who are knowledgeable, competent and confident with IABP, NIV, IFNO2 and arterial lines, and troubleshoot when problems arise, keeping disruption to a minimum and maintaining a peaceful environment.	Encourage staff, and Jean, to create an environment that reminds Michael of home. Check staff have a sound evidence base and competency level.
Embodiment/ reductionist body	Michael's attention is dominated by his bodily needs which constantly remind him of restrictions as a result of the MI.	Staff are focused on Michael's physical signs, symptoms, technical observations and blood results.	Inspire staff to view Michael in a broader meaningful context which includes psychological, environmental, social and spiritual matrices.

capacity is founded on openness and how some practices, such as taking direction from superiors without expressing fear or lack of knowledge, may be based on historical traditional roles and the postmodern separation of science, art and morality. A detailed discussion on this is offered in Chapter 9 of Galvin and Todres (2013), as they explore what they call 'the creativity of "unspecialisation"'and how the head, heart and hand of practices are possibly becoming obscured by the compartmentalisation of specialist tasks – i.e. CCU and ITU roles in HFNO2 and IABP management. So as a reflective point consider if that is what was occurring in the care of Michael maybe.

CHAPTER SUMMARY

Michael's illness was complex and had a profound effect on him and Jean as they both fought for meaning and understanding of the ever changing situation. There were many complications that staff faced as they too attempted to understand the illness and treatments alongside helping Michael and Jean make sense of meaning. Yet these unique experiences provide further opportunities for learning and growth in our understanding of what it means to humanise the care we give critically ill patients. An illness or problem/need is different from one person to another and staff need to develop skills to see outside of the immediacy of the illness and what may be hidden and as such request early help from specialist staff to prevent pressure ulcer development or undernourishment.

The leadership and management skills of staff at all levels need to be developed, as does their motivation for these. Self-development and some of the questions set in this chapter may help in part to develop these and the professional gaze and humanising dimensions of healthcare delivery.

FURTHER READING

Banning, A., Baumbach, A., Blackman, D., Curzen, N., Devadathan, S., Fraser, D., Ludman, P., Norell, M., Muir, D., Nolan, J. and Redwood, S. (2015) Percutaneous coronary intervention in the UK: recommendations for good practice 2015, *Heart*. 101: 1–13.

Biology Boundless (2018) 'Dead Space: V/Q Mismatch.' Available at: http://oer2go.org/mods/en-boundless-static/www.boundless.com/biology/textbooks/boundless-biology-textbook/the-respiratory-system-39/breathing-221/dead-space-v-q-mismatch-840-12085/images/pulmonary-edema/index.html

McCance, K.L. and Huether, S.E. (2014) Chapter 31: The cardiovascular and lymphatic systems.

Sullivan, E.J. and Garland, G. (2013) Chapter 11: Leading and managing change and transition.

Watch YouTube video

Ventilation Perfusion (VQ) Mismatch Explained Clearly by MedCram.com
https://www.youtube.com/watch?v=RJ-H8_0-8wk

REFERENCES

Adams, J.S. (1963) Towards an understanding of inequality, *Journal of Abnormal and Social Psychology, 67*: 422–36.

Alderfer, C.P. (1972) *Existence, Relatedness and Growth*. New York: Free Press.

Benner, P. (1984) *From Novice to Expert: Excellence and Power in Clinical Nursing Practice*. Palo Alto, CA: Addison-Wesley.

Bradshaw, A. and Merriman, C. (2008) Nursing competence 10 years on: fit for practice and purpose yet? *Journal of Clinical Nursing, 17*(10): 1263–9.

British Heart Foundation (BHF) (2016) *Eating Well*. Available at: www.bhf.org.uk/publications/ healthy-eating-and-drinking/eating-well

Care Quality Commisison (CQC) (2014) *Fundamental Standards*. Available at: https://www.cqc. org.uk/news/stories/our-fundamental-standards

Coles, C. and Fish, D. (1997) *Developing Professional Judgement in Health Care: Learning through the critical appreciation of practice* (2nd edn). London: Butterworth-Heinemann.

Contino, D.S. (2004) Leadership competencies: knowledge, skills, and aptitudes nurses need to lead organizations effectively, *Critical Care Nursing, 24*(3): 52–64.

Copstead, L.E. and Banasik, J.L. (2007) *Pathophysiology. Biological and Behavioural Perspectives* (3rd edn). London: Saunders.

Corley, A., Caruana, L.R., Barnett, A.G., Tronstad, O. and Fraser, J.F. (2011) Oxygen delivery through high-flow nasal cannulae increase end-expiratory lung volume and reduce respiratory rate in post-cardiac surgical patients, *British Journal of Anaesthesia, 107*: 998–1004.

Delclaux, C., L'Her, E. and Alberti, C. (2000) Treatment of acute hypoxemic nonhypercapnic respiratory insufficiency with continuous positive airway pressure delivered by a face mask: a randomized controlled trial, *Journal of the American Medical Association, 284*: 2352–60.

Department of Health (2000) *Comprehensive critical care: a review of adult critical care services, and levels of critical care for adult patients*. London: UK Government.

Department of Health (2015) *NHS Constitution*. London: UK Government. Available at: www.gov.uk/government/uploads/system/uploads/attachment_data/file/480482/NHS_ Constitution_WEB.pdf

Desai, S.V., McClave, S.A. and Rice, T.W. (2014) Nutrition in the ICU: An Evidence-Based Approach, *Chest, 145*(5): 1148–57.

Drakos, S.G., Bonios, M.J., Anastasiou-Nana, M.I., Tsagalou, E.P., Terrovitis, J.V., Kaldara, E., Maroulidis, G., Nanas, S.N., Kanakakis. J. and Nanas, J.N. (2009) Long-term survival and outcomes after hospitalization for acute myocardial infarction complicated by cardiogenic shock, *Clinical Cardiology, 32*(8): 4–8.

Esteban, A., Frutos-Vivar, F. and Muriel, A. (2013) Evolution of mortality over time in patients receiving mechanical ventilation, *American Journal of Respiratory Critical Care Medicine 188*: 220–30.

Fajadet, J. and Chieffo, A. (2012) Current management of left main coronary artery disease, *European Heart Journal, 33*: 36–50.

Ferrer, M., Esquinas, A., Leon, M., Gonzalez, G., Alarcon, A. and Torres, A. (2003) Non-invasive ventilation in severe hypoxemic respiratory failure: a randomized clinical trial, *American Journal of Respiratory Critical Care Medicine, 168*: 1438–44.

Galvin, K. and Todres, L. (2013) *Caring and Well-being. A Lifeworld Approach*. Abingdon: Routledge.

Gopee, N. and Galloway, J. (2014) Opinions of families, staff, and patients about family participation in care in intensive care units, in *Leadership and Management in Health Care* (2nd edn). London: Sage.

Grossman, S. and Porth, C.M. (2013) *Porth's Pathophysiology: Concepts of Altered Health States* (9th edn). Philadelphia: Lippincott Williams and Wilkins.

Health and Safety Executive (2017) *What Is Competence?* Available at: www.hse.gov.uk/competence/what-is-competence.htm

Herzberg, F., Mausner, B. and Snyderman, B. (1959) *The Motivation of Work*. New York: Wiley.

Kendall-Gallagher, D., Reeves, S., Alexanian, J.A., and Kitto, S. (2016) A nursing perspective of interprofessional work in critical care: findings from a secondary analysis, *Journal of Critical Care, 38*: 20–26.

Krijthe, B.P., Heeringa, J., Kors, J.A., Hofman, A., Franco, O.H., Witteman, J.C., and Stricker, B.H. (2013) Serum potassium levels and the risk of atrial fibrillation: The Rotterdam Study, *International Journal of Cardiology, 168*: 5411–15.

Krishna, M. and Zacharowski, K. (2009) Principles of intra-aortic balloon pump counterpulsation, *Continuing Education in Anaesthesia, Critical Care and Pain, 9*(1): 24–8.

Lee, J.H., Rehder, K.J., Williford, L., Cheifetz, I.M. and Turner, D.A. (2013) Use of high flow nasal cannula in critically ill infants, children and adults: a critical review of the literature, *Intensive Care Medicine, 39*(2): 247–57.

Locke, E.A. (1968) Toward a theory of task motivation and incentives, *Organizational Behaviour and Human Performance, 3*: 157–89.

Martin, T.J., Hovis, J.D. and Costantino, J.P. (2000) A randomized, prospective evaluation of noninvasive ventilation for acute respiratory failure, *American Journal of Respiratory Critical Care Medicine, 161*: 807–813.

Maslow, A.H. (1943) A theory of human motivation, *Psychological Review, 5*: 370–96.

Maslow, A.H. (1987) *Motivation and Personality* (3rd edn). London: Harper & Row.

McCance, K.L. and Huether, S.E. (2014) *Pathophysiology: The Biologic Basis for Disease in Adults and Children* (7th edn). Canada: Elsevier.

Miner, J.B. (2005) *Organizational Behaviour 2: Essential Theories of Process and Structure*. London: Routledge.

Nursing and Midwifery Council (2015) *Standards for Competence for Registered Nurses*. Available at: www.nmc.org.uk

NICE (2006) *Nutrition Support for Adults: Oral Nutrition Support, Enteral Tube Feeding and Parenteral Nutrition.* Clinical guideline [CG32]. Available at: www.nice.org.uk/Guidance/CG32

NICE (2013) *Myocardial Infarction with ST-Segment Elevation: Acute Management.* Clinical guideline [CG167]. Available at: www.nice.org.uk/guidance/cg167

Nishimura, M. (2015) High-flow nasal cannula oxygen therapy in adults, *Journal of Intensive Care,* 3(1): 15.

Patel, B.K., Wolfe, K.S., Pohlman, A.S., Hall, J.B. and Kress, J.P. (2016) Effect of non-invasive ventilation delivered by helmet vs face mask on the rate of endotracheal intubation in patients with Acute Respiratory Distress Syndrome: a randomized clinical trial, *JAMA (Journal of American Medical Association),* 315(22): 2435–41.

Patersen, A. and Bunton, R. (1997) *Foucault, Health and Medicine.* London: Routledge.

Radcliff, M. (2000) Doctors and nurses: new game, same result, *British Medical Journal,* 320: 1085.

Rathore, F.A., Ahmad, F. and Zahoor, M.U. (2016) Case report of a pressure ulcer occurring over the nasal bridge due to a non invasive ventilation facial mask, *Open Access Case Report.* Available at: http://assets.cureus.com/uploads/case_report/pdf/5246/1484855792-20170119-3063-10n9l9y.pdf

Sica, D.A., Struthers, A.D., Cushman, W.C., Wood, M., Banas, J.S, and Epstein, M. (2002) Importance of potassium in cardiovascular disease, *Journal of Clinical Hypertension,* 4, 198–206.

Skinner, B.F. (1953) *Science and Human Behaviour.* New York: Free Press.

Sullivan, E.J. and Garland, G. (2013) *Practical Leadership and Management in Healthcare for Nurses and Allied Health Professionals* (2nd edn). London: Pearson.

Thompson, D. (2005) A critical review of the literature on pressure ulcer aetiology, *Journal of Wound Care,* 1: 87–90.

Vital, F.M., Ladeira, M.T. and Atallah, A.N. (2013) Non-invasive positive pressure ventilation (CPAP or bilevel NPPV) for cardiogenic pulmonary oedema, *Syst Rev. 2013*(5):CD005351.

Vroom, V.H. (1995) *Work and Motivation.* San Francisco: Jossey-Bass Classics.

Wahr, J.A., Parks, R., Boisvert, D., Comunale, M., Fabian, J., Ramsay, J., and Mangano, D.T. (1999) Preoperative serum potassium levels and perioperative outcomes in cardiac surgery patients. Multicenter study of perioperative ischemia research group, *Journal of the American Medical Association,* 281: 2203–10.

Watson, R. (2002) Clinical competence: Starship Enterprise or straitjacket? *Nurse Education Today,* 22(6): 476–80.

Weitsman, T. and Meerkin, D. (2013) Primary Percutaneous Coronary Intervention devices to prevent no-reflow phenomenon, *Intervention Cardiology,* 5(3): 289–300.

WHO (2003) *Diet, Nutrition and the Prevention of Chronic Diseases.* Available at: http://apps.who.int/iris/bitstream/10665/42665/1/WHO_TRS_916.pdf?ua=1

Yalcin, N., Cihan, A., Gundogdu, H. and Ocakci, A. (2013) Nutrition knowledge level of nurse, *Health Science Journal*, 7(1): 99–108.

Yanhua, C. and Watson, W. (2011) A review of clinical competence assessment in nursing, *Nurse Education Today*, 31(8): 832–6.

CHAPTER 6

Acute Kidney Injury

Case Study: Brian

DESIREE TAIT

━━ **CHAPTER AIMS** ━━━━━━━━━━━━━━━━━━━ ✔ ━━

1 To critically examine the factors that influence clinical decision making and the 'clinical gaze' of nurses involved in risk assessing and nursing people with acute kidney injury and related co-morbidities.
2 To explore perceptions of expertise and how this may impact on patient outcome.
3 To discuss the concept of hope when a person experiences clinical deterioration following a diagnosis of metastatic cancer and acute kidney injury.

INTRODUCTION

In Chapter 2 the complex and interrelated nature of the triggers that lead to critical illness were analysed in the context of holism and person-centred practice. In this chapter the complexity of holistic understanding is further analysed in the context of personal, cultural and structural factors described by Thompson (2016) that can influence how the person as the patient is understood and how this may impact on nurses' 'clinical gaze' and the clinical decisions made. The person at the centre of this chapter is Brian Bennett, a 45-year-old man who was admitted to hospital with a provisional diagnosis of sepsis and acute kidney injury. Brian's co-morbidities on admission included a diagnosis of metastatic melanoma with spread to his inguinal nodes for which he had been prescribed oral chemotherapy.

▰▰▰ CASE STUDY: BRIAN'S STORY ▰▰▰▰▰▰ ○▰▰▰

Brian Bennet is a 45-year-old man who until recently lived in the English Midlands where he worked as a publican for 10 years until he was diagnosed with cancer. Brian has never married and has not been in a relationship with another person for two years. He lived in a flat above the public house and considered himself lucky that the company had kept him on after his partner left. Brian smoked 20 cigarettes a day and drank socially in the bar most evenings. Following his diagnosis of metastatic melanoma and commencement of chemotherapy, Brian found that he was unable to continue in his role as pub manager and within the space of a few weeks he found himself without an income and a home. The only option that he felt was available to him was to ask his mother to take him in while he was receiving treatment. Brian's mother, Mary, lived alone near the south coast, after divorcing Brian's father 20 years ago. She also worked in hospitality, mainly in pubs and restaurants until she retired three years ago and was happy to share her two-bedroom house with Brian. Since moving in with his mother, Brian had been feeling stronger and decided to enrol in the local college part-time, on a management course.

When Brian received his diagnosis of metastatic melanoma (see Bite Size Knowledge 6.1: Pathogenesis of metastatic melanoma) he was referred to a specialist oncologist in the Midlands, close to where he was living at the time. The oncologist prescribed a package of oral combination chemotherapy including Trametinib and Dabrafenib (see Bite Size Knowledge 6.2: Dabrafenib and Trametinib, their actions and side effects, for the related pharmacology). Brian continued to take the chemotherapy when he moved to the south of England. The specialist cancer nurse in the Midlands had a meeting with him before he left and provided him with a resource pack which included information about the drugs he was taking, side effects and a check list for him and his mother to use in order to diagnose any complications early and how they should seek help when needed. In the south of England palliative care services were organised by Mary's and now Brian's GP. Brian remained under the care of the specialist oncology consultant in the Midlands who liaised with Brian directly and via his GP. In the period between his diagnosis of cancer and his admission to hospital (approximately 7 months) Brian had gained 30 kg so that his weight on admission was 105 kg and height 1.8 metres. Brian continued with his cancer medication as prescribed and had completed six cycles of Dabrafenib together with two cycles of Trametinib. Bite Size Knowledge 6.1: Pathogenesis of metastatic melanoma and Bite Size Knowledge 6.2: Dabrafenib and Trametinib, their actions and side effects, provide you with a summary of the pathogenesis and related innovations in the treatment of metastatic melanoma. On the morning of his admission to the emergency department, Brian had gone to see his GP complaining of feeling unwell, shivery and tired, with a 24-hour history of diarrhoea. His respirations were 23/minute, heart rate was 130/minute, BP 123/93 and a core temperature of 40°C. According to the primary care risk assessment tool developed jointly by the Oncology Nursing Society and Macmillan (2016) Brian was presenting with red and amber flags for chemotherapy toxicity (core temperature of 40°C, shortness of breath and diarrhoea). The GP referred him directly to the emergency department, suspecting neutropenic sepsis as a consequence of chemotherapy (NICE, 2012).

Assessing the Degree of Risk for Patients Receiving Palliative Chemotherapy

The risk of adverse effects associated with cancer chemotherapy has been widely published (Brooks et al., 2014; Hassett et al., 2011) and has triggered a number of initiatives that focus on risk assessment and triage of patients with life-threatening side effects (Oncology Nursing Society and Macmillan, 2016) and mobile applications that encourage the patient to feel empowered to risk assess and manage their own symptoms (Maguire et al., 2009). Several studies of mortality within 30 days of chemotherapy have been undertaken using a national database and findings indicate that those patients receiving systemic anti-cancer therapy are at a high risk of experiencing side effects of both high and low severity of risk to mortality (Pearce et al., 2017; Wallington et al., 2016; Mort et al., 2008; O'Brien et al., 2006). High severity side effects leading to risk of mortality within 30 days have been associated with neutropenic sepsis (O'Brien et al., 2006). Recommendations based on evidence of mortality within 30 days have offered information about the degree of risk associated with increasing age, cancer type, whether the patient is receiving curative or palliative cancer therapy, and the organisational and communication factors that can impact on clinical decision making. In Brian's case, he had been receiving systemic anti-cancer therapy for several months, his therapy was palliative rather than curative and there were particular factors associated with location and access to a specialist oncologist that impacted on his care and the clinical decisions made. These factors will be explored later in the chapter.

BITE SIZE KNOWLEDGE 6.1

Pathogenesis of metastatic melanoma

Incidence: The incidence of melanoma worldwide has shown a steady but rapid increase compared to other types of cancer such as breast and colon cancer. In the UK, melanoma is the fifth most common type of cancer with approximately 16,000 new cases diagnosed in 2015 (Cancer Research UK, 2017). The incidence of melanoma varies considerably between countries and according to Leonard et al. (2018) is related to factors such as variations in racial skin phenotype, economy and pattern of skin exposure to the sun, in particular to ultraviolet (UV) light radiation in the UV-B spectrum. They go on to highlight that the incidence of melanoma is prevalent in the young and middle aged population, with incidence increasing after the age of 25 years until the age of 50. There is also a high incidence in 85-89 age group possibly associated with long-term chronic exposure to the sun. Therefore,

(Continued)

(Continued)

in addition to intense intermittent skin exposure to the sun, a chronic continuous pattern of exposure, or UV light from mainly sunbeds, congenital and genetic susceptibility are all identified as risk factors (Leonard et al., 2018).

Pathogenesis: Melanocytes are cells found in the basal epidermis of the skin, the eye and in hair follicles. Their function is to produce and release melanin: a pigment that acts as a shield for UV radiation. In melanomas associated with intermittent sun exposure in the age range of <55 years, the main genetic drivers associated with the initial mutation are the B-Raf proto-oncogenes (BRAF), the most common of which is BRAF[V600E]. These benign melanocytes can remain inactive for years (managed by immune surveillance) until changed by exposure to UV rays leading to further genetic mutations (related to the mitogen-activated protein kinase, MAPK, pathways [MEK1 and MEK2]) and malignant transformation of the benign cells in a birthmark or mole to a malignant melanoma. In summary the key pathways identified in the genesis of malignant melanoma in the majority of cases are the BRAF[V600E] pathway and MAPK pathways. Current innovations in cancer research have therefore focused on developing drugs that inhibit the pathways that lead the development of malignant melanoma and its subsequent spread. These drugs, their actions and side effects are summarised in Bite Size Knowledge 6.2: Dabrafenib and Trametinib, their actions and side effects.

Hope and Survival

The population of people living with cancer is increasing as improvements in early diagnosis, treatment and monitoring continue to grow (Loonen et al., 2018). For example, the estimated number of people living in England with cancer in 2012 was 1.8 million, by 2030 this figure is estimated to be over 3 million (Independent Cancer Task Force, 2015). There is evidence however that many people who survive cancer struggle with the consequences and side effects of treatment (Treanor et al., 2013; Santin et al., 2012). Brian has been given an opportunity to live with and survive cancer because of innovations in treatment (see Bite Size Knowledge 6.2: Dabrafenib and Trametinib, their actions and side effects), although his care remains palliative. In this context it can be argued that hope is fundamental to life (Felder, 2004; Benzein et al., 2001). Mok et al. (2010) argue that hope is both a coping strategy and a factor that enhances a person's quality of life. Benzein et al. (2001) in their study of the lived experience of hope in palliative care found that the patients described 'taking each day as it comes', the participants never lost hope that there may be a cure, hope that today would be better than yesterday and that they had to have hope because if it disappeared there was nothing. This was a small study that cannot be generalised but the consistency and depth of feeling around hope have been found in similar studies (Hall, 1990; Herth, 1989).

In Brian's case his sense of hope had been reinforced by the medical oncologist and the local palliative care team. This sense was reinforced when after he became unwell, his GP recognised his situation as an emergency and facilitated his emergency admission to hospital. Brian knew there were risks, he was anxious, he had lost his home and his job but the reward of cancer survivorship was worth fighting for.

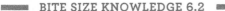 BITE SIZE KNOWLEDGE 6.2

Dabrafenib and Trametinib, their actions and side effects

Actions: BRAF inhibitors such as Dabrafenib, are drugs that shrink or slow the growth of cancer cells in people with metastatic melanoma associated with $BRAF^{V600E}$ cell mutations. Clinical trials undertaken in the last five years have demonstrated that when oral BRAF inhibitors are prescribed in combination with oral MEK inhibitors such as Trametinib, there are significant improvements in quality of life and survival at two years (Long et al., 2016; Grob et al., 2015; Long et al., 2015; Robert et al., 2015). MEK inhibitors are drugs that inhibit the mitogen-activated protein kinase (MAPK) pathways by inhibiting the enzymes MEK1 and/or MEK2 (Leonard et al., 2018). Overall these drugs target mutated BRAF proteins and MEK enzymes that stimulate growth and spread of mutated cells thereby inhibiting growth and spread.

Side effects: Both drugs have a considerable list of side effects and include the following:

- Dabrafenib (according to British National Formulary (2017) and Long et al. (2015)):
  - Common side effects include: Acinitic keratosis (rough patches of skin), alopecia, arthralgia, basal cell carcinoma, constipation/diarrhoea, cough, reduced appetite, decreased left ventricular fraction, dry skin, hand-foot syndrome (reddening, swelling and numbness of hands and feet), headache, hyperglycaemia, hypophosphataemia, flu like symptoms such as malaise, pyrexia, myalgia and nausea and vomiting.
  - Less common side effects include: Nephritis, pancreatitis, prolonged QT interval, renal failure.

- Trametinib (according to British National Formulary (2017) and Long et al. (2015)):
  - Common side effects include: Abdominal pain, alopecia, haemorrhage, anaemia, bradycardia, constipation/diarrhoea, cough, cellulitis, dyspnoea, and hypertension, left ventricular dysfunction, nausea and vomiting, hand-foot syndrome, malaise, pyrexia, rash, > aspartate aminotransferase (AST), > alanine aminotransferase (ALT) and hypoalbuminemia.

(Continued)

(Continued)

    o Less common side effects include: risk of gastrointestinal perforation and colitis, interstitial lung disease, retinal detachment and rhabdomyolysis and > alkaline phosphatase.

- Additional side effects are noted when these drugs are used in combination and these include:

    o Dizziness, hyponatremia, hypotension, leucopenia, neutropenia, thrombocytopenia, muscle spasms and night sweats.

When Brian was admitted for emergency care he looked anxious and frightened. He described feeling confused about why everything was so urgent all of a sudden! On clinical examination he presented with the following:

- Apart from being anxious he was alert and orientated to time and place. He was complaining of a dry cough and was tachypnoeic at a rate of 25/minute. His oxygen saturations were recorded as 97% and he was receiving 2 litres of nasal oxygen. Otherwise Brian's airway and breathing were within prescribed normal parameters according to the Royal College of Physicians (2017).
- Brian's heart rate was elevated at 135/minute, in sinus tachycardia, and his BP was 123/93. He was shivering and had a fever of 40°C. Brian was complaining of flu-like symptoms, aching all over, loss of appetite and general malaise. At that time Brian had not passed urine and he had a history of diarrhoea in the last 24 hours.
- On examination he was sweating profusely and complaining of general tenderness in his abdomen. There was some pitting oedema around his ankles.

In light of Brian's medical history and medication, the admitting team supported a provisional diagnosis of neutropenic sepsis. This was evidenced by heart rate >130/minute, respiratory rate equal to 25/minute, supplemented by oxygen in order to maintain saturations of 97%, and recent chemotherapy as highlighted by UK Sepsis Trust (2017), NICE (2016) and NICE (2017). Brian was for full resuscitation and the Sepsis 6 pathway, according to the UK Sepsis Trust Toolkit (2017, was initiated in conjunction with the NICE (2012) guidance on the management of neutropenic sepsis. Table 6.1 provides a summary of the core investigations and interventions undertaken in the emergency department prior to his transfer to an acute medical admissions unit.

It is significant to note at this point that Brian was not considered for urinary catheterisation and hourly monitoring of urine output. According to the UK Sepsis Trust (2017) and NICE (2017) there is not a specific requirement to monitor urine output hourly with

Table 6.1 Summary of Brian's investigations and interventions undertaken in the emergency room (ER)

Biochemistry and haematology	Biochemistry and haematology cited as out of normal range	Possible causes of abnormal biochemistry	Interventions initiated in ER	Rationale
Sodium (Na): 132 mmol/l Potassium (K): 3.9 mmol/l			Isotonic saline administered IV Monitor Chloride	Brian has elevated chloride levels
Chloride (Cl): 176 (95–105 mmol/l)	Cl: 176 mmol/l	Elevated, related to a change in acid-base balance		
Urea: 9.0 (2.5–7.8 mmol/l)	Urea: 9.0 mmol/l	Elevated, indicative of impaired renal function	Maintain SpO$_2$ >94% with oxygen	Indicative of stage 2 AKI
Creatinine: 204 (55–105 µmol/l)	Creatinine: 204 µmol/l	Elevated, marker for AKI Could be associated with side effects of Dabrafenib and Trametinib	Use of isotonic crystalloids to maintain an equal fluid balance	
Urinalysis of urine passed in ER: Blood ++++ Protein ++	Urinalysis of urine passed in ER: Blood ++++ Protein ++		Urine sample sent for culture and sensitivity Blood and stool samples sent for culture and sensitivity Flu swabs Empiric antibiotics	Identify source of possible infection according to the Sepsis 6 protocol
Glucose: 9.7 (3.5–8 mmol/l)	Glucose: 9.7 mmol/l	Elevated as part of the stress response		

(Continued)

Table 6.1 (Continued)

Biochemistry and haematology	Biochemistry and haematology cited as out of normal range	Possible causes of abnormal biochemistry	Interventions initiated in ER	Rationale
Venous blood gas: pH: 7.44 HCO_3: 24.8 mmol/l Lactate: 1.6 mmol/l			Continue to monitor for evidence of respiratory and/or metabolic deterioration	All appear to be within the normal range No indication metabolic acidosis
Alanine aminotransferase (ALT): 152 (10–40 U/l)	ALT: 152 U/l	Elevated as a side effect of Trametinib Indicative of liver damage		
Alkaline phosphatase 95 U/l				
Albumin 39 g/l				
Amylase 154 U/l				
C- reactive protein (CRP): 204 mg/l (<10mg/l)	C- reactive protein (CRP): 204 mg/l	Elevated, indicative of an acute infection, inflammation or tissue injury	Identify source of inflammation or injury	
White blood cell (WBC): 5.5 x10⁹/l (3.7–9.5x10⁹/l in Males)				White blood cells within the normal range
Neutrophils 4.9x10⁹/l (2.0–7.5 x10⁹/l)				No evidence of neutropenia, therefore not neutropenic sepsis
Platelets 57x 10⁹/l (150–400x 10⁹/l)	Platelets 57 10⁹/l	Thrombocytopenia is a side effect of Trametinib Can also be associated with sepsis		

the aid of a urinary catheter and it is the responsibility of the clinical team to decide its appropriateness based on the patient's clinical picture. Acute kidney injury (AKI) is defined as an increase in serum creatinine of 26 μmol/l or greater within 48 hours; a 50% rise in serum creatinine over an estimated period of seven days; or a fall in urine output to < 0.5ml/kg/hour for more than 6 hours (Kellum and Lamiere, 2013; NICE, 2013). The importance of monitoring trends in urine output over hours and days was significant and in Brian's case (see Table 6.3), he was already presenting with elevated serum creatinine levels that were indicative of a 50% rise over a period of several days and an accurate estimation of hourly urine output over 6 hours would have added to the data confirming the presence and severity of AKI. According to Kellum et al. (2015) following an analysis of 23,866 critically ill patients' electronic health records, those patients who meet the criteria for both an elevated serum creatinine and oliguria had a 50% increase in the requirement for renal replacement therapy and hospital mortality, than those patients who met a single criterion.

It can also be argued that for patients with increased risk of AKI complicated by the use of nephrotoxins, and/or with a deteriorating clinical picture and/or evidence of chronic kidney disease the requirement for a detailed assessment of the patient's clinical and social history, as well as an A to E assessment, is paramount (Kellum and Lamiere, 2013; NICE, 2013). This approach is supported by Hertzberg et al. (2017) who argue that without the identification and utilisation of valid and reliable kidney injury biomarkers, the use of serum creatinine and urine output criteria viewed in the clinical context of the patient are the best ways to inform clinical decision making leading to a diagnosis of AKI. In Brian's case the provisional diagnosis of neutropenic sepsis and associated AKI appear to have been linked to the most obvious cause, that of cancer chemotherapy induced neutropenic sepsis (NICE, 2012) and other factors that may have been impacting on his clinical condition were not reported.

Acute Kidney Injury Incidence, Triggers and Pathophysiology

According to Aitken et al. (2013) and Kanagasundaram (2015) there has been a steady increase in the incidence of AKI compared to 20 years ago, although it is pertinent to note that the population data from the papers studied did not use a standard operational definition for AKI and cannot be compared. In 2012 at the Kidney Disease Improving Global Outcomes (KDIGO) conference a consensus was reached that combined the existing definitions of AKI into a common classification system and this has now been integrated into international clinical guidelines for care and a standardisation of definition, prevention, diagnosis and management (KDIGO, 2012).

Table 6.2 A summary of the severity criteria for AKI based on guidance from KDIGO (2012) and NICE (2013)

Stage of severity for AKI based on either SCr or urine output	Increase in serum creatinine (SCr)	Urine output
1	• ≥26.5 µmol/l within 48 hours • Or: 1.5 - 1.9 times the baseline SCr within 7 days	• <0.5mls/kg/hour for 6 - 12 hours
2	• 2.0 - 2.9 times the baseline within 7 days	• <0.5mls/kg/hour for ≥12 hours
3	• ≥3.0 times the baseline within 7 days • Or: ≥354 µmol/l increase with 7 days • Or: initiation of renal replacement therapy	• <0.3mls/kg/hour for ≥24 hours • Or: anuria ≥12 hours

The KDIGO definition of AKI focuses on clinical diagnosis and estimation of severity rather than on cause or pathogenesis. Historically the classification of AKI has focused on causal triggers associated with where and how they impact on the renal system. Kanagasundaram (2015) describes these as:

- Pre-renal azotaemia: evidence of renal dysfunction such as elevated creatinine caused by a decrease in blood flow to the kidneys and a corresponding reduction of glomerular filtration rate.
- Post renal AKI: where there is an obstruction to urinary blood flow caused by renal calculi or neurological causes as in multiple sclerosis.
- Renal AKI (intrinsic): where there is evidence of renal cellular damage, the causes of which can be sub-divided into:
  o glomerular causes such as glomerular nephritis
  o vascular causes such as scleroderma renal crisis in systemic sclerosis
  o tubulointerstitial disease (involving the tubules and/or interstitium of the kidney) predominately described as ischaemic acute kidney injury. Associated triggers include nephrotoxins such as x-ray contrast media, medications, allergic reactions, ischaemia, sepsis and local infection.

Kanagasundaram (2015) goes on to argue that in many cases pre-renal and renal AKI can exist concurrently and AKI may occur in sepsis without evidence of renal hypo-perfusion. The causes and pathogenesis of AKI are therefore often multifactorial and are associated with a number of factors such as: reduced circulating volume, nephron toxic agents, renal

1. **INITIATION AND EXTENSION PHASE**

Renal injury is evolving and continues to be propagated into the extension phase where there is evidence of intense ischaemia-reperfusion injury

Caused by: Reduced perfusion, toxicity/sepsis

Characterised by one or more of:

A period of renal hypo-perfusion

Evidence of clinical deterioration

Recent history of a nephron-toxic event

Leading to reduced glomerular filtration rate

Duration: 24-36 hours

2. **MAINTENANCE OR OLIGURIC PHASE**

Period of established renal injury and dysfunction

Characterised by:

Oliguria

Elevated serum creatinine and urea

Continued reduction in glomerular filtration rate

Elevated serum potassium

Metabolic acidosis

Overload of body sodium and water

Duration: Weeks or months

3. **RECOVERY PHASE**

Period of renal repair, recovery and return of renal function

Characterised by:

Urinary diuresis

Reduced serum creatinine and urea

Increased creatinine clearance

Risk of reduced levels of sodium and potassium and dehydration associated with polyuria

Duration: Several weeks

Figure 6.1   Phases of AKI (Doig and Huether, 2014; Molitoris, 2003)

vascular disease and sepsis. Doig and Huether (2014) describe AKI as progressing through three phases and these include: an initiation phase associated with renal hypo-perfusion and or toxicity that lasts 24–36 hours before evidence of moving to the maintenance or oliguric phase associated with established renal injury and dysfunction that lasts weeks or months, leading to a recovery phase associated with renal repair and return of renal function that may last several weeks (illustrated in figure 6.1). According to Molitoris (2003) the period between the initiation phase and maintenance phase includes an extension phase during which the effects of the initial insult are propagated and can include a period of intense ischaemia-reperfusion injury leading to the decline in renal function manifested in the maintenance phase. Brian's story focuses on his journey through the initiation and maintenance phases of AKI before his transfer to a specialist renal unit.

It is during the initiation and extension phase that damage to renal function occurs. According to Kanagasundaram (2015) and Patschan and Muller (2015) the pathophysiological factors that lead to renal cellular damage include: haemodynamic factors, renal cellular endothelial injury, tubular epithelial cell injury and the immune response that is associated with the corresponding inflammatory response. These factors will be examined in the order they occur, beginning with haemodynamic factors. It is interesting to note that the focus of this factor is not to consider renal perfusion as a whole but to explore how renal perfusion and the unitisation of energy occurs at different locations in the kidney. For example one area of the kidney that has a high demand for oxygen and energy is the outer medulla where energy is required to maintain the counter-current exchange system in the loop of Henle (Brezis and Rosen, 1995). Any reduction in blood flow and oxygenation of this area will impact on the movement of sodium and water as well as urea (Doig and Huether, 2014). A second area of importance is the effective functioning of the glomeruli. Glomerular filtration rate is normally maintained by ensuring an effective mean arterial pressure and this is achieved by the use of negative feedback mechanisms in human physiology, such as stimulation of the sympathetic nervous system, the renin angiotensin aldosterone system and cellular vasodilatory mechanisms including prostaglandins and nitric oxide. Glomerular filtration is driven by hydrostatic pressure within the capillary bed of each glomerulus. The afferent arterioles leading into the glomeruli are vasodilated in order to allow good flow into the capillary bed and this is achieved by the release of prostaglandins and nitric oxide. The efferent arterioles, in comparison, are vasoconstricted in order to maintain effective glomeruli filtration pressure and this is achieved by the use of angiotensin II. There are a number of factors that can lead to the disruption of these processes and these include: old age, atherosclerosis, chronic hypertension, chronic kidney disease, sepsis, renal artery stenosis, radio-contrast agents and nephrotoxic drugs. Some commonly used drugs that affect glomerular blood flow are non-steroidal anti-inflammatory drugs (NSAIDS) and angiotensin converting enzyme inhibitors (ACE inhibitors). NSAIDS block the cyclooxygenase pathway and the subsequent release of prostaglandins (Rang et al., 2015). As a consequence they can affect vasoactive function at the afferent arterioles of the glomeruli. ACE inhibitors block the effects of angiotensin II and thereby affect vasoactivity at the efferent arteriole (ibid.). Kanagasundaram (2015) argues that NSAIDs and ACE inhibitors are rarely the sole cause of AKI; their effect on glomerular filtration however can exacerbate the risk of AKI on the presence of other factors.

The second pathological factor is endothelial injury in response to renal ischaemia-reperfusion injury. This leads to swelling of the endothelial cells and leakage of fluid into the renal interstitial space. The initial ischaemic effect of ischaemia-reperfusion injury activates the inflammatory response and the associated clotting cascade, leading to the formation of micro thrombi in the lumen of vessels and impaired vascular reactivity to changes in blood pressure. The continued production of cytokine pro-inflammatory mediators (see Chapter 2, Figure 2.3) continues the damage to the micro-vascular lumen.

The third pathological factor is the damage that occurs to epithelial cells in the tubular lumen that can be found in the affected areas such as in the outer medulla of the kidney in the proximal tubules located immediately before the loop of Henle. Histologically the damage may be seen as loss of epithelial brush border in the affected tubules, sloughing of tubular epithelial cells, the formation of tubular casts and potentially some areas of cellular regeneration associated with recovery.

The fourth pathological factor is associated with the immune response triggered by pro-inflammatory cytokines and chemokines leading to increased vascular permeability, an increase in reactive oxygen species (ROS) (see Bite Size Knowledge 2.3: Oxidative stress and reactive oxygen species in critical illness), cell injury and leucocyte recruitment leading to necrosis, phagocytosis and T-lymphocyte infiltration of damaged renal cells (Basile et al., 2012). These factors continue to be maintained until anti-inflammatory cytokines are released (interleukins 4 and 10) which suppress the production of pro-inflammatory cytokines and promote repair and recovery (see Chapter 2, Figure 2.5: The role of some of the key cytokines involved in the acute inflammatory response).

RETURNING TO BRIAN'S STORY

For Brian the evidence of AKI was overwhelming and within 24 hours the clinical picture demonstrated signs of elevated creatinine, oliguria and reduced glomerular filtration (see Table 6.3: A summary of Brian's renal function in the 48 hours prior to admission to intensive care). The damage to Brian's kidneys during the initial and extension phase meant he had moved into the maintenance phase of AKI. According to Basile et al. (2012) the length of time a patient such as Brian would remain in this phase and the potential for renal repair and regeneration are determined by the proportion of cells destroyed or severely damaged and the reduction of any toxic triggers associated with continued damage to renal integrity.

Table 6.3 A summary of Brian's renal function in the 48 hours prior to admission to intensive care

Biochemistry and urine output	On admission	First 24 hours	Second 24 hours
SCr in μmol/l (baseline 81 μmol/l)	176	198	551
Urea in mmol/l	9.0	11.7	18.2
Estimated Glomerular filtration rate (e-GFR) in mls/minute	No record	20	10
Arterial pH	No sample (venous pH = 7.33)	7.31	7.29
Base excess	No sample (venous = -3.2)	−3.7	−6.7
Calculated bicarbonate ($_cHCO_3$) in mmol/l	No sample (venous = 21.4)	21	18.3
Weight	105Kg	Not weighed	Not weighed
Urine output (mls)	50	186	0
Calculated urine output in 24 hours based on KDIGO criteria (Table 6.2)	Insufficient data	7.75mls/hour (For Brian 0.5mls/Kg/ hr = 52.5 mls)	Anuria
AKI severity score	SCr equates to stage 2 severity AKI	SCr and Oliguria equates to stage 2 severity AKI	SCr and Oliguria equates to stage 3 severity AKI
Evidence of failing renal function by e-GFR	No record	Severely reduced renal function	Renal failure

In summary Brian was admitted to emergency care via an urgent GP referral with a provisional diagnosis of neutropenic sepsis secondary to cancer chemotherapy and a subsequent diagnosis of AKI. This provisional diagnosis was modified within 24 hours based on the results of his white cell and neutrophil count which remained within the normal range. A second provisional diagnosis of sepsis with unknown cause was agreed and he remained on the pathway for managing sepsis (Rhodes et al., 2017). After spending 48 hours in an acute care setting Brian's deteriorating clinical picture (see Table 6.4: Summary of Brian's clinical and biochemical picture form the day of his admission to ICU until his discharge on **Day 12**) triggered his admission to intensive care (ICU) where he was commenced on continuous venovenous haemodiafiltration (CVVHF) via cannulation of the right internal jugular vein. Brian continued on CVVHF for 12 days before his eventual transfer to a regional dialysis unit. During this period, Brian continued to take his oral chemotherapy drugs on the recommendation of the oncologist who had initially prescribed the regime. Brian had not been referred to an oncologist in the local area and so in spite of his severe clinical deterioration, he had not been assessed

Table 6.4 Summary of Brian's clinical and biochemical picture from the day of his admission to ICU until his discharge on Day 12.

Biochemistry, haematology and clinical signs and symptoms	On admission to ICU	On Day 3	On Day 6	On Day 9	On Day 11
Sodium (Na) (133 - 146 mmol/l)	132	131	135	133	128
Potassium (K) (3.5 - 5.3 mmol/l)	5.1	4.3	4.4	3.9	4.1
Estimated glomerular filtration rate (eGFR) (>90)	10 from 20	7	11	12	13
Urea: (2.5-7.8 mmol/l)	18.2	22.2	15.3	10.8	15.1
Creatinine: (55 - 105 µmol/l)	551 from 298	693	494	324	473
Urine output (0.5ml/Kg/Hr)	Anuria for previous 10 hours	Anuria	Anuria	Anuria	Anuria
CVVHF	Commenced	Continues	Continues	Continues	Continues
Elimination (Bristol stool chart)	Vomit x1 Type 6 x 2	Bowels open Type 5	Bowels open Type 6	Bowels open Type 5	Bowels open Type 5
Glucose: (3.5-8) mmol/l	8.2	8.0	6.8	6.4	5.6
Arterial blood gas: (pH: 7.35 - 7.45 paO_2:10.6 - 13.3 kPa $paCO_2$: 4.7 - 6.0 kPa HCO_3^-: 22 - 28 mmol/l Base excess (BE) +/-2 Lactate: 0.5 - 2 mmol/l)	pH: 7.34 paO_2: 13.5 $paCO_2$: 4.23 BE -7.9 Lactate: 1.3	pH 7.36 paO_2 12.8 $paCO_2$ 5.2 BE: -0.5 Lactate 1.0	pH 7.37 paO_2 12.5 $paCO_2$ 5.84 BE: 0.0 Lactate 0.5	pH 7.37 paO_2 12.8 $paCO_2$ 4.82 BE: -0.8 Lactate 0.5	pH 7.41 paO_2 13.1 $paCO_2$ 5.42 BE: -0.7 Lactate 0.8
Alanine aminotransferase (ALT), (10 - 40 U/l)	145	213	284	77	53
Alkaline phosphatase (30 - 50 U/L)	83	137	295	298	272
Albumin (35 - 50 g/l)	29	27	No record	No record	25
Amylase <200 U/l	194	1028	1431	1026	727
C- reactive protein (CRP): (<10mg/l)	376	331	87	131	74

(Continued)

Table 6.4 (Continued)

Biochemistry, haematology and clinical signs and symptoms	On admission to ICU	On Day 3	On Day 6	On Day 9	On Day 11
White blood cell (WBC): (3.7 – 9.5 x10⁹/l in Males)	7.8	8.8	11.5	6.2	5.5
Neutrophils (2.0 – 7.5 x10⁹/l)	7.4	7.9	8.0	7.0	7.1
Cultures	No urine or faecal infection	No obvious focus for infection	Ultrasound scan is negative for focus of infection	Echocardiogram Normal – no sign of endocarditis	No changes
Platelets (150 – 400x 10⁹/l)	57	14 (one unit platelets transfused)	136	222	290
Hb (13 – 17 g/dl)	12.3	11.9	8.0	7.9	7.7
Respiratory rate/minute	20	22 Audible wheeze	18	16	18
Oxygen saturation %	95	93	97	97	96
Oxygen therapy	2l nasal cannula	3l nasal cannula	3l nasal cannula	2l nasal cannula	Air
Heart rate/minute	118	128	98	80	100
Blood pressure	96/60	155/89	109/83	110/87	145/82
Temperature °C	36.8	36.8	39.0	36.7	36.8
Fluid balance	Positive 6,000 mls	Negative 500 mls	Positive 668 mls	Negative 359	Positive 11
Mental status	Alert, anxious	Feels tired	Feels tired and shivery	Feeling less tired	Feeling less tired
Pain	No pain	Abdomen tender left side	Abdomen tender left side	No abdominal tenderness	No abdominal tenderness
Antibiotics	Tazocin (day 1)	continues	continues	Antibiotics now discontinued	Antibiotics now discontinued
Dabrafenib and Trametinib	Daily dose	continues	continues	continues	To be discontinued on the advice of oncologist

by his oncology team although they had been in contact by telephone. During this time the provisional diagnosis of sepsis remained despite no evidence of infection in his lungs, blood cultures, stool specimen, urine sample, during a computerised tomography scanning of his abdomen and renal system and an echocardiogram of his heart.

Brian's pattern of tachypnoea, wheezy cough, tachycardia, abdominal pain, diarrhoea and an unstable temperature with spiking pyrexia up to 39°C, continued throughout his period in ITU, together with evidence of raised inflammatory markers and thrombocytopenia. The medical diagnosis remained as sepsis and AKI and it was not until the medical team managed to speak to Brian's consultant oncologist that detailed questions were asked about the side effects of Dabrafenib and Trametinib. It was at this point that the consultant oncologist confirmed that the side effects of these drugs could mimic the signs and symptoms of sepsis, pancreatitis and also cause glomerulonephritis. He recommended an immediate cessation of the chemotherapy and the commencement of steroids to manage the inflammatory effects of the medication. Following a review of the nursing and medical notes the chemotherapy medication had been administered daily without comment and the documented nursing and medical care focused on the care of Brian's AKI and related symptoms.

The triggers and causes of AKI are multifactorial, as discussed earlier in the chapter and there may not be a single trigger leading to the manifestation of this condition. It is important to consider a number of factors and review these during the process of planning care, in Figure 6.2: A summary of the conditions necessary for nurses' clinical decision making in Brian's care and the factors that affected them, the conditions necessary for clinical decision making (introduced in Chapter 1) have been identified and some of the factors that may have influenced the process of nurses' clinical decisions when caring for Brian have been presented. Of these there are a number of issues that will be explored in the context of Thompson's PCS model (see Bite Size Knowledge 2.4). They include the following:

- structural and political factors that drive practice in the NHS such as NICE guidance and a strong emphasis on single system specialisation in a society that lives with polypharmacy and multi-morbidity
- organisational and cultural factors that inhibit effective communication
- the impact of personal and professional knowledge and expertise on assessment and management of care.

Personal, Cultural and Structural Factors Affecting Nurses' Clinical Decision Making During Brian's Care in ICU

In 2009 following a national confidential inquiry into the care of patients who died in hospital in England with a primary diagnosis of AKI, a number of factors that influenced

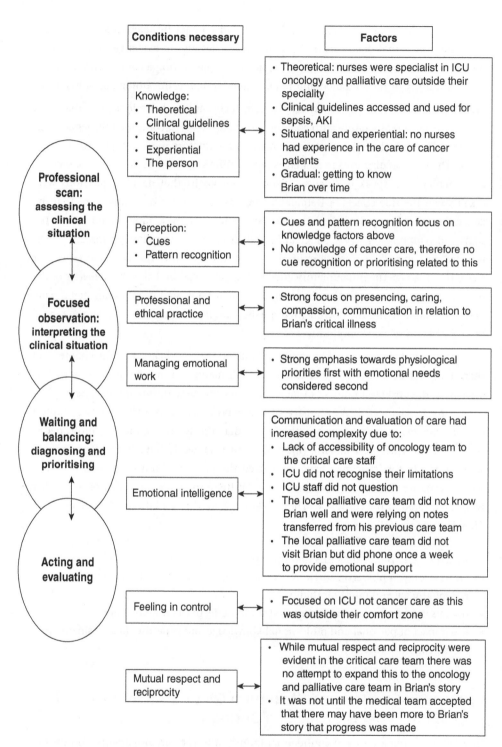

Figure 6.2 A summary of the conditions necessary for nurses' clinical decision making in Brian's care and the factors that affected them

the quality of care were identified. These included factors related to assessment, investigation and management of AKI, where they identified evidence of delays in diagnosis and poor assessment of the complications related to AKI; junior members of the health care team were unable to recognise a deteriorating patient and severity of illness; and organisational factors such as inconsistencies in the availability of referral and support to specialist teams, the availability of renal scanning equipment and inconsistencies in the provision of renal replacement therapy. The recommendations and work following this report have produced a large number of related national and international clinical guidelines aimed at improving the quality of care for people with AKI (NICE, 2013; NICE 2016; UK Sepsis Trust, 2017).

Evidence based practice, described by the Evidence-based Medicine Working Group (1992: 2420) has the potential to:

> de-emphasise[s] intuition, unsystematic clinical experience, and pathophysiologic rationale as sufficient grounds for clinical decision making.

According to White (2016) the increasing complexity of healthcare systems has challenged all members of the healthcare team, particularly nurses, to seek and use evidence based practice. She identifies five factors that have driven this process and these include: safety and quality assurance, the growth and expansion of new knowledge, the delay in transitioning new knowledge in clinical practice, the acknowledgement of the necessity for continuing professional development, and finally empowerment of the service user to question their management. In Brian's case the development of evidence based practice and the adoption of clinical guidelines improved the speed and safety of his care in the context of his critical illness and the evidence based guidance used to support the management of his AKI and possible sepsis was valid and reliable.

According to Benner et al. (2011) evidence based practice, as illustrated in Brian's story, is not sufficient to ensure safe and effective practice. They argue that although clinical forethought, situational experience and thinking in action have less emphasis in evidence based practice, they are still valuable tools in the nurses' clinical decision making itinerary. It is these skills used in clinical decision making that help the nurse to see the patient holistically, ask questions and seek answers. The challenge faced by the nurses caring for Brian was that their clinical situational knowledge and experience focused on his critical illness alone and they lacked the specialist knowledge required to understand the wider picture portrayed.

According to the Academy of Medical Sciences (2018) there is international recognition of the wider challenges associated with multimorbidity. These include recognition that in our increasingly specialised health care there is valid and reliable evidence to support the diagnosis, management and treatment of a single condition in isolation but not how

Table 6.5 The relationship between humanised care, critical illness triggers and the role of the nurse in Brian's story

Humanising dimensions	Critical illness triggers	Managing stressors and coping strategies	Role of expert nurse in support strategies
Insiderness/ objectification	Brian's diagnosis of cancer and his chemotherapy have led to him losing his home and work. His physiological stress response related to these factors would have increased his vulnerability to immune-suppression, and delayed recovery from illness and infection.	For Brian this would have been related to his strategies for maintaining hope.	• To see beyond the diagnosis and use active listening to hear Brian's story. • To collaborate with the palliative care team and ensure consistency of practice.
Agency/passivity	Brian has lost control of his life story. He has had to rely on his mother after managing his own independent life for 25 years. He is at risk of becoming a passive recipient of care rather than a partner in his care.	For Brian this would have been related to his strategies for maintaining hope.	• Work collaboratively with Brian when possible. • Agree short-term goals.
Uniqueness/ homogenisation	Brian's feelings of loss and his coping strategies will be unique to him.	Fostering a sense of safety and comfort.	• Work collaboratively with Brian when possible. • To collaborate with the palliative care team and ensure consistency of practice. • To work with Brian and his family in order to create a sense of safety.
Togetherness/ isolation	Brian has been isolated from his previous life in order to find comfort and safety. Now because of his critical illness he has become further isolated and his life is contained within the ICU environment.	Coping with isolation and loneliness.	• Encourage openness and partnership.
Sense making/ loss of meaning	Brian is unsure of how he has become critically ill and why his kidneys have failed.	Managing information to foster empowerment.	• Provide information to both Brian and his family so that they can understand what has happened and why.
Personal journey/ loss of personal journey	Brian's diagnosis of cancer and his chemotherapy have led to him losing his home and work. His life journey has been interrupted.	For Brian this would have been related to his strategies for maintaining hope.	• Work collaboratively with Brian when possible. • Agree short-term goals.
Sense of place/ dislocation	Brian feels as though he is in transition. He no longer has a sense of home.	For Brian this would have been related to his strategies for maintaining hope.	• Work collaboratively with Brian when possible. • Agree short-term goals.
Embodiment/ reductionist	Brian is in danger of losing his sense of self as disease and its management take priority.	He is more than sepsis, AKI and a recipient of cancer care.	• See the person behind the disease.

each single condition impacts on the diagnosis, management and treatment of another. In Brian's case the treatment for malignant melanoma was relatively new (Long et al., 2016) and had changed his prognosis from poor to good, although still palliative. Equally the chemotherapy drugs were specialised and related specifically to a particular tumour type. As White (2016) reminds us, the delay in transitioning evidence based practice to clinical practice is always evident, and this would have required the nurses to question and think in action in order to provide evidence based care.

The nurses in Brian's story were exposed to a number of structural and organisational challenges in the context of his care; however, professional practice requires the nurse to continually learn and question their practice in order to provide safe, person-centred and clinically effective care (Nursing and Midwifery Council, 2015). According to McCormack and McCance (2017) in order to achieve person-centred practice nurses should develop their self-awareness, clarify their values and beliefs, and have the commitment and inter-personal skills required to provide safe and compassionate care (factors illustrated in Figure 6.2: A summary of the conditions necessary for nurses' clinical decision making in Brian's care and the factors that affected them). There are a number of authors who argue that for person-centred and humanised care to exist there is a need for the local and wider organisation to be working collaboratively with shared values and beliefs and shared decision making (McCormack and McCance, 2017; Stirk and Sanderson, 2012). The challenge for the nurses and intensivists involved in Brian's care was that the special-ist oncology team were distant and unable to visit. Part of Brian's care, his palliative care, had been transferred but decisions regarding the progression of his cancer and ongoing active treatment were still being managed by a team some miles away and integration of the care was limited.

The net effect of these issues was that critical aspects of Brian's care were not considered until the other causes of Brian's condition related to sepsis were ruled out. Brian's care was not considered holistically and in context, meaning that although compassionate and safe care were achieved within the boundaries of critical care practice, the wider picture of Brian's experience of living with and trying to survive cancer in the context of palliative care were not addressed. A summary of how Brian's care could have been man-aged and documented is illustrated in Table 6.5.

REFLECTIVE EXERCISE 6.1

In your practice of managing care in ICU how many of your patients have co-morbidity and are receiving polypharmacy? Select one patient example and reflect on the following:

- How much did you and your team know about the multiple conditions the patient was living with?

(Continued)

(Continued)

- How did you plan the patient's care to prioritise both the critical and chronic aspects of his/her care?
- How did the patient's chronic conditions impact of his/her recovery and discharge from the unit?
- Did this patient have a high risk of readmission to ICU? If so, why?
- Were there any strategies that you could have used to risk assess and prevent a patient's likely return to critical illness?

The answers and action plan generated from this exercise can be used as discussion points for developing your own practice.

CHAPTER SUMMARY

In this chapter we have examined the care of Brian who was admitted with a provisional diagnosis of neutropenic sepsis and AKI. As the story unfolded the complexities of caring for a person with multiple pathology began to emerge and with that an identification of the requirement for person-centred and collaborative clinical decision making. Personal, cultural and structural factors that impacted on Brian's care have been identified and explored in the context of the conditions necessary for clinical decision making.

FURTHER READING

NCEPOD (2009) Adding Insult to Injury: A Review of the Care of Patients Who Died in Hospital with a Primary Diagnosis of Acute Kidney Injury. London. NCEPOD. Available at: www.ncepod.org.uk/2009report1/Downloads/AKI_report.pdf

REFERENCES

Aitken, E., Carruthers, C., Gall, L., Kerr, L., Geddes, C. and Kingsmore, D. (2013) Acute kidney injury: outcomes and quality of care, *Quarterly Journal of Medicine, 106*(4): 323–32

Basile, D., Anderson, M. and Sutton, T. (2012) Pathophysiology of acute kidney injury, *Comprehensive Physiology, 2*(2): 1303–53.

Benner, P., Hooper Kyriakidis, P. and Stannard, D. (2011) *Clinical Wisdom and Interventions in Acute and Critical Care – A Thinking in Action Approach* (2nd edn). New York: Springer Publishing Company.

Benzein, E., Norberg, A. and Saveman, B. (2001) The meaning of the lived experience of hope in patients with cancer in palliative home care, *Palliative Medicine, 15*: 117–26.

Brezis, M. and Rosen, S. (1995) Hypoxia of the renal medulla – its implications for disease, *New England Journal of Medicine, 332*: 647–55.

British National Formulary (2017) *BNF 74, September 2017–March 2018*. London: BMJ Group and Pharmaceutical Press.

Brooks, G., Abrams, T., Meyerhardt, J., Enzinger, P.C., Sommer, K., Dalby, C.K., Uno, H., Jacobson, J.O., Fuchs, C.S. and Schrag, D. (2014) Identification of potentially avoidable hospitalizations in patients with GI cancer, *Journal of Clinical Oncology*, *32*(6): 496–503.

Cancer Research UK (2017) Skin cancer statistics, available at: www.cancerresearchuk.org/health-professional/cancer-statistics/statistics-by-cancer-type/skin-cancer [accessed 8 April 2018].

Doig, A. and Huether, S. (2014) Alterations of renal and urinary tract function, in McCance, K. and Huether, S. *Pathophysiology: the biological basis for disease in adults and children* (7th en). St Louis, MO: Elsevier Mosby.

Evidence-based Medicine Working Group (1992) Evidence-based medicine: a new approach to teaching the practice of medicine, *Journal of the American Medical Association*, *268*(17): 2420–5.

Felder, B. (2004) Hope and coping in patients with a cancer diagnosis, *Cancer Nurse*, *27*: 320–4.

Grob, J.J., Amonkar, M.M., Karaszewska, B., Schachter, J., Dummer, R., Mackiewicz, A., Stroyakovskiy, D., Drucis, K., Grange, F., Chiarion-Sileni, V., Rutkowski, P., Lichinitser, M., Levchenko, E., Wolter, P., Hauschild, A., Long, G.V., Nathan, P., Ribas, A., Flaherty, K., Sun, P., Legos, J.J., McDowell, D.O., Mookerjee, B., Schadendorf, D. and Robert, C. (2015) Comparison of dabrafenib and trametinib combination therapy with vemurafenib monotherapy on health-related quality of life in patients with unresectable or metastatic cutaneous BRAF Val600-mutation-positive melanoma (COMBI-v): results of a phase 3, open-label, randomised trial, *Lancet Oncology*, *16*: 1389–98.

Hall, B. (1990) The struggle of the diagnosed terminally ill person to maintain hope, *Nursing Science Quarterly*, *3*: 177–84.

Hassett, M., Rao, S., Brozovic, S., Stahl, J.E., Schwartz, J.H., Maloney, B. and Jacobsond, J.O. (2011) Chemotherapy-related hospitalization among community cancer centre patients, *Oncologist*, *16*(3): 378–87.

Herth, K. (1989) Hope and coping in patients with cancer diagnosis, *Oncology Nursing Forum*, *16*: 67–72.

Hertzberg, D., Ryden, L., Pickering, J.W., Sartipy, U. and Holzmann, M.J. (2017) Acute kidney injury – an overview of diagnostic methods and clinical management, *Clinical Kidney Journal*, *10*(3): 323–31.

Independent Cancer Task Force (2015) *Achieving World Class Cancer Outcomes: A Strategy for England 2015–202*. Available at: www.cancerresearchuk.org/sites/default/files/achieving_world-class_cancer_outcomes_-_a_strategy_for_england_2015-2020.pdf

Kanagasundaram, N. (2015) Pathophysiology of ischaemic acute kidney injury, *Annals of Clinical Biochemistry*, *52*(2): 193–205.

Kellum, J and Lameire, N., for the KDIGO AKI working group. (2013) Diagnosis, evaluation and management of acute kidney injury: a KDIGO summary (Part 1), *Critical Care*, *17*(204): 1–15.

Kellum, J., Sileanu, F., Murugan, R., Lucko, N., Shaw, A.D., and Clermont, G. (2015) Classifying AKI by urine output versus serum creatinine level, *Journal of the American Society of Nephrology, 26*: 2231–8.

KDIGO (2012) KDIGO Clinical Practice Guidelines for Acute Kidney Injury. *Kidney International 2 (supplement), 2*(1): 1–138.

Leonard, G., Falzone, L., Salemi, R., Zanghi, A., Spandidos, D.A., McCubrey, J.A., Candido, S., and Libra, M. (2018) Cutaneous melanoma: from pathogenesis to therapy (review), *International Journal of Oncology, 52*: 1071–80.

Long, G., Grob, J., Nathan, P., Ribas, A., Robert, C., Schadendorf, D., Lane, S.R., Mak, C., Legenne, P., Flaherty, K.T. and Davies, M. (2016) Factors predictive of response, disease progression and overall survival after dabrafenib and trametinib combination treatment: a pooled analysis of individual patient data from randomised trials, *Lancet Oncology, 17*: 1743–54.

Long, G.V., Stroyakovskiy, D., Gogas, H., Levchenko, .E., de Braud, F., Larkin, J., Garbe, C., Jouary, T., Hauschild, A., Grob, J.J., Chiarion-Sileni, V., Lebbe, C., Mandalà, M., Millward, M., Arance, A., Bondarenko, I., Haanen, J.B., Hansson, J., Utikal, J., Ferraresi, V., Kovalenko, N., Mohr, P., Probachai, V., Schadendorf, D., Nathan, P., Robert, C., Ribas, A., DeMarini, D., Irani, J.G., Swann, S., Legos, J.J., Jin, F., Mookerjee, B. and Flaherty, K. (2015) Dabrafenib and trametinib versus dabrafenib and placebo for Val600 BRAF mutant melanoma: a multicentre, double blind, phase 3 randomised controlled trial, *Lancet, 386*: 444–51.

Loonen, J., Blijlevens, N., Prins, J., Dona, D., Den Hartogh, J., Senden, T., van Dulmen-Den Broeder, E, van der Velden, K. and Hermens, R. (2018). Cancer suvivership care: person centred care in a multidisciplinary shared model. *International Journal of Integrated Care, 18*(1): 4.

Maguire, R., Cowie, J., Leadbetter, C., McCall, K., Swingler, K., McCann, L. and Kearney, N. (2009) The development of a side effect risk assessment tool (ASyMS (c)-SERAT) for use in patients with breast cancer undergoing adjuvant chemotherapy, *Journal of Research in Nursing, 14*(1): 27–40.

McCormack, B. and McCance, T. (2017) *Person-centred Practice in Nursing and Health Care: Theory and Practice* (2nd edn). Chichester: Wiley Blackwell.

Mok, E., Lau, K. and Lam, W. (2010) Health care professional's perspective on hope in the palliative care setting, *Journal of Palliative Medicine, 13*(7): 877–83.

Molitoris, B. (2003) Transitioning to therapy in ischaemic acute renal failure [comment], *Journal of the American Society of Nephrology, 14*: 265–7.

Mort, D., Lansdown, M., Smith, N., Protopapa, K. and Mason, M. (2008) *Systemic Anti-cancer Therapy: For Better, for Worse?* National Confidential Inquiry into Patient Outcomes and Death. Available at: www.ncepod.org.uk/2008sact.html [accessed 18 April 2018].

National Institute for Health and Care Excellence (NICE) (2012) *Neutropenic Sepsis: Prevention and Management in People with Cancer: Clinical Guideline 151*. Available at: www.nice.org.uk/guidance/cg151 [accessed 15 April 2018].

National Institute for Health and Care Excellence (NICE) (2013) *Acute Kidney Injury: Prevention, Detection and Management: CG169*. Available at: www.nice.org.uk/guidance/qs76 [accessed 15 April 2018].

National Institute for Health and Care Excellence (NICE) (2016) *Sepsis Recognition, Diagnosis and Early Management: NG 51*. Available at: www.nice.org.uk/guidance/ng51 [accessed 15 April 2018].

National Institute for Health and Care Excellence (NICE) (2017) *Sepsis Risk Stratification Tools*, Available at: www.nice.org.uk/guidance/ng51/resources/algorithms-and-risk-stratification-tables-compiled-version-2551488301 [accessed 15 April 2018].

Nursing and Midwifery Council (2015) *The Code for Nurses and Midwives*. Available at: www.nmc.org.uk/globalassets/sitedocuments/nmc-publications/nmc-code.pdf [accessed 23 April 2018].

O'Brien, M., Borthwick, A., Rigg, A., Leary, A., Assersohn, L., Last, K., Tanm, S., Milan, S., Tait, D. and Smith, I.E. (2006) Mortality within 30 days of chemotherapy: a clinical governance benchmarking issue for oncology patients, *British Journal of Cancer, 95*: 1632–6.

Oncology Nursing Society and Macmillan (2016) *Oncology/Haematology 24 Hour Triage: Rapid Assessment and Access Tool Kit*. Oncology Nursing Society and Macmillan.

Patschan, D. and Muller, G. (2015) Acute kidney injury, *Journal of Injury and Violence Research, 7*(1): 19–26.

Pearce, A., Haas, M., Viney, R., Pearson, S., Haywood, P., Brown, C. and Ward, R. (2017) Incidence and severity of self-reported chemotherapy side effects in routine care: a prospective cohort study, *PLOS ONE, 12*(10): 1–12.

Rang, H., Dale, M., Ritter, J., Flower, R.J. and Henderson, G. (2015) *Rang and Dale's Pharmacology* (8th edn). Edinburgh: Elsevier, Churchill Livingstone.

Rhodes, A., Evans, L.E., Alhazzani, W., Levy, M.M., Antonelli, M., Ferrer, R., Kumar, A., Sevransky, J.E., Sprung, C.L., Nunnally, M.E., Rochwerg, B., Rubenfeld, G.D., Angus, D.C., Annane, D., Beale, R.J., Bellinghan, G.J., Bernard, G.R., Chiche, J.D., Coopersmith, C., De Backer, D.P., French, C.J., Fujishima , S., Gerlach, H., Hidalgo, J.L., Hollenberg, S.M., Jones, A.E., Karnad, D.R., Kleinpell, R.M., Koh, Y., Lisboa, T.C., Machado, F.R., Marini, J.J., Marshall, J.C., Mazuski, J.E., McIntyre, L.A., McLean, A.S., Mehta, S., Moreno, R.P., Myburgh, J., Navalesi, P., Nishida, O., Osborn, T.M., Perner, A., Plunkett, C.M., Ranieri, M., Schorr, C.A., Seckel, M.A., Seymour, C.W., Shieh, L., Shukri, K. A., Simpson, S.Q., Singer, M., Thompson, B.T., Townsend, S.R., Van der Poll, T., Vincent, J.L., Wiersinga, W.J., Zimmerman, J.L. and Dellinger, R.P. (2017) Surviving Sepsis Campaign: international guidelines for management of sepsis and septic shock: 2016, *Intensive Care Medicine, 43*: 304–77.

Robert, C., Karaszewska, B., Schachter, J., Rutkowski, P., Mackiewicz, A., Stroiakovski, D., Lichinitser, M., Dummer, R., Grange, F., Mortier, L., Chiarion-Sileni, V. and Druci, K. (2015) Improved overall survival in melanoma with combined dabrafenib and trametinib, *New England Journal of Medicine, 372*(1): 30–9.

Royal College of Physicians (2017) *National Early Warning Score (NEWS) 2: Standardising the Assessment of Acute Illness Severity in the NHS*. London: Royal College of Physicians, Available at: www.rcplondon.ac.uk/projects/outputs/national-early-warning-score-news-2 [accessed 15 April 2018].

Santin, O., Mills, M., Treanor, C. and Donnelly, M. (2012) A comparative analysis of the health and wellbeing of cancer survivors to the general population, *Support Care Cancer, 20*: 2545–52.

Stirk, S. and Sanderson, H. (2012) *Creating Person-centred Organisations: Strategies and Tools for Managing Change in Health and Social Care and the Voluntary Sector*. London: Jessica Kingsley Publishers.

The Academy of Medical Sciences (2018) *Multi-morbidity: A Priority for Global Health Research*. London: Academy of Medical Sciences.

Thompson, N. (2016) *Anti-discriminatory Practice* (6th edn). London: Palgrave.

Treanor, C., Santin, O., Mills, M. and Donnelly, M. (2013) Cancer survivors with self-reported late effects: their health status, care needs and service utilisation, *Psycho Oncology, 22*: 2428–35.

UK Sepsis Trust (2017) Education and clinical tools Available at: https://sepsistrust.org/education/clinical-tools/ [accessed 21 June 2018].

Wallington, M., Saxon, E., Bomb, M., Smittenaar, R., Wickenden, M., McPhail, S., Rashbass, J., Chao, D., Dewar, J., Talbot, D., Peake, M., Perren, T., Wilson, C. and Dodwell, D. (2016) 30 day mortality after systemic anti-cancer treatment for breast and lung cancer in England: a population based, observational study, *Lancet Oncology, 17*: 1203–16.

White, K. (2016) *Evidence-based Practice, in Translation of Evidence into Nursing and Health Care* (2nd edn). New York: Springer.

CHAPTER 7

Gastrointestinal Disorder

Case Study: Rebecca

SARA J. WHITE AND FLEUR LOWE

CHAPTER AIMS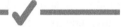

1 To understand Rebecca's experiences of Inflammatory Bowel disease, GI bleeding, Colitis and pelvic pain.
2 To explore how IBD affects sleep, anxiety and mood.
3 To appreciate how multiple ward transfers and moving patients at night impacts on recovery.
4 To realise the impact of caregiving on the family.

INTRODUCTION

This chapter explores how Rebecca, a 45-year-old lady, and her partner (Simon) manage chronic ill health and multiple needs, predominantly focusing on her gastric health needs. It will also explore how multiple ward transfers have the potential for missed care and how moving patients at night is detrimental to their sleep quality; it also explores the impact on the caregiver.

Before we introduce Rebecca's story let us first remind ourselves of risk factors associated with Gastrointestinal bleeding (GI).

GASTROINTESTINAL (GI) BLEED RISK FACTORS

Upper or lower GI bleeding is a symptom of many conditions. Non-variceal upper gastrointestinal bleeding (UGIB) is a significant problem worldwide despite decreasing numbers. NICE (2016) highlights that peptic ulcer disease is the most common pathology underlying upper gastrointestinal bleeding and occurs in 35–50% of cases, with acute UGIB having a

10% hospital mortality rate. A significant risk factor for non-variceal upper GI bleed is medications such as nonsteroidal anti-inflammatory drugs (NSAIDs), aspirin, selective serotonin reuptake inhibitors, and other antiplatelet and anticoagulant medications. Other risk factors include: Peptic ulcers, Gastritis, Oesophageal varices, Mallory-Weiss tear, Cancer, Helicobacter pylori infection. In patients with cardiovascular disease and kidney disease, UGIB tends to be more severe and has greater morbidity. UGIB carries significant morbidity and mortality. NICE (2017a) states that in approximately a fifth of cases no cause for UGIB is found. One of the most common causes of lower GI bleeding (LGIB) is diverticulosis. Griffiths (2017) quotes figures for Western countries being 5% of the population by the age of 40, 25% by the age of 60 and 65% at 85 years. In England and Wales this is over 5 million people. It affects men and women equally. Most people who have diverticulosis do not have any symptoms. When diverticulosis causes symptoms, diverticular disease symptoms include constipation, cramps, bloating, and painless bleeding from the rectum. Diverticular disease also includes diverticulitis (when diverticula become inflamed or infected) and symptoms include abdominal pain (usually left sided), fever, nausea, vomiting, cramps and constipation. Possible complications include Abscess, Stricture, Perforation, Peritonitis, Fistula (between the colon and the bladder, small intestine, vagina, or skin) (Thompson, 2016). Other risk factors are Inflammatory Bowel Disease (Ulcerative Colitis, Crohn's disease, microscopic colitis, and pouchitis), Angiodysplasia, Intestinal polyps, Haemorrhoids. (NB: several conditions that can cause similar symptoms to IBD but are not IBD include: infections, drug-induced colitis, coeliac disease and irritable bowel syndrome). The natural history of IBD is complicated and requires frequent hospital admissions and surgery. IBD has major impact on health-related quality of life as it impacts on individuals' relationships, career and mental health. Below we shall discuss sleep, anxiety and mood. First however, let's have an overview of Rebecca.

CASE STUDY 7.1: REBECCA

Rebecca is a 45-year-old lady who lives with her long-term partner and main carer, Simon. She is a non-smoker and drinks minimal alcohol. Due to a weak left leg she uses a wheelchair. She receives a one morning per week care package. Rebecca's past medical history is in Box 7.1 below.

BOX 7.1

Rebecca's past medical history

- diverticular disease/ulcerative colitis
- stroke
- asthma
- myocardial infarction

- coronary artery bypass graft
- hypertension
- prinz metal angina
- hypercholesterolaemia
- high BMI
- low mood
- posterior pelvic floor repair for rectocele (3 weeks ago).

Rebecca's Polypharmacy

- amlodipine
- bumetanide
- clopidogrel
- lansoprazole
- mirtazapine
- monomax
- rosuvastatin
- solifenacin.

Allergies = morphine and penicillin.

Two weeks ago Rebecca was diagnosed with Ulcerative Colitis (see Bite Size Knowledge 7.1: Colitis causes and signs and symptoms) and she presented to ED with sudden onset of vomiting and left iliac fossa pain radiating through to her back since the morning, and worse on eating and movement. A longstanding supra pubic catheter was draining well and she had normal bowel motions until the onset of pain. Observations are within normal parameters. On admission, bloods showed several abnormalities (see Box 7.2: Abnormal Blood Results on Admission).

▬▬ BOX 7.2 ▬▬

Abnormal blood result on admission

- Lactate: 2.4 mmols/L
- Base excess: -6.2
- pH: 7.591.
- HCO_3: 20.9 mmols/L
- CO_2: 2.29 kPa
- WCC: 16.3 x 10^9/L
- Neutrophilia: 14.5 x 10^9/L
- GGT: 209 IU/L.

On examination the abdomen was generally tender, soft, non-peritonitic and bowel sounds are heard. A rectal examination revealed an empty rectum with no blood present. A small amount of yellow discharge from around the catheter site was noted and a swab sent for microscopy culture and sensitivities. Differential diagnoses included exacerbation of diverticular disease, ischaemic colitis, renal colic and complication from the pelvic floor repair.

She was referred to the general surgical and gynaecological teams and admitted to a surgical ward with an ongoing plan of analgesia, intravenous antibiotics and fluids.

A CT showed abnormal right hemi-colon with features in keeping with colitis. Aetiology could have been inflammatory, infective or ischaemic. A few diverticular were seen in the large bowel. She developed type 7 diarrhoea and was reviewed by a consultant surgeon and was commenced on oral metronidazole; a stool sample was sent for C.diff, salmonella and shigella.

A consultant gynaecologist review noted that Rebecca was sexually active; that she had irregular periods but had not had a recent smear test; a vaginal examination was normal – however, due to the pain a swab was sent to exclude sexually transmitted disease such as chlamydia. Because of the diarrhoea Rebecca was admitted to a side room on an orthopaedic ward.

On **Day 2** Rebecca was reviewed by the consultant surgeon; her diarrhoea was settling but she still had intermittent pain and bilious vomiting.

On **Day 3** Rebecca still had intermittent acute pain. She was reviewed by a gastroenterology specialist registrar and the gastric team took over her care. Her hypotension was treated with IV fluids and antihypertensive medication was omitted. Her stool culture returned a negative result.

A CT angiogram performed on **Day 5** was normal and she was prescribed IV steroids. By **Day 7** Rebecca's pain and diarrhoea settled and her appetite returned and she was transferred to a gastroenterology ward. Here she was reviewed (on **Day 8**) by a clinical nurse specialist for irritable bowel disease and was prescribed Mesalazine.

On **Day 10** Rebecca experienced sharp inspiratory pain radiating to posterior shoulder and was short of breath (SOB). A treatment dose of low molecular weight heparin was commenced and a CT pulmonary angiography booked. Later that evening she passed approximately 500mls of malaena; she felt clammy and dizzy and was hypotensive. Her Blatchford score was 11 and Rockall score was 4. Later that night she developed cramping abdominal pain, had three more episodes of malaena with fresh clots; she had central chest pain, nausea and was SOB, she was clammy, pale, hypotensive and her pulse was thready. Her ECG was normal. The Haematology consultant suggested treating with 3 litres of IV crystalloid, 2 units of RBC, 2 units of platelets, Tranexamic acid, Vitamin K and Protamine Sulfate. Clopidogrel was withheld. (See Box 7.3: Blood Results on Day 10).

BOX 7.3

Blood results on Day 10

- K 2.8 mmol/L
- Na 138 mmol/L
- Urea 7.7 mmol/L
- Creat 61 mmol/L
- eGFR 106
- Hb 89
- MCV 76
- Plt 477 g/L x 10^9/L
- WBC 18.9 x 10^9/L
- Troponin <13
- Lactate 2.3 mmols/L.

On **Day 11**, following two episodes of large volume malaena with an HB drop to 75, Rebecca was treated with 3 units of RBC. Central venous access was obtained and she was admitted to intensive care for invasive monitoring. An Oesophago-Gastro Duodenoscopy (OGD) and computed tomography pulmonary angiogram (CTPA) were normal. A contrast abdominal CT showed a thickening of the wall of the caecum and proximal colon, but no obvious bleeding point. Following this treatment **Days 12–14** were uneventful and although weak and lethargic she was comfortable and was transferred to a surgical ward. However on **Day 15** she was transferred back to the gastro ward and was rehabilitated and discharged home.

BITE SIZE KNOWLEDGE 7.1

Colitis causes and signs and symptoms

Colitis is inflammation of the inner lining of the colon. It may be an acute short-term condition or chronic and life-long.
Causes include:

- infection
- inflammatory bowel disease such as crohn's and ulcerative colitis (UC)
- ischaemic colitis
- allergic reactions
- microscopic colitis (Wedro, 2017).

(Continued)

(Continued)

Symptoms and associated symptoms include:

- abdominal pain
- bloating, cramping
- diarrhoea with or without blood in the stool
- fever
- chills
- fatigue
- dehydration.

UC and Crohn's symptoms can also include:

- iritis
- joint swelling
- aphthous mouth ulcer
- pyoderma gangrenosum.

Infective causes include:

- C. Difficile
- campylobacter
- shigella
- E.coli
- Yersinia
- salmonella
- viruses
- parasites.

Risk factors: Ischaemia caused by:

- decreased blood supply from hypotension
- mechanical obstruction
- anaemia
- age
- heart disease
- non-anticoagulated atrial fibrillation (AF)
- stroke
- peripheral artery disease such as diabetes
- HTN
- high cholesterol and smoking.

INFLAMMATORY BOWEL DISEASE / COLITIS / ULCERATIVE COLITIS

Although not proven, the cause of inflammatory bowel disease is thought to be an auto-immune response (NICE, 2017a). Microscopic colitis results from invasion of the layers of the colon wall with lymphocytic white blood cells or collagen. There is no blood in the stool and the primary cause is thought to be an autoimmune response (Münch et al., 2012; Rasmussen and Munck, 2012;, Park et al., 2015), although non-steroidal anti-inflammatory drugs (NSAIDS) may also be a factor (Milman and Kraa, 2010). Colitis can be caused by allergies including cow or soy milk and antibiotics (BMA/RPS, 2016). According to the National Institute for Care Excellence (NICE, 2017a), UC is the most common type of inflammatory disease of the bowel. The incidence in the UK is approximately 10 per 100,000 people annually, and a prevalence of approximately 240 per 100,000. This amounts to around 146,000 people. The cause is unknown and it can develop at any age, but peak incidence is between the ages of 15 and 25 years.

UC usually affects the rectum, and a variable extent of the colon proximal to the rectum. The inflammation is continuous in extent. Inflammation of the rectum is referred to as proctitis, and inflammation of the rectum and sigmoid as proctosigmoiditis. Left-sided colitis refers to disease involving the colon distal to the splenic flexure. Extensive colitis affects the colon proximal to the splenic flexure, and includes pan-colitis, where the whole colon is involved.

Symptoms of active disease or relapse include bloody diarrhoea, an urgent need to defaecate and abdominal pain. It is a lifelong disease, associated with significant morbidity, and affects a person's social and psychological wellbeing, particularly if poorly controlled. Typically, it has a relapsing–remitting pattern.

According to NICE, current medical approaches focus on treating active disease to address symptoms, to improve quality of life, and thereafter to maintain remission. The long-term benefits of achieving mucosal healing remain unclear. The treatment chosen is likely to depend on clinical severity, extent of disease and the person's preference, and may include the use of aminosalicylates, corticosteroids or biological drugs. These drugs can be oral or topical (into the rectum), and corticosteroids may be administered intravenously in people with acute severe disease. Surgery may be considered as emergency treatment for severe relapses that do not respond to drug treatment. People may also choose to have elective surgery for unresponsive or frequently relapsing disease that is affecting their quality of life.

CHRONIC PELVIC PAIN IN WOMEN

Chronic pelvic pain (CPP) is commonly described as pain felt below the umbilicus, which lasts for at least 6 months. It is a debilitating condition that impairs quality of life. According to Latthe et al. (2006) its prevalence ranges from 2.1% to 24% worldwide. Zondervan et al. (1999) found that in the UK 38 per 1000 women are affected annually; a rate comparable to asthma and back pain (37 and 41 per 1000 respectively). Symptoms include dysmenorrhoea and dyspareunia. Secondary dysmenorrhoea describes period pain associated with a physical cause, whereas in primary dysmenorrhoea no underlying cause is identified. One of the most common causes of CPP is endometriosis. Tissue that is normally found lining the inside of the uterus is also present outside the uterus, usually in the pelvic cavity. Definitive diagnosis is usually by laparoscopy or laparotomy. Other causes include pelvic inflammatory disease, pelvic congestion syndrome, nerve entrapment, neuropathic pain and postsurgical pain. In some patients a cause cannot be found. Several neural paths within the pelvis transmit pain from the reproductive organs, but these nerve fibres may also refer pain to somatic receptors and manifest as chronic pelvic pain (Alsom et al., 2009). Changes to inflammatory cytokines observed in patients with interstitial cystitis, irritable bowel syndrome, and vulvar vestibulitis might indicate neurogenic inflammation (Wesselmann, 2001).

Treatment depends on the underlying cause. Social and psychological factors are strongly associated with CPP, making effective treatment a challenge (Daniels and Khan, 2010). According to NICE (2017b) strategies for endometriosis depend on the patient's age, symptoms, whether the patient wants to have children and whether there is associated subfertility. Hormonal treatments aim to stop ovulation, allowing the endometrial deposits to regress. Conservative surgery via laparoscopy or laparotomy aims to remove the endometrial deposits, usually by laser or electrocautery. Hysterectomy, with or without removal of the ovaries, may be considered for severe symptoms that do not respond to conservative treatment. When the cause of the pain remains unknown, conservative treatments include non-steroidal anti-inflammatory drugs or a trial of the oral contraceptive pill. Surgical treatment options include vaginal uterosacral ligament resection, presacral neurectomy (PSN) involving total removal of the presacral nerves, and uterine nerve ablation (UNA) involving transection of the uterosacral ligaments at their insertion into the cervix (NICE, 2007a).

As one reads Rebecca's case study it can be clearly seen that she had several ward transfers and the aforementioned information about inflammatory bowel disease and chronic pelvic pain may not have been known by the multiple staff looking after her. Even if they did have the knowledge about the conditions they would not have had specific knowledge about the triggers and how Rebecca managed her illnesses and associated stressors and coping strategies. This chapter will now focus on multiple ward transfers.

THE IMPACT OF MULTIPLE WARD TRANSFERS

In 2015 a report commissioned by the Foundation Trust Network (National Health Service Providers) highlighted the risks associated with poorly managed patient transfers. They urged all healthcare providers to consider how to better provide patients with the right treatment at the right time, in the right place and by the right person. The primary goal of adopting the model of specialist ward care is to provide clinical medical and nursing knowledge and skills that better meets patient need. However, due to the dynamic ever increasing specialisation of UK healthcare systems, increasing demand, government targets and scarcer resources, patients are frequently transferred between departments and wards. Sometimes these transfers are for sound clinical reasons including provision of specialist clinical care; specific investigations; infection control and to avoid mixed sex breaches. Unfortunately patients are also often transferred to facilitate patient flow and placed in wards not equipped or staffed for their specialised needs. A survey of patients' views undertaken by Kings Fund (Patterson, 2012) highlighted that frequent ward transfers left patients feeling as if they were moved around like a parcel and resulted in a lack of confidence in the person in charge of their care. According to Stylianou et al. (2017) this phenomenon is more common in publicly funded healthcare systems such as New Zealand, Australia and some European countries including the United Kingdom; however, there is minimal research evidence into the effects on patient care.

Patient-centred care should take into account patients' individual needs and preferences, and continuity of care and patient safety are widely regarded as core values. Patient transfers are fraught with potential problems and can lead to adverse events (see Box 7.4: Risk Factors Associated with Transfers). Early research, such as Daly et al. (2001), highlighted that the discharge mortality of 'at risk patients' may be reduced by 39% if they remained in intensive care units for a further 48 hours and consequently they devised a discharge triage model to identify patients at risk from too early and inappropriate discharge from intensive care. The Kings Fund report (Patterson, 2012) quotes doctors as saying 'It is common for patients to move four or five times during their stay . . .particularly afflicting elderly patients moved to outlying wards during the night' with 10 out of 12 being moved after 20:00. Indeed one of their recommendations was that 'once a patient reached a ward after assessment in the acute medical unit, they should not move again, unless there are exceptional circumstances', yet as we can see in Rebecca's story she was moved many times.

■■■ BOX 7.4 ■■

Risks associated with transfers include

- Loss of information leading to fragmentation of and gaps in patient care (Cook et al., 2000).
- Difficulty in identifying and contacting the correct clinician responsible for the patient's care (Evanoff et al., 2005).
- Medication errors some of which may lead to patient deaths (Beach, 2006), incomplete or lost medical records, delay in essential investigations and treatment, medication errors, key information not handed over, increased risk of delirium in vulnerable patients (Ellis et al., 2011).
- Increased length of stay (Patterson, 2012).

As managers we also need to consider not only the impact on the patient and their family but the associated cost. Back in 2005 Hendrich and Lee highlighted that the inefficient movement of patients within the hospital led to a wasteful cost to the health service with increased length of stay; and the National Health Service Litigation Authority (2013) requires that each Trust has an approved process describing the management of risks associated with the transfer of patients. It sets out minimum requirements for the transfer procedure and approved documentation specific to each patient group.

Reflection

Could Rebecca's transfers be considered exceptional due to circumstances? And do your staff know the trust transfer process?

Key Priorities for Transferring Acutely Ill Patients

In 2007 the National Institute for Health Care Excellence (NICE, 2007b) set out key priorities relating to the transfer of acutely ill patients. Although these are aimed at step down transfers from a level two facility to a ward, these principles should also be applied to inter-ward transfers. The principles include:

- Avoiding transfers between 22.00 and 07.00. If they do occur document as an adverse incident. To ensure continuity of care a formal structured handover by medical and nursing staff should be supported by a written plan.
- Ensure the ward can deliver the plan, with support from critical care if required.
- The handover of care should include:
  - a summary of the stay including diagnosis and treatment
  - a monitoring and investigation plan
  - a plan for ongoing treatment including drugs and therapies, nutrition plan, infection status and any agreed limitations of treatment
  - physical, rehabilitation, psychological, emotional, specific communication and language needs.

Discharge from Critical Care

Recovery from critical illness is highly individual and therefore care needs to be patient-centred and personalised (NICE, 2009). For many, discharge from critical care is the start of an uncertain journey to recovery characterised by weakness, loss of energy, physical difficulties, vivid or disturbing dreams, sleep deprivation, anxiety, depression, post-traumatic stress phenomena and a loss of cognitive and social functioning (Jones et al., 2006). Family members become informal caregivers causing relationships to alter and uncertain financial security (McKinney and Deeny, 2002; Jones et al., 2004; Paul et al 2004; Young et al., 2005; Combe, 2005; Strahan and Brown, 2005). Further inappropriate transfers may jeopardise this recovery and increase length of stay.

Multiple transfers of acutely ill patients with complex needs between wards, whilst daunting for patients, can be equally frightening for their family. With each transfer, the risk to patient safety increases as does the discontinuity of care. Information deterioration known as funnelling may occur (Poletick and Holly, 2010); this is where information is being compressed to make it manageable and this in turn leads to a progressive loss of information, which may contribute to an adverse patient outcome. Consequently in the period immediately before discharge from critical care, NICE recommends that patients are re-assessed (NICE, 2009) and that patients should be reviewed after discharge from critical care, by Critical Care Outreach Team (see Chapter 3 for information about the development of CCOT and principle roles).

There is no doubt that not only was Rebecca's condition affected by the transfers but that when these occurred at night it affected her sleep and sleep quality.

SLEEP, ANXIETY AND MOOD

Sleep is a complex biological rhythm and an essential human need and the consequences of chronic sleep loss are profound. There are many factors which affect sleep and sleep quality including physical illnesses, environment, lifestyle, emotional stress, drugs and alcohol, smoking and medications. For clients with inflammatory bowel diseases (IBD) pain is a common disturbance of sleep. This is often a result of increased gastric secretions that occur during Rapid Eye Movement (REM) sleep. REM usually occurs every 90 minutes and lasts 5–30 minutes. During REM the brain is highly active and metabolism may increase by up to 20%; Non-rapid Eye Movement (NREM) has four stages during which the depth of sleep and the length of time at each stage varies. During the III & IV stages (deep or delta sleep) the heart rate and respiratory rate drop by 20–30%, swallow and saliva production reduce and energy is restored and growth hormones released. The loss of NREM sleep causes immunosuppression, slows tissues repair, lowers pain tolerance, triggers profound fatigue and increases susceptibility to infection (McChance and Huether, 2010). Graff et al. (2011) in a study of over 300 people with IBD, found that 23% had elevated CRP; 12% were anaemic; 72% of those with active and 30% with inactive disease were fatigued; 49% experienced poor sleep quality and perceived stress. They concluded that fatigue and poor sleep were highly prevalent in active disease and significant for many with inactive disease; thus psychological factors are associated with fatigue in IBD. Patel et al. (2016) studied the effects of sleep disturbances on patients with gastrointestinal symptoms and pain and concluded that the impact on IBS and pain caused distress and poor quality of life. Stevens et al. (2017) studied sleep and mood in people with IBD. They also found that poor sleep, anxiety and depression are common with patients with IBD and that these were associated with a relapse. They found that there was significant improvement in sleep and mood after patients with IBS took anti-TNF (tumour necrosis factor) agents or vedolizumab. A TNF inhibitor suppresses the physiologic response to TNF and is part of the inflammatory response. TNF is involved in autoimmune and immune-mediated disorders such as inflammatory bowel diseases and therefore TNF inhibitors may part of the treatment.

Tang and Sanborn (2014) and Andrews et al. (2014) studied the effects of poor sleep and chronic pain. They agreed that physical activity helped with sleep promotion and enhanced mood, but they found that people with inflammatory conditions needed to finely balance the amount of physical activity because it could make the inflammation, and thus the pain, worse. Consequently sustained poor, or lack of, sleep leads to anxiety, depression and chronic fatigue; and for patients with IBD pain is a contributing factor.

CHRONIC ILLNESS AND IMPACT ON FAMILY

There is no doubt that a chronic illness affects the individual and this in turn affects their mental health; indeed there is research that shows how certain health conditions are associated with depression (see Box 7.5: Health Conditions Associated with Depression). However the amount of social support has an impact on this and Ahn et al. (2017) give a very good overview of the research related to how positive support from family and friends helps to reduce depression whereas negative social support leads to higher levels of depression. However this chapter will focus on the effects of the chronic ill-health on the family.

BOX 7.5

Health Conditions Associated With Depression

- heart disease: Skala et al. (2006)
- hypertension: Bogner and de Vries (2008)
- stroke: Knapp and House (2011)
- diabetes: Nouwen et al. (2010)
- cancer: Husson et al. (2010)
- osteoarthritis: Jämsen et al. (2013)
- chronic obstructive pulmonary disease: Cully et al. (2006)
- IBD: Walker et al. (2008)

The effects of chronic illness can substantially affect family members and having an ill relative and the burden on family as caregivers is well documented (Sautter et al., 2014; Wittenberg and Prosser, 2013; Wittenberg et al., 2013). Research shows that family caregivers suffer not only from physical and mental ill-health with increased mortality risks, strain and other negative outcomes but the relationships between the family member and other relatives changes too. Our case study focuses on Rebecca, and her spouse Simon is the caregiver. Caregiving is multi-tasked and can include buying groceries, cooking meals, cleaning, assistance with bathing or personal care, making and driving Rebecca to medical appointments, dispensing medicine, helping her get in or out of bed. Many of these Rebecca would have done once but as she became more chronically ill Simon took over, which left very little time for his own personal recreations. This may have caused a strain not only on his relationship with Rebecca but with other members of the family. Relationship strain can be perceived as criticism and negative or lack of support. Perceptions of criticism from family members can cause a spouse to become depressed, have a decreased quality of life and life satisfaction as well as an increase in their own ill health. Indeed research reveals that the needs of the spouse are often overlooked at a time when s/he needs the strength to support a partner in new ways (Carson et al., 2016; Gerson and Gerson, 2012; Roslan et al., 2011; Wittenberg et al., 2013). Research also shows that quality spousal care not only helps recipients cope with their chronic health needs and symptoms, success of chronic illness management and better patient outcomes (such as reducing pain and depression) but this in turn helps the spouse cope too as they see their loved one more positive (Lavelle et al., 2014). Roslan et al.'s (2011) systematic review of a significant amount of literature identified that many studies highlighted that their results were consistent with self-determination theory (Ryan and Deci, 2000). Self-determination theory is a theory of human motivation. It is concerned with supporting our natural or intrinsic tendencies to behave in effective and healthy ways and how humans adopt the conditions that foster these in a positive way. However criticisms from spouses or health professionals can adversely affect the ability to cope. Consequently health professionals must remember that healthcare professionals are educated in health, generally to degree level as a minimum, and as such cannot expect a non-trained informal care giver (family member) to give the specialist level of care professionals can provide. Health professionals must also remember that the non-trained informal caregivers are often a similar age to the patient and as this may make them elderly too they will also have normal age-related health needs and symptomologies.

Reflection

Reflect on your communication with a relative who is giving health care to a loved one and consider if this has been positive or critical. Ask a peer for their opinion and consider whether it is the same as your perception and if not what you can learn from this.

HUMANISING CARE

This chapter has not only considered the care of Rebecca but also the impact of her illness on Simon, consequently the humanising dimensions will focus on both. Table 7.1 applies these to Rebecca and Table 7.2 to Simon. Human sensitive care we believe not only considers the patient but the family too. A lifeworld approach to care (explored in Chapter 1) encourages us to think about who we are as humans and how we relate to others around us. We need to consider if Rebecca and Simon were asked about their feelings of care (insiderness), remembering that they are both unique individuals who should be looked at individually with their own issues and preferences, and if they feel they can ask questions when they do not understand what is occurring (sense making) they need to feel connected not only to each other but also to the staff (togetherness).

Now read Table 7.1 and 7.2, add your thoughts and consider where they overlap and formulate a comprehensive humanising care table which incorporate both Rebecca and Simon. The Burdett Trust commissioned a Humanising Care tool kit (2016) to help staff explore humanising care and you may like to refer to that too.

Table 7.1 Humanising care for Rebecca

Humanising dimensions	Critical illness triggers	Managing stressors and coping strategies	Role of expert nurse in support strategies
Insiderness/ objectification	Rebecca has multiple chronic illnesses and triggers include: • Chronic inflammatory response to diverticular disease • Psychological stress – causing raised BP • Delayed cellular recovery.	Rebecca is reliant on care from Simon; she is worried about the stress this is causing him.	Enable connectedness by helping staff understand that it is good to take time to listen to Rebecca's anxieties.
Agency/ passivity	Rebecca is out of her comfort zone and feels unable to decide on a positive way forward as her health history is complicated.	Rebecca needs a full understanding of the ward routine and staff roles and how they can help her understand her multiple conditions and associated treatments.	Ensure staff give Rebecca a sound evidence based rationale re why it is important to focus on the present care. Discuss her recovery time and return home.

Humanising dimensions	Critical illness triggers	Managing stressors and coping strategies	Role of expert nurse in support strategies
Uniqueness/ homogenisation	Rebecca fears that the life she has had with Simon may be lost. She has a sense of loss of role and the responsibilities she once had as wife and how Simon is now undertaking these roles.	Rebecca has a unique view of the world she now lives in and this must be recognised if staff are to help her overcome her fears.	Ensure staff are not being judgemental or critical about Rebecca's lifestyle and how Simon is caring for her. Challenge staff assumptions and any poor behaviour being demonstrated, enabling staff to learn and reflect.
Togetherness/ isolation	Rebecca does not fully understand the present state of her gastric problems and neither does Simon.	Rebecca loves Simon and wants him to understand her health needs as much as she does so they can explore ways of coping together.	Involve them both in helping to adjust to new lifestyle choices that they may need to make.
Sense making/ loss of meaning	Not understanding what her present gastric needs are and the trigger factors that may make it worse.	Staff need to provide Rebecca with adequate knowledge of the world she is in at present so she and Simon can make sense of the care.	Enable staff to recognise that what is 'normal' to them is frightening for Rebecca. Help staff form questions and answers that are not perceived as being critical.
Personal journey/loss of personal journey	Rebecca has gastric pain and has reduced intake as bowel motions make the pain worse.	Rebecca needs a comprehensive understanding of the bowel and the need to keep hydrated with adequate nutrition if she is to keep strong and heal.	Enable staff to ensure Rebecca has a working knowledge of bowel anatomy and physiology and how one has affected the other and the associated care and treatment.
Sense of place/ dislocation	Rebecca is frightened that she may die and leave Simon alone. She wants to go home.	Rebecca might like to talk through her fears with a counsellor or chaplain or a healthcare professional.	Ensure staff have a sound evidence base regarding what fears chronic gastric problems may bring and can offer coping strategies.
Embodiment/ reductionist body	Rebecca is concerned because she has so many health needs and medications and she does not wish to tell nurses of these fears in case she is thought to be feeble.	Rebecca may like to talk to a specialist nurse for support.	Ensure staff are enabling Rebecca to make choices. Ensure they have a good working knowledge of support structures that Rebecca can access.

Table 7.2 Humanising care for Simon

Humanising dimensions	Illness triggers	Managing stressors and coping strategies	Role of expert nurse in support strategies
Insiderness/ objectification	Perceptions of criticisms from family members and health professionals. Not focusing on his own healthcare needs.	Simon is a full time carer and does not hold a paid job and he is concerned about criticisms; he is also worried that his and Rebecca's standard of living is reducing.	Enable connectedness by helping staff understand that it is good to take time to listen to Simon and his worries.
Agency/ passivity	Simon feels unable to decide what healthcare needs Rebecca requires and if he is undertaking them correctly.	Simon needs to understand the care he gives and how to perform it well. He also needs to understand things such as healthy diet, medication, exercise, etc. He needs help to understand the roles of healthcare professionals and who best to seek advice from.	Ensure staff give Simon a sound evidence based rationale re why it is important to focus on the present care. Discuss recovery time and Rebecca's and his physical, emotional and spiritual needs when she returns home.
Uniqueness/ homogenisation	Simon fears that the life he had and which he enjoys is being lost because of the time Rebecca needs.	The world in which Simon lives and his fears of what may change due to Rebecca's chronic illness must be recognised if staff are to help him overcome his fears.	Ensure staff are not judgemental about Simon's lifestyle. Challenge any assumptions being displayed. Enable staff to reflect and learn from any negative behaviour they show.
Togetherness/ isolation	Simon and Rebecca do not fully understand the gastric problems.	Simon loves Rebecca and fears being without her.	Enable Simon and Rebecca to explore trigger factors which make the gastric illness worse and help them to adjust style choices.
Sense making/ loss of meaning	Not understanding the trigger factors affecting the gastric problems.	Staff need to provide Simon with adequate knowledge of Rebecca's chronic illnesses so he can make sense of the care needs.	Enable staff to recognise that what is 'normal' to them causes Simon to feel fear. Help staff form questions and answers that are not critical.
Personal journey/loss of personal journey	Simon witnesses Rebecca's gastric pain and does not understand what makes it worse or how to relieve it.	Simon needs a comprehensive understanding of the bowel and its functioning so he can understand what is causing the pain.	Enable staff to ensure Simon has a working knowledge of bowel anatomy and physiology and the associated care and treatments.

Humanising dimensions	Illness triggers	Managing stressors and coping strategies	Role of expert nurse in support strategies
Sense of place/ dislocation	Simon knows that Rebecca is frightened of death but does not know how to help her.	Simon might like to talk through his fears with a counsellor or chaplain or healthcare professional.	Ensure staff have a sound evidence base regarding what fears Simon may have and can offer coping strategies.
Embodiment/ reductionist body	Simon is concerned because Rebecca has so many health needs and medications and he wants to appear strong and capable of caring for her.	Simon may like to talk to a specialist nurse for support.	Ensure staff enable Simon to help Rebecca make choices. Ensure they have a good working knowledge of support structures that can be accessed.

REFLECTIVE EXERCISE 7.1

1 What do your staff understand about sleep quality and its effect on anxiety levels and mood? What do they do to assess sleep and how do they promote good quality sleep?
2 Consider how you can help your staff consider how chronic illness has an impact on family members.
3 What strategies have you implemented to ensure the handover of information ensures patient safety and the delivery of quality health care?
4 Explore the human factors that play a role in the transfer of patients and the safe handover of information. How do you develop your staff to acquire the key skills needed for safe handover? Explore skills such as:

- interpersonal communication
- knowledge and experience
- documentation that is accurate, legible, comprehensive yet succinct and relevant
- strategies to minimise interruptions
- physical and emotional pressures
- electronic data access
- effective strategies that protect against information decay and funnelling.

CHAPTER SUMMARY

This chapter has explored how gastric disturbances, such as Inflammatory Bowel disease, GI bleeding, Colitis and pelvic pain, have significant impact on the client and their family. It has looked at how ward transfers need to be carefully considered as they impact on the client's sleep and have a cost to the organisation. We have also considered how chronic health needs impact not only on the client but their caregiver and therefore advise that humanising care be considered for both.

FURTHER READING

Dayton, E. and Henriksen, K. (2007). Communication failure: basic components, contributing factors, and the call for structure. *Joint Commission Journal On Quality And Patient Safety/ Joint Commission Resources, 33*(1), 34–47.

Gosbee, J. (1998) Communication among health professionals, *British Medical Journal, 316*(7132): 642.

Leonard, M., Graham, S. and Bonacum, D. (2004) The human factor: The critical importance of effective teamwork and communication in providing safe care, *Quality and Safety in Health Care, 3*(1): 85–90.

McQuillan, P., Pilkington, S., Allan, A., Taylor, B., Short, A. and Morgan, G. (1998) Confidential inquiry into quality of care before admission to intensive care, *British Medical Journal, 316*(7148): 1853–8.

NHS Providers (2015) *Right Place, Right Time. Better Transfers of Care: A Call for Action.* Foundation Trust Network. Available at: http://nhsproviders.org/media/1258/nhsp-right-place-lr.pdf

O'Toole, A. (2016) Optimal management of collagenous colitis: a review, *Clinical and Experimental Gastroenterology, 9*: 31–9.

Sherwood, G and Barnsteiner, J (eds) (2017) *Quality and Safety in Nursing: A Competency Approach to Improving Outcomes* (2nd edn). London: Wiley Blackwell.

REFERENCES

Ahn, S., Kim., S. and Zhang, H. (2017) Changes in depressive symptoms among older adults with multiple chronic conditions: role of positive and negative social support, *International Journal of Environmental Research and Public Health, 14*(16): 1–11.

Alsom, N., Harrison, G., Khan, K.S. and Patwardhan, S. (2009) Visceral hyperalgesia in chronic pelvic pain, *British Journal of Obstetrics and Gynaecology, 116*: 1551–5.

Andrews, N.E., Strong, J. and D'Arrigo, P. (2014) Association between physical activity and sleep in adults with chronic pain: a momentary within-person perspective, *Physical Therapy, 94*(4): 499–510.

Beach, C. (2006) Morbidity and mortality rounds: Lost in transition. *Agency for Healthcare Research and Quality.* Available at: https://psnet.ahrq.gov/webmm/case/116/Lost-in-Transition [accessed 20 January 2018].

Bogner, H.R and de Vries, H.F. (2008) Integration of depression and hypertension treatment: a pilot, randomised controlled trial, *Annual of Family Medicine, 6*: 295–301.

British Medical Association (BMA)/Royal Pharmaceutical Society (RPS) (2016) *British National Formulary.* Issue September 2015–March 2016. Available at: www.bnf.org/

Burdett Trust. (2016) *The Humanising Care Toolkit.* Available at: www.btfn.org.uk/library/directory_listings/337/Humanising%20Care%20Toolkit.pdf

Carson, S., Cox, C., Wallenstein, S., Hanson, L., Danis, M., Tulsky, J., Chai, E and Nelson, J. (2016) Effects of palliative care-led meetings from families of patients with chronic critical illness: a randomized clinical trial, *Journal of the American Medical Association, 316*(1): 51–62.

Combe, D. (2005) The use of patient diaries in an intensive care unit, *Nursing in Critical Care*, *10*: 31–4.

Cook, R.I., Render, M. and Woods, D. (2000) Gaps in the continuity of care and progress on patient safety, *British Medical Journal*, *320*(7237): 791–794.

Cully, J.A., Graham, D.P., Stanley, M.A., Ferguson, C.J., Sharafkhaneh, A., Souchek, J. and Kunik, M.E. (2006) Quality of life in patients with Chronic Obstructive Pulmonary Disease and Comorbid Anxiety or Depression, *Psychosomatics*, *47*(4): 312–19.

Daly, K., Beale, R. and Chang, R.W. (2001) Reduction in mortality after inappropriate early discharge from intensive care unit: logistic regression triage model, *British Medical Journal*, *322*(7297):1274–6.

Daniels, J.P. and Khan, K.S. (2010) Chronic pelvic pain in women, *British Medical Journal*, *341*; c4834.

Ellis, G., Whitehead, M., Robinson, D., O'Neill, D. and Langhorne, P. (2011) Comprehensive geriatric assessment for older adults admitted to hospital: meta-analysis of randomised data, *British Medical Journal*, *343*: d6553.

Evanoff, B., Potter, P., Wolf, L., Grayson, D., Dunagan, C. and Boxerman, S. (2005) Can we talk? Priorities for patient care differed among health care providers, in Henriksen, K., Battles, J.B., and Mark, E., et al. (eds) *Advances in Patient Safety: From Research to Implementation 1*, 5–14. Agency for Healthcare Research and Quality. Available at: www.ncbi.nlm.nih.gov/books/NBK20468/

Gerson, M. and Gerson, C. (2012) The importance of relationships in patients with Irritable Bowel Syndrome: a review, *Gastroenterology Research and Practice*, 1–5.

Graff, L.A., Vincent, N., Walker, J.R., Clara, I., Carr, R., Ediger, J., Miller, N., Rogala, L., Rawsthorne, P., Lix, L. and Bernstein, C.N. (2011) A population-based study of fatigue and sleep difficulties in inflammatory bowel disease, *Inflammatory Bowel Diseases*, *17*(9): 1882–9.

Griffiths, M. (2017) A personal look at diverticular disease. Available at: www.mydiverticulitis.co.uk/

Hendrich, A.L. and Lee, N. (2005) Intra-unit patient transports: time, motion, and cost impact on hospital efficiency, *Nurse Economics*, *23*(4): 157–64.

Husson, O., Mols, F. and van de Poll-Franse, L.V. (2010) The relation between information provision and health related quality of life, anxiety and depression among cancer survivors: a systematic review, *Annals of Oncology*, *22*: 761–72.

Jämsen, E., Peltola, M., Eskelinen, A. and Lehto, M.U.K. (2013) Comorbid diseases as predictors of survival of primary total hip and knee replacements: a nationwide register-based study of 96,754 operations on patients with primary osteoarthritis, *Annals of the Rheumatic Diseases*, *72*(12): 1975–82.

Jones, C., Skirrow, P., Griffiths, R.D., Humphri, G., Ingleby, S., Eddleston, J., Waldmann, C. and Gager, M. (2004) Post-traumatic stress disorder related symptoms in relatives of patients following intensive care, *Intensive Care Medicine*, *30*: 456–60.

Jones, C., Griffiths, R.D., Slater, T., Benjamin, K.S. and Wilson, S. (2006) Significant cognitive dysfunction in non-delirious patients identified during and persisting following critical illness, *Intensive Care Medicine*, *32*: 923–6.

Knapp, P. and House, A. (2011) Depression after Stroke. Chapter 82 in Abou-Saleh, M.T., Katona, C. and Kumar, A. (2011) *Principles and Practice of Geriatric Psychiatry* (3rd edn). John Wiley and Sons, Ltd.

Latthe, P., Latthe, M., Say, L., Gulmezoglu, M. and Khan, K.S. (2006) WHO systematic review of prevalence of chronic pelvic pain: a neglected reproductive health morbidity, *Biomedical Central Public Health*, 6: 177.

Lavelle, T., Wittenberg, E., Lamarand, K. and Prosser, A. (2014) Variation in the spillover effects of illness on parents, spouses and children of the chronically ill, *Applied Health Economical and Health Policy*, 12: 117– 24.

McChance, K.L and Huether, S.E. (2010) *Pathophysiology. The Biologic Basis for Disease in Adults and Children* (7th edn). Canada: Elsevier Mosby.

McKinney, A. and Deeny, P. (2002) Leaving the intensive care unit: a phenomenological study of the patient's experience, *Intensive and Critical Care Nursing*, 18: 320–31.

Milman, N and Kraa, G. (2010) NSAID-induced Collagenous Colitis, *The Journal of Rheumatology*, 37(11): 2432–43.

Münch, A., Aust, D., Bohr, J., Bonderup, O., Fernández Bañares, F. and Hjortswang. H. (2012) Microscopic colitis: current status, present and future challenges: statements of the European Microscopic Colitis Group, *Journal of Crohns and Colitis*, 6(9): 932–45.

National Health Service Litigation Authority (2013) *Risk Management Standards 2013–14 for NHS Trusts providing Acute, Community, or Mental Health and Learning Disability Services and Non-NHS Providers of NHS Care*. Available at: www.NHSLA.com

National Institute for Health Care Excellence (NICE) (2007a) *Laparoscopic Uterine Nerve Ablation (LUNA) for Chronic Pelvic Pain. Interventional Procedures Guidance 234*. Available at: www.nice.org.uk/guidance/ipg234

National Institute for Health Care Excellence (NICE) (2007b) *Acutely ill adults in hospital: recognising and responding to deterioration*. Available at: www.nice.org.uk/guidance/cg50

National Institute for Health Care Excellence (NICE) (2009) *Rehabilitation after Critical Illness in Adults*. Available at: www.nice.org.uk/guidance/cg83

National Institute for Health Care Excellence (NICE) (2016) *Acute Upper Gastrointestinal Bleeding in over 16s: Management*. Available at: www.nice.org.uk/guidance/cg141/resources/ acute-upper-gastrointestinal-bleeding-in-over-16s-management-pdf-35109565796293

National Institute for Health Care Excellence (NICE) (2017a) *Ulcerative Colitis: Management. Clinical guideline 166*. Available at: www.nice.org.uk/guidance/cg166

National Institute for Health Care Excellence (NICE) (2017b) *Endometriosis: Diagnosis and Management. NG73*. Available at: www.nice.org.uk/guidance/ng73

Nouwen, A., Winkley, K., Twisk, J., Lloyd, C. E., Peyrot, M., Ismail. K. and Pouwer, F. (2010) Type 2 diabetes mellitus as a risk factor for the onset of depression: a systematic review and meta-analysis, *Diabetologia*, 53: 2480–6.

Park, T., Cave, D. and Marshall, C. (2015). Microscopic colitis: a review of aetiology, treatment and refractory disease, *World Journal of Gastroenterology*, 21(29): 8804–10.

Patel, A., Hasak, S., Cassell, B., Ciorba, M.A., Vivio, E.E., Kumar, M., Prakash Gyawali, C. and Sayuk, G.S. (2016) Effects of disturbed sleep on gastrointestinal and somatic pain symptoms in irritable bowel syndrome, *Alimentary Pharmacology & Therapeutics*, 44: 246–58.

Patterson, L. (2012) Wrong bed, wrong ward. *Kings Fund*. Available at: www.kingsfund.org.uk/ sites/default/files/linda-patterson-wrong-bed-wrong-ward-poor-transitional-care-patient- outcomes-kingsfund-dec12.pdf

Paul, F., Hendry, C. and Cabbrelli, L. (2004) Meeting patient and relatives' information needs upon transfer from an intensive care unit: the development and evaluation of an information booklet, *Journal of Clinical Nursing*, 13(3): 396–405.

Poletick, E.B. and Holly, C. (2010) A systematic review of nurses' inter-shift handoff reports in acute care hospitals, *JBI Library of Systematic Reviews*, 8(4): 121–72.

Rasmussen, M.A. and Munck, L.K. (2012) Systematic review: are lymphocytic colitis and collagenous colitis two subtypes of the same disease – microscopic colitis? *Aliment Pharmacology Therapy*, 36(2): 79–90.

Roslan, A., Heisler, M. and Piette, J. (2011) The impact of family behaviours and communication patterns on chronic illness outcomes: a systematic review, *Journal of Behavioural Medicine*, 35: 221–39.

Ryan, R. and Deci, E. (2000) Self-determination theory and facilitation of intrinsic motivation, social development and wellbeing, *American Psychologist*, 55: 68–78.

Sautter, J., Tulsky, J., Johnson, K., Olsen, M., Burton-Chase, A., Hoff Lindquist, J., Zimmerman, S. and Steinhauser, K. (2014) Caregiver experience during advanced chronic illness and last year of life, *Journal of American Geriatrics*, 62(6): 1082–90.

Skala, J.A., Freedland, K.E. and Carney, R.M. (2006) Coronary heart disease and depression: a review of recent mechanistic research, *Canadian Journal of Psychiatry*, 51: 738–45.

Stevens, B.W., Borran, N.Z., Velonias, G., Conway, G., Cleland, T., Andrewes, E., Khalili, H., Garber, F.G., Xavier, R.J., Yajnik, V. and Ananthakrishnan, A.N. (2017) Vedolizumab Therapy is associated with an improvement in sleep quality and mood in Inflammatory Bowel Diseases, *Digestive Diseases and Sciences*, 62: 197–206.

Strahan, E. and Brown, R. (2005) A qualitative study of the experiences of patients following transfer from intensive care, *Intensive and Critical Care Nursing*, 21: 160–71.

Stylianou, N., Fackrell, R. and Vasilakis, C. (2017) Are medical outliers associated with worse outcomes? A retrospective study within a regional NHS hospital using routine data, *British Medical Journal Open*, 7: e015676.

Tang, N. and Sanborn, A. (2014) Better quality sleep promotes daytime physical activity in patients with chronic pain? A multilevel analysis of the within-person relationship, *PLoS ONE*. 9(3): 1–9. Available at: http://journals.plos.org/plosone/article?id=10.1371/journal.pone.0092158

Thompson, A.E. (2016) Diverticulosis and Diverticulitis, *Journal of the American Medical Association*, 316(10): 1124.

Walker, J.R., Ediger, J.P., Graff, L.A., Greenfeld, J.M., Clara, I., Lix, L., Rawsthorne, P., Miller, N., Rogala, L., McPhail, C.,and Bernstein, C.N. (2008) The Manitoba IBD Cohort Study: a population-based study of the prevalence of lifetime and twelve-month anxiety and mood disorders, *American Journal of Gastroenterology*, 103: 1989–97.

Wedro, B. (2017) *What is Colitis?* Available at: www.medicinenet.com/colitis/article.htm

Wesselmann, U. (2001) Neurogenic inflammation and chronic pelvic pain, *World Journal of Urology*, 19: 180–5.

Wittenberg, E and Prosser, L. (2013) Disutility of illness for caregivers and families: a systematic review of the literature, *Pharmaco- economics*, 31: 489–500.

Wittenberg, E., Saada, A. and Prosser, L. (2013) How illness affects family members: a Qualitative Interview Survey, *Patient*, 6: 257–68.

Young, E.I., Eddleston, J., Ingleby, S., Streets, J., McJanet, L., Wang, M. and Glover, L. (2005) Returning home after intensive care: a comparison of symptoms of anxiety and depression in ICU and elective cardiac surgery patients and their relatives, *Intensive Care Medicine*, 31: 86–91.

Zondervan, K.T., Yudkin, P.L., Vessey, M.P., Dawes, M.G., Barlow, D.H. and Kennedy, S.H. (1999) Prevalence and incidence of chronic pelvic pain in primary care: evidence from a national general practice database, *British Journal of Obstetrics and Gynaecology*, 106: 1149–55.

CHAPTER 8

Endocrine Disorders

Case Study: Conner

SARA J. WHITE AND FLEUR LOWE

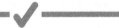

CHAPTER AIMS

1 To explore the care and management of diabetes, pancreatic cancer and gastric exocrine problems.
2 To discuss the clinical decision making related to the care and management of diabetes for the patient acknowledged in the case study and the role of the Diabetic Specialist Nurse (DSN).
3 To consider humanising care needs of the patient, his next of kin and family.

INTRODUCTION

This chapter offers a case study of a client with multiple co-morbidities. It offers a discussion regarding how pathophysiology of one condition can cause complications when trying to manage another. It will also explore why specialist nurses are potentially needed 24 hours per day. Finally it will explore how role ambiguity, distrust and fear can cause family friction at a time of heightened anxiety.

CASE STUDY 8.1: CONNER

Conner is a 75-year-old retired accountant who lives with his wife. He has a PMH of COPD (Asthma), Congestive Cardiac Failure, Chronic Kidney Disease (large polycystic kidneys) and Type 2 Diabetes Mellitus (T2DM) (see Bite Size Knowledge 8.1: Diabetes).

In March, Conner was admitted complaining of lethargy, pruritus, intermittent nausea and vomiting, pale stools, dull abdominal pain and jaundice. Having had an Endoscopic Retrograde

(Continued)

(Continued)

Cholangiopancreatography (ERCP) a stent was inserted. He was discharged after 6 days to be followed up in outpatients; however, he was readmitted 10 days later with worsening symptoms. He was hypotensive, short of breath, his jaundice and pruritus were worsening and his blood sugars were erratic. He had had an acute deterioration in the last 5 weeks, and lost 2.5 stone (15.87 Kilograms) in 2 months and had a poor appetite. He maintained independence and stayed in hospital for another 10 days.

The plan was to: manage the Obstructive Jaundice (see Bite Size Knowledge 8.2: Obstructive Jaundice) and establish the cause; reinsert a larger bore stent; undertake an ultrasound with contrast when Conner was more stable; manage the Acute Kidney Injury (see Chapter 6); regulate blood glucose level and reduce hyperglycaemia.

▬▬▬ BOX 8.1 ▬▬▬

Blood Results on Admission

Conner's blood results showed abnormalities (normal values for the trust caring for Conner are given in brackets):

Urea - 229 (2.5-7.8 mmol/l)

Creatinine - 926 (80 - 115umol/l)

CRP - 94 (0 - 4 mg.l)

Platelets - 190 (150 - 400 mmol)

WCC - 8.2 (4 - 11.0)

GFR - 663 mL/min/1.73m2 (120ml/min)

Glucose - 18.3 (3.85 - 6.05 nmol/l)

pH - 7.28 (7.35 - 7.45)

Globulin - 35 (21 - 37g/l)

Albumin - 34 (35 - 50 g/l)

Bilirubin - 205 (0 - 21 umol/l)

ALT - 212 (10 - 40 IU/l)

ALP - 951 (30 - 130 IU/l)

INR - 1.2 (0.8 - 1.2 ratio)

Hba1C (on 21st Feb) - 83 mmol/mol (20 - 42 mmol/mol).

Discussion Point

Explore what these blood results mean and what they indicate.

Blood Sugar Measurements (BM)

On admission Conner's Blood Glucose (BM) was 48.3 mmol/L; this was managed by variable rate of insulin. Over his time in hospital Conner's BM ranged from 2.0 to 30.6 mmol/l. Conner tended to have hypoglycaemic episodes at bed time. The Diabetic Specialist Nurse (DSN) saw Conner every week day and adjusted his insulin accordingly. On admission Conner was taking Novomix 30 in the morning and evening and after initial IV management this was continued subcutaneously. The number of units varied from 8–56 units in the morning to 4–56 units in the evening. On his first admission in March Conner's BM's ranged from 2.0 to 13.8. On his second admission in March–April they ranged from 0.9 to 30.6.

On a night in early April Conner was unresponsive and a resuscitation call was made. He was found to have a BM of 0.9 and this was managed as per protocol with IV 20% and 10% glucose.

Due to his pancreatic insufficiency and his nausea and vomiting Conner was prescribed Creon – a pancrelipase which is a combination of lipase, protease, and amylase. One of the side effects of Creon is changes in blood sugar – hence the difficulty in Conner's BM management.

During March Conner's wife had a conversation with the senior medic regarding the likely diagnosis of pancreatic cancer (see Bite Size Knowledge 8.3: Pancreatic Cancer) and the prognosis was 8 months' survival. She was unhappy that she had initially heard of this possible diagnosis from one of Conner's sons (her stepson) prior to discussion with the doctor.

BITE SIZE KNOWLEDGE 8.1

Diabetes

Diabetes is a lifelong condition. Over 4 million people in the UK live with diabetes.

Type 1 diabetes is an immune mediated or idiopathic disorder where there is beta cell destruction leading to absolute insulin deficiency and therefore glucose is unable to enter muscle or adipose tissue.

Type 1 symptoms include: thirst; tiredness; muscle and weight loss; frequent micturition.

Type 1 diabetes is an autoimmune condition, where the immune system attacks the pancreas, leading to inability to produce insulin. Symptoms occur over a few days or weeks for

(Continued)

(Continued)

young people and a few months for adults. It can be inherited/genetic. It is not known exactly what triggers the immune system to attack the pancreas, but some researchers have suggested it may be a viral infection.

Treatment is insulin, monitoring, healthy diet and lifestyle.

Type 2 diabetes is where there is resistance to the action of insulin on peripheral tissue and where there is a secretory deficit in insulin production and insulin resistance as the beta cells do not produce enough insulin or the body's cells do not react to insulin.

Type 2 symptoms: frequent micturition – particularly at night; thirst; tiredness; unexplained weight loss; itching around the penis or vagina, or frequent episodes of thrush; wounds heal slowly; blurred vision.

Treatment is monitoring, healthy diet and lifestyle, oral blood glucose lowering therapy.

Other types of diabetes include genetic defects in beta cell function, genetic defects, drug or chemically induced beta cell dysfunction, gestational.

Diagnosis is based on:

- glycosylated haemoglobin (HbA1c) levels
- fasting plasma glucose
- two hour plasma glycose during oral glucose tolerance test (OGTT)
- random glucose test.

(After: NICE, 2016a; NICE, 2015; McCance and Huether, 2014; Copstead and Banasik, 2000)

===== BITE SIZE KNOWLEDGE 8.2 ===== =====

Obstructive Jaundice (OJ)

OJ occurs when the outflow of bile from the liver is obstructed. This results in an overflow of bile and its by-products into the blood and bile excretion from the body is incomplete. Causes include: gallstones, malignant tumour of the gallbladder or pancreas, biliary stricture, cholangitis, congenital structural defects, choledochal cysts, lymph node enlargement, pancreatitis, parasitic infection and trauma.

There are four types according to the Benjamin classification:

1 complete obstruction
2 intermittent obstruction
3 chronic incomplete obstruction
4 segmental obstruction.

Hepatic function is compromised resulting in deranged liver function tests (LFTs). Jaundice is the yellowish pigmentation of the skin, sclera and conjuctival membranes caused by hyperbilirubinaemia. It usually occurs when bilirubin level is > 30mg/L. Deposits of bile salts in the skin causes pruritus.

Treatment of OJ is based on the cause:

- endoscopic Retrograde Cholangio-pancreatography (ERCP) followed by cholecystectomy
- in malignancy, surgery depends on the stage of the tumour and may include removal of the bile ducts, partial liver resection and Whipple resection
- endoscopic sphincterotomy and stenting in non-operable cases.

(After Miller, 2014; NICE, 2016b)

Reflection

Visit: www.liverandpancreas.co.uk/the-management-of-obstructive-jaundice.php

---

BITE SIZE KNOWLEDGE 8.3

Pancreatic cancer

Pancreatic adenocarcinomas may present with abdominal pain or, when they occur in the head of the pancreas, are more likely to develop jaundice as they block the pancreatic and common bile ducts. More than 95% of all pancreatic cancers arise from the exocrine elements (digestive elements) and 60–70% of exocrine pancreatic cancers are localised to the head (Pancreatic Cancer UK, 2018).

Diabetes increases the risk of developing pancreatic cancer.

Very early cancers may be treated by wide excision of the pancreas, duodenum and related structures (called a Whipple procedure).

Reflection

Visit:

Pancreatic Cancer Research Fund: www.pcrf.org.uk
Pancreatitis – Acute: NICE (2016c): https://cks.nice.org.uk/pancreatitis-acute#!scenario
Acute Liver Failure (Sood, 2017): https://emedicine.medscape.com/article/177354-overview

DISCUSSION: DIABETES

Diabetes is a serious and potentially life-threatening lifelong condition (see Bite Size Knowledge 8.1: Diabetes) and over the last 10 years statistics show a significant rise in the number of people with diabetes. The International Diabetes Federation (2015) estimated that there were 415 million people, between the ages of 20 and 70, worldwide with diabetes and that by 2040 this could potentially rise to 642 million (i.e. 1 in 10). They also estimate that globally 1 in 2 adults with T2DM are undiagnosed. In the UK there are an estimated 4.5 million people living with diabetes. Diabetes UK (2016) states that since 1996, the number of people diagnosed with diabetes in the UK has more than doubled from 1.4 million to almost 3.5 million and they estimate that 1.1 million are undiagnosed. A Health Survey for England undertaken by Public Health England (2015) estimated that 10.7% of the English population (approximately 5 million people) are at increased risk of T2DM. Diabetes UK also state that in the UK there are about 31,500 children and young people under the age of 19 with diabetes.

Good diabetes management has been shown to reduce the risk of complications (Diabetes Care, 1999; Stratton et al., 2000; Diabetes UK, 2016). Key to management and patient education is the Diabetic Specialist Nurse (DSN). Yet whilst diabetes is known to be the most common long-term metabolic condition affecting older people (Sinclair, 2009) and the number of people with diabetes is increasing. the number of UK Diabetic Specialist Nurses is static. Indeed at the time of writing one third of NHS hospitals in the UK now have no specific DSN. It is also anticipated that about half of the DSNs will retire in the next 10 years (i.e. by 2027) and the NHS is not recruiting enough DSNs to keep pace with the growing number of people with diabetes (RCN, 2010; TREND-UK, 2015). Another complicating factor is that many of the DSN positions in the UK are Monday to Friday 9.00–17.00 albeit the NHS is operational for 24 hours per day and as such patients need specialist care during their stay.

The role of the DSN and how he helped Conner and his wife is discussed later in this chapter. First adherence and concordance to diabetic treatment is discussed.

Adherence, Concordance or Compliance to Diabetic Management and Treatment

Extensive literature reviews show that in developed countries adherence to therapy averages 50% (World Health Organisation, 2003; Carter et al., 2005; National Institute for Health and Care Excellence (NICE) 2009). The cause for approximately half of this non-adherence is patients being unaware that they are not taking medication as prescribed or the regimen is too complex. The consequences are waste, morbidity and hospital admissions (WHO, 2003). Non-adherence is common in diabetes treatment, where patients often alter or abandon therapy without telling their doctor (WHO, 2003).

Adherence, the term used to describe compliance with a treatment regimen, focuses on the patient's behaviour and is affected by a multitude of factors. A better understanding of these factors has led to the evolution of concordance. This term describes a partnership between the patient and the healthcare provider in terms of shared decision making, by encouraging the patient to participate in developing a treatment regime which, in theory, should result in optimal medicines management. However, in practice, this may not always be the case as the patient may simply follow the practitioner's advice or, after considering all the options, decide not to adhere to the prescribed therapy. The latter may be viewed as a disadvantage, but this approach allows the practitioner to be informed of the patient's views and decision rather than assuming that the patient is taking their medication when they are not.

Conner's case history demonstrates the risk associated with assuming adherence to a treatment regimen at home. Admission to hospital led to life-threatening unstable blood glucose levels as it was wrongly assumed that the patient was taking insulin at the correct time of day and with food. In addition, Conner relinquished control of his diabetes treatment regimen to his wife. On questioning it was apparent that she did not understand the association between the type of insulin and food intake. This had led to hypoglycaemia at night, which she was self-managing by giving her husband an additional snack at bedtime. As Conner's clinical condition deteriorated over the course of five weeks, he became more dependent on his wife. Neither of them had sought advice from the General Practitioner (GP) to discuss the difficulties they faced. Older adults have more chronic health conditions and consume more prescription medications, and utilise more healthcare resources, than any other patient population (Noureldin and Plake, 2017). Consequently, caregiving can be exhausting as carers perform many tasks which they may not be trained to offer – medicines management being one.

Rankin et al. (2011) discuss how many patients and family members struggle to self-manage diabetes because they have a poor knowledge and understanding and because the health services have not adequately examined the reasons. Their research highlighted that knowledge deficits were influenced by various life course events which included diagnosis at a young age and decision making responsibility of parents, lack of engagement with information when well, inconsistent information provision and lack of awareness that knowledge was poor or incomplete.

This leads us to question why patients and caregivers are passive and not more forthcoming and seek help and support. There are potentially a number of reasons for this. Health service targets and the increasing pressures on GPs have led to consultations being cut back to ten minutes. With a condition as complicated as diabetes, this may not be adequate to elicit the patient's full participation, explore the problem in detail, and check the patient's (and potentially their next of kin or/and carer's) understanding of the agreed course of action (Edwards and Elwyn, 2004). In addition, the prevailing, traditional asymmetric power in the doctor–patient relationship, where the doctor controls the consultation and the patient acts deferentially can result in the patient agenda not being fully explored in an attempt to avoid potential disagreement and conflict (Royal College of General Practitioners, 2013; Pollock and, Grime 2002). In this scenario the balance of control was heavily weighted towards Conner's wife. Conner was passive and had lost the sense of agency as his wife held very firm views on how to manage her husband's diabetes and was not easily dissuaded from her set course of action – a coping strategy for managing her various roles.

During Conner's stay in hospital, the DSN faced two key challenges: advising nurses and doctors how to treat the patient's unstable blood sugars in the short term, until the underlying cause of his deterioration was ascertained, and educating the patient and his wife how to maintain stable blood glucose levels in the longer term.

Conner's erratic blood sugar levels were causing his wife increasing anxiety about her husband's diabetic management in hospital. She could not understand why his blood sugar was so difficult to control in hospital when he was normally very stable at home. This caused significant conflict between her and the healthcare professionals attempting to treat her husband. The nurses noted he frequently ate sweets and although he claimed to be eating normally it became clear during further consultations that he was eating significantly less as an inpatient. An in-depth consultation with his wife shed further light on the situation. He was having hypos at night and she managed these by giving him another meal pre-bedtime. He had also lost 2 stone in weight over recent months. He had insulin at breakfast time and again at 20.00, but not always with food. This management led to him having chronic hyperglycaemia. This is caused by decreased beta cell production of insulin and increased glucagon secretion and results in complications such as retinopathy and cataracts, neuropathy, hypertension, peripheral vascular disease, stroke, heart disease, steatohepatitis biliary disease, gastroparesis, nephropathy, glomerulosclerosis, Chronic kidney disease, oxidative stress, immunosuppression, infection, cancer and decreased cognition.

However in hospital Conner's diabetic management followed protocol, which could be perceived as objectification, as he was given insulin at breakfast (08.00) and supper (18.00) with food and he did not have a meal pre-bedtime. In addition he was eating less and on occasion declined to eat most of his food. Consequently his blood sugars remained erratic. Further investigations eventually led to the diagnosis of exocrine pancreatic insufficiency resulting in malabsorption of glucose.

Exocrine pancreatic insufficiency develops when the pancreas is no longer able to make the enzymes that help the body to digest food into nutrients. These enzymes are lipase which breaks down fat, protease which breaks down proteins and amylase which breaks down carbohydrates. Unabsorbed food can lead to diarrhoea, weight loss, bloating and abdominal pain due to damage to sensory nerves and scarring and obstruction of the pancreatic duct. In diabetes the patient is at risk of hypoglycaemia as the gut fails to absorb glucose. Therefore insulin and anti-diabetic drugs are either reduced or stopped (Pancreatic Cancer UK, 2018). Supplements of pancreatin are also given to compensate for reduced or absent exocrine secretion. They assist the digestion of starch, fat and protein. Because pancreatin is inactivated by gastric acid, it is best taken with each meal, either whole or mixed with slightly acidic fluid, such as apple juice, or soft food (Joint Formulary Committee, 2017). In diabetes the patient is at risk of hyperglycaemia as the gut is enabled to absorb glucose. Therefore insulin and anti-diabetic drugs are needed.

Once Conner's exocrine pancreatic insufficiency was treated by the addition of Creon, his blood sugars stabilised and he was able to go home on a much reduced dose of insulin. The therapeutic relationship and insiderness that the DSN had built with Conner and his wife during this time helped them to understand the relationship between insulin and food and enabled them to better manage his condition, take control and have agency. They were also reassured by the knowledge that with ongoing telephone consultations with the DSN to help them titrate the insulin regime as required, they would be able to manage at home, where they would feel safe and secure in the diabetes management (sense of place).

Nutrition and Diabetes

An extensive literature review was undertaken by Evert et al. (2014) to determine nutritional therapy recommendations for those with diabetes. Whilst they found that no 'one-size-fits-all', they also found that a healthful eating pattern, regular physical activity, pharmacotherapy and good support from a knowledgeable healthcare team enables those with diabetes to manage their condition well and live healthily. So whilst patients may ask what the optimal calorie, carbohydrate, protein and fat intake is there is no one ideal. Consequently goals for nutrition therapy should be developed collaboratively with the patient and based on an assessment of their eating pattern, preferences and metabolic goals.

The American Diabetes Association recommended goals are as follows:

- A1C ,7%
- blood pressure, 140/80 mmHg
- LDL cholesterol ,100 mg/dl; triglycerides,150 mg/dl; HDL cholesterol .40
- mg/dl for men; HDL cholesterol .50 mg/dl for women.

Key principles of healthy eating were explored in Chapter 5 and the same applies to those with diabetes. As such when helping patients with diabetes eat healthily, by reducing the amount of sugar and fat, nurses need to offer help to choose carbohydrate and protein containing foods, nutrient-dense, high-fibre foods and avoid processed foods which contain added sodium, fat, and sugars, recognising that the amount of carbohydrates and available insulin may be the most important factor influencing glycaemic response after eating. Wherever possible involvement with the dietitian is best practice. Ball et al. (2016) identified that dietitians are significant in enhancing the nutritional care provided to patients with diabetes. Here they tailor dietary guidelines to individuals, they utilise supportive counselling and open communication styles, to facilitate care for patients in order that they achieve and maintain healthy dietary behaviours. Yu et al's. (2017) systematic analysis explored the effectiveness of lifestyle interventions offered by qualified dieticians verses non-qualified healthcare staff. Here they identified that better body weight and glucose-related outcomes were better achieved by dietitian-delivered interventions.

The Role of the Diabetic Specialist Nurse

The role of the Diabetic Specialist Nurse (DSN) (also called Diabetic Nurse Adviser or Consultant) was introduced over 50 years ago in response to the increasing number of people with diabetes (Pickup and Williams, 2003). Gradually the role of the DSN became complex as the complexity and number of those with diabetes itself became more multifaceted. The DSN typically has expertise in diabetes, performing advanced nursing roles which include improving the quality of care, consultation, collaboration, education, research, prescribing and transformational leadership, all aiming to enhance patient care and satisfaction. The quality improvement from an organisational perspective is to also enhance integrated care and multidisciplinary services and management of scarce resources (Williams, 2011) and ensure that the infrastructure of systems and processes are in place.

Authors, such as Avery and Butler (2008), James et al. (2009), Gosden et al, (2009) and Middleton (2012), discuss how the role of the DSN has evolved and how specialist nurses are under scrutiny because of the need for efficiency savings and the financial austerity of the NHS. However the lack of funds for specialist nurses is causing a crisis as DSNs are having less patient contact, less time to attend training, a reduction in the grade of the nurse (Keogh, 2014) all of which are having an impact on the quality of care despite the desire of Lord Darzi (Department of Health, 2008) for practitioners to place quality at the heart of the NHS.

Literature reviewed clearly highlighted that the DSN should lead diabetes care alongside medical consultants providing expert clinical support and this certainly occurred in the care of Conner. However the literature also speaks of the potential harm coming to patients over the weekend as there is a reliance on junior doctors and a lack of specialist services (Aylin et al., 2010) coupled with inexperienced staff working without sufficient training during unsocial hours. This was evidenced by the fact that Conner's diabetes control was worse at weekends.

Role Ambiguity and Loss of Meaning

As highlighted, Conner's wife appeared to be uncertain of her role in diabetes management and she had a knowledge deficit as well as a loss of meaning. When Conner was in hospital his wife could see that his care and treatment was not as she would do it, and that his diabetes management was being affected so she was struggling with this; at the same time her role as wife seemed to be diminished when the consultant spoke to Conner's son. So she was being pulled in various directions as she tried to respond to her status and this came over as confrontational. Indeed the presence of family members and carers in the hospital setting can present challenges to nurses. On one hand the caregiver can offer vital knowledge about the patient's needs and routine and potentially fill a gap in the knowledge of hospital nursing staff but on the other hand provision of high-quality evidence based care may be in conflict with this as low health literacy of caregivers may be a barrier to effective diabetic care (Yuen et al., 2018). Schubart (cited Mostofsky 2014: 1051) suggests that 'the psychosocial strains on a person caring for a family member with a chronic or life threatening condition can rival the physical strains on the patient, yet the challenges of these family caregivers are often hidden from the medical community'.

There was also a strained relationship between Conner's wife and Conner's son and this came to the forefront when the doctor had a conversation with Conner's son about the potential pancreatic cancer diagnosis – Conner's son was visiting when the consultant visited so this was a chance meeting. Partnerships and marriages are glued together with uncertain and shifting bonds and sometimes insecurity occurs when the second wife feels powerless when facing the children of the first wife and consequently conflict occurs. Role conflict occurs when there are incompatible demands placed upon a person such that compliance with both would be difficult. Family cohesion is important when there is a chronically sick adult in the family. Rosland et al.'s (2011) systematic review found that critical, overprotective, controlling, and distracting family responses to illness management were associated with negative patient outcomes, whereas Fisher and Weihs (2000) found that family encouragement of self-reliance was associated with better disease-related quality of life among people with diabetes. However for interventions to be effective the patient and significant other must have trust in the service, have a sense of belonging and kinship (togetherness).

Distrust and Fear

Trust is at the heart of effective compliance with treatments and therapies and paramount to the delivery of health care (Mohseni and Lindstrom, 2007). Trust is a fundamental ethical goal for nurses as perceiving, enhancing and justifying trust are embedded in law and policy. Indeed the absence of trust might have harmful effects for the health of patients, as it could delay consultation by a patient, or patients may withhold necessary information (Ahnquist et al., 2010). Armstrong et al.'s (2006) research showed that patients with high levels of distrust in health care are more likely to avoid health care and less likely to maintain continuity of care. Distrust also occurs due to social, political, racial and economic factors, and events such as trauma, mental illness, stigma and risk taking behaviours, all of which have been linked with poorer adherence to medication regimens and strongly associated with worse self-reported health (Shoff and Yang, 2012; Whetten et al., 2008; Mohseni and Lindstrom, 2007; Armstrong et al., 2006). Winn et al. (2015) also showed that the relationship between patients' preferences concerning health outcomes and/or their treatments are key to concordance. Taber et al. (2014) suggested that mistrust in medicine today is escalating as people judge the medical care and system based on misinformation and perceptions. Gille et al. (2015) highlight that several researchers have pointed towards a contemporary crisis of trust in healthcare systems and that there have been many examples that show the severe effects of mistrust. They emphasise that patients are often trusting misleading information, which they perceived to be trustworthy (i.e. found on the internet) and that this could have negative health effects and prolong recovery. Helping patients and their family make sense of situations is fundamental to health care and requires clinicians to encounter each situation and each conversation with a sense of uniqueness and newness and an appreciation that this situation is different for each and every person. Ahmad et al. (2013) found that patients, very early on in a conversation, make assessments about the care they are being offered based on the perceived competency of the healthcare professional and their intention. Good clinicians and health staff have extraordinary, complex and difficult conversations as a routine part of their interactions and consequently must be multi-skilled in this (Browning, 2012). Indeed, this is an important role as a DSN as they help patients and family make sense of the condition, treatment and care being offered.

However one could suggest that trust is often taken for granted and healthcare professionals do not afford the time to explore perceptions of trust with the patient and their family (homogenisation). Building trust is based on active listening, respectful interaction and compassionate dialogue and is crucial for important conversations to occur so that clients and their family have a sense of wellbeing and make sense of the situation they are facing/due to face. The DSN formed a relationship with Conner and his wife and provided comfort through the connection and relationship, which was to be vital during Conner's time in hospital and once discharged. During this time of crisis and fear of the unknown the DSN enabled Conner's wife to voice her concerns and fears. He took time to explain the treatments to her and escalated her fears to the consultants looking after Conner. In essence he faced Conner and his wife as other human beings who had needs that he could help with; he humanised the care for them and helped them make sense through their personal journey which gave them understanding and agency.

As highlighted above there were several consultants caring for Conner's needs and the art and skill of understanding these multiple perspectives for Conner and his family fell upon the DSN; here he offered clarity of their specialist roles, understanding of the clinical situation and language used and where breakdown occurred mending the situation. The fast pace of change and nature of critical care crisis situations are susceptible to breakdown and the 'skilled know-how' (Benner et al., 1999), clinical reasoning in, and of, the situation is a key component of the DSN role as they hold the specialist knowledge of the individual diabetic patient's problems and needs.

Discussion Point

Conner's wife was feeling hopeless and vulnerable. What could healthcare professionals have done to (a) prevent it occurring and (b) manage it when it did?

There have been many studies that have explained how whilst competent nurses are very good in their understanding and critical thinking related to the clinical problems that they encounter in practice, they are less successful when trying to explain what they are doing and why to patients and families and more importantly in the case study of Conner when meeting hostility. Empowerment and autonomy help reduce or minimise hostility.

Empowerment, Autonomy and Advocacy

We doubt if there is a qualified nurse who disputes that diabetes education is essential but knowledge alone does not predict behaviour. Literature clearly indicates that poor knowledge prevents good diabetes control but good knowledge does not automatically ensure good control, and that attitudes were more strongly related and psychosocial factors have a stronger relationship to behavioural outcomes and health belief (Dunning, 2014; Jerreat, 2000; Pickup and Williams, 2003; Lockington et al., 1988). Consequently many authors discuss empowerment and empowerment models (also termed patient-centred models) which recognise that to modify behaviours and encourage patients to take responsibility for their own health the patient needs to *want* to make choices, *control* their care and *understand* the consequences. A nurse cannot empower a patient as it is not something that one person can just give to another; patients have to be helped and advised to have self-efficacy and become empowered. An evidence review by Woodall et al. (2010) highlighted that practitioners use the term 'empowered' casually. They note that healthcare practitioners appreciate that empowerment is a central principle of care as it enables patients to take greater active control of their health needs, that it has a positive impact on their self-efficacy, self-esteem, sense of control, an increase in knowledge and awareness which leads to a behaviour change and improved quality of life. Rogers (1967 and 1978) describes how healthcare practitioners' (HCP) need to have key qualities such as respect, empathy, genuineness and reassurance. He notes that *respect* is having a positive regard for the humanity of the patient and to do this HCPs need to have an unconditional positive regard for the humanity of the patient and be aware of their own prejudices and biases to ensure the patient is not adversely affected. Rogers describes *empathy* as the ability to identify with patients' experiences and feelings; *genuineness* is being honest and *reassurance* is promoting patient confidence in self and in their treatment. Consequently for empowerment to be truly felt there needs to be a collaborative approach to health care where the management of diabetes is designed to help the patient make choices, maximise their knowledge and become self-aware is vital.

One needs to recognise that Conner chose to relinquish responsibility to his wife and this could have been either because he had an external locus of control or/and due to anxiety and stress about his illness (and he did not want to take control) or/and because his wife was dominant in their relationship, that is for them to know. However, Conner's wife was hostile because she did not feel empowered. Sofhauser (2015) presents the scholarly literature on hostility and identifies that one theme is hostility due to overt or covert challenges to belief or behaviour. Conner's wife felt she was managing his diabetes well but this was challenged when he was in hospital. The DSN recognised this and encouraged questions and dialogue by using active listening allowing her time to discuss any concerns about Conner's treatment (not only about his diabetes control); he provided clear constant information and therefore developed a trusting relationship which enabled Conner's wife to feel in control and empowered. Once this was established he could start to enable her to change behaviour and make necessary changes to her management of Conner's diabetes as he helped her to develop more knowledge about diabetes and associated management.

▬▬ REFLECTIVE EXERCISE 8.1 ▬▬▬▬▬▬▬▬▬ ▬▬▬▬

Explore the knowledge of diabetes within your own team and the risk factors – i.e. social issues such as deprivation and obesity, macrovascular and microvascular foot complications, cardiovascular disease (heart disease, stroke, peripheral vascular disease, atherosclerosis), retinopathy, nephropathy, sexual dysfunction, neuropathy, depression.

- What knowledge do you and your team have regarding the relationship between insulin and food?
- Discuss feelings of fear, hopelessness and vulnerability and associated prevention and management based on trust, empowerment and advocacy.
- Explore pancreatic cancer and what the NHS could do to improve early diagnosis.
- Watch: Pancreatic carcinoma – causes, symptoms, diagnosis, treatment and pathology: www.youtube.com/watch?v=XFxMOiJRZQg
- What is the impact of having multiple specialists involved in patient care and what is the nurse's role?
- Revisit Chapters 1 and 2 and complete Table 8.1: Humanising health care for Conner.

Table 8.1 Humanising health care for Conner

Humanising dimensions	Bio-psychosocial triggers	Managing stressors and coping strategies	Role of expert ward nurse in support strategies
Insiderness/ objectification	Conner was an accountant and led an active life despite his complex medical history.		
Agency/ passivity	During early admission Conner was limited in his ability to voice his needs due to his erratic blood sugars and he relinquished responsibility of diabetes management to his wife.		
Uniqueness/ homogenisation	Conner is aware of his long-term medical diagnosis but limited in his knowledge of treatments and life expectancy related to diabetes and pancreatic cancer.		
Togetherness/ isolation	Conner's wife and his two sons from his first wife's relationship is strained and at times causes friction.		
Sense making/ loss of meaning	Conner's diabetes is not managed well. He has been referred for specialist treatment of his pancreatic cancer and is cared for by different consultants for his diabetes, COPD, CCF and pancreatic insufficiency.		
Personal journey/ loss of personal journey	Conner wishes to make a meaningful recovery, manage his diabetes and cancer and other health conditions and live the last few months of his life to the full.		
Sense of place/ dislocation	The hospital is a strange and frightening environment for Conner and his wife and policies and processes that are not his normal daily routine are affecting his diabetes management causing his wife to feel fear and distrust.		
Embodiment/ reductionist body	Conner has lost a lot of weight recently and is chronically tired and feels unwell, and this is affecting his ability to eat, interact and voice his needs and opinions.		

CHAPTER SUMMARY

This chapter has used the complicated case study of Conner to explore how healthcare providers can play a proactive role in engaging caregivers in discussion about knowledge of the underlying illness and management of the condition. It has explored how diabetes is a life-threatening condition and how the DSN has expertise not only in diabetes management but in assessing the patient and family needs and in providing timely support and education which aid patient care. It has stressed how there is a need for the DSN and how healthcare providers need to consider the infrastructures in specialist care provision.

REFERENCES

Ahmad, R., Ferlie, E. and Atun, R. (2013) How trustworthiness is assessed in health care: a sensemaking perspective, *Journal of Change Management*, *13*(2): 159–78.

Ahnquist, J., Wamala, S. and Lindstrom, M. (2010) What has trust in the health-care system got to do with psychological distress? Analyses from the national Swedish survey of public health, *International Journal of Qualitative Health Care*, *22*: 250–8.

Armstrong, K., Rose, A., Peters, N., Long, J., McMurphy, S. and Shea, J. (2006) Distrust of the health care system and self-reported health in the United States, *Journal of General Internal Medicine*, *21*(4): 292–7.

Avery, L. and Butler, J. (2008) An evaluation of the role of diabetes nurse consultants in the UK, *Journal of Diabetes Nursing*, *12*(3): 58–63.

Aylin, P., Yunus, A., Bottle, A., Majeed, A., and Bell, D. (2010) Weekend mortality for emergency admissions. A large, multicentre study, *British Medical Journal – Quality and Safety in Health Care*, *19*: 3.

Ball, L., Davmor, R., Leveritt, M., Desbrow, B., Ehrlich, C. and Chaboyer, W. (2016) The nutrition care needs of patients newly diagnosed with type 2 diabetes: informing dietetic practice, *Journal of Human Nutrition and Dietetics*, *29*(4): 487–95.

Benner, P., Hooper-Kyriakidis, P. and Stannard, D. (1999) *Clinical Wisdom and Interventions in Critical Care. A Thinking-in-action Approach*. London: W.B. Saunders Co.

Browning, D. (2012) Sturdy for common things: cultivating moral sensemaking on the front lines of practice, *Journal of Medical Ethics*, *38*: 233–5.

Carter, S., Taylor, D. and Levenson, R. (2005) *A Question of Choice-compliance in Medicine Taking. From Compliance to Concordance* (2nd edn.). London: Medicines Partnership.

Copstead, L. and Banasik, J. (2000) *Pathophysiology. Biological and Behavioural Perspectives* (2nd edn). London: W.B. Saunders Co.

Department of Health (2008) *High-Quality Care for All. NHS Next Stage Review*. London: Department of Health.

Diabetes Care (1999) Epidemiology of Diabetes Interventions and Complications (EDIC). Design, implementation, and preliminary results of a long-term follow-up of the Diabetes Control and Complications Trial cohort, *Diabetes Care*, *22*(1): 99–111.

Diabetes UK (2016) Facts and Stats. Available at: www.diabetes.org.uk/Documents/
Position%20statements/DiabetesUK_Facts_Stats_Oct16.pdf

Dunning, T. (2014) *Care of People with Diabetes: A Manual of Nursing Practice* (4th edn). Oxford:
Wiley Blackwell.

Edwards, A. and Elwyn, G. (2004) Involving patients in decision making and communication
risk: a longitudinal evaluation of doctors' attitudes and confidence during a randomised
trial, *Journal of Evaluation in Clinical Practice, 3*: 431–7.

Evert, A., Boucher, J., Cypress, M., Dunbar, S., Franz, M., Mayer-Davis, E., Neumiller, J.,
Nwankwo, R., Verdi, C., Urbanski, P., Williams, S. and Yancy, W. (2014) Nutrition
therapy recommendations for the management of adults with diabetes, *Diabetes Care, 37*:
Supplement 1.

Fisher, L. and Weihs, K.L. (2000) Can addressing family relationships improve outcomes in
chronic disease? Report of the national working group on family-based interventions in
chronic disease, *Journal of Family Practice, 49*: 561–6.

Gille, F., Smith, S. and Mays, N. (2015) Why public trust in health care systems matters
and deserves greater research attention, *Journal of Health Services Research and Policy,
20*(1): 62–4.

Gosden, C., James, J., Winocour, P., Turner, B., Walton, C., Nagi, D., Williams. R, and Holt, R.
(2009) Leading the way: the changing role of the diabetes specialist nurse, *Journal of
Diabetes Nursing, 13*(9): 330–7.

International Diabetes Federation (2015) *Diabetes Atlas* (7th edn). Available at: www.
diabetesatlas.org

James, J., Gosden, C. and Winocour, P. (2009) Diabetes specialist nurses and role evolvement:
a survey by Diabetes UK and ABCD of specialist diabetes services 2007, *Diabetes Medicine,
26*: 560–5.

Jerreat, L. (2000). *Diabetes for Nurses*. London: Whurr.

Joint Formulary Committee (2017) *BNF 73*. London: British Medical Association and Royal
Pharmaceutical Society.

Keogh, K. (2014) Lack of funds for specialist nurses 'causing a crisis in diabetes care', *Nursing
Standard, 28/29*: 11.

Lockinton, T.J., Farrant, S., Meadows, K.A., Dowlatshahi, D and Wise, P.H. (1988). Knowledge
profile and control in diabetic patients. *Diabetic Medicne.* 5; 381-386.

McCance, K. and Huether, C. (2014) *Pathophysiology: the Biological Basis for Disease*. St Louis,
MO: Elsevier/Mosby.

Middleton, N. (2012) The role of the DSN in providing quality diabetes care within
constrained finance, *Journal of Diabetes Nursing, 16*(5): 188–98.

Mohseni, M. and Lindstrom, M. (2007) Social capital, trust in the health-care system and self-
rated health: the role of access to health care in a population-based study, *Social Science
Medicine, 64*: 1373–83.

Mostofsky, D. (ed.) (2014) *The Handbook of Behavioral Medicine*. Oxford: Wiley-Blackwell.

NICE (2009) *Medicines Adherence*. London: NICE.

NICE (2015) *Type 2 Diabetes in Adults: Management*. Available at: www.nice.org.uk/guidance/
ng28/resources/type-2-diabetes-in-adults-management-pdf-1837338615493

NICE (2016a) *Type 1 Diabetes in Adults: Diagnosis and Management*. Available at: www.nice. org.uk/guidance/ng17/resources/type-1-diabetes-in-adults-diagnosis-and-management-pdf-1837276469701

NICE (2016b) *Jaundice in Adults*. Available at: https://cks.nice.org.uk/jaundice-in-adults

NICE (2016c) *Pancreatitis – Acute*. Available at: https://cks.nice.org.uk/pancreatitis-acute #!scenario

Noureldin, M. and Plake, K. (2017) Correlates of caregivers' involvement in the management of older adults' medications, *Research in Social and Administrative Pharmacy, 13*(4): 840–8.

Pancreatic Cancer UK (2018) Available at: https://www.pancreaticcancer.org.uk/information-and-support/facts-about-pancreatic-cancer/types-of-pancreatic-cancer/

Pickup, J. and Williams, G. (eds) (2003) *Textbook of Diabetes 2* (3rd edn). Oxford: Blackwell.

Pollock, K. and Grime, J. (2002) Patients' perceptions of entitlement to time in general practice consultations for depression: qualitative study, *British Medical Journal, 325*: 687–92.

Public Health England (2015) NHS Diabetes Prevention Programme (NHS DPP) Non-diabetic hyperglycaemia. Produced by: National Cardiovascular Intelligence Network (NCVIN).

Rankin, D., Heller, S. and Lawton, J. (2011) Understanding information and education gaps among people with type 1 diabetes: a qualitative investigation, *Patient Education and Counseling, 83: 1*, 87–91.

Rogers, C. (1967) *On Becoming a Person: A Therapist's View of Psychotherapy*. London: Constable.

Rogers, C. (1978) *Carl Rogers on Personal Power*. London: Constable.

Rosland, A., Heisler, M. and Piette, J. (2011) The impact of family behaviors and communication patterns on chronic illness outcomes: a systematic review, *Journal of Behavioural Medicine, 35*: 221–39.

Royal College of General Practitioners (2013) *The 2020 GP. Compendium of Evidence*. London: Royal College of General Practitioners.

Royal College of Nursing (RCN) (2010) *Clinical Nurse Specialist: Adding Value to Care*. London: RCN.

Shoff, C. and Yang, T. (2012) Untangling the associations among distrust, race, and neighbourhood social environment: A social disorganization perspective, *Social Science and Medicine, 74*(9):1342–52.

Sinclair, A.J. (2009) *Diabetes in Old Age* (3rd edn). Chichester: John Wiley and Sons.

Sofhauser, C. (2015) Hostility patterns: implications for nursing practice, *Nursing Science Quarterly, 28*(3): 202–8.

Sood, G.K. (2017) *Acute Liver Failure*. Available at: https://emedicine.medscape.com/article/177354-overview

Stratton, I.M., Adler, A.I. and Neil, H. (2000) Association of glycaemia with macrovascular and microvascular complications of Type 2 diabetes (UKPDS 35): prospective observational study, *British Medical Journal, 321*: 405–12.

Taber, J., Leyva, B. and Peroskie, A. (2014) Why do people avoid medical care? A qualitative study using national data, *Journal of General Internal Medicine, 30*(3): 290–7.

TREND-UK (2015) *An Integrated Career and Competency Framework for Diabetes Nursing* (4th ed). *TREND-UK*. SB Communications group. London. Available at: www.panpeninsuladiabetes. org/user_uploads/competency-framework.pdf

Whetten, K., Reif, S., Whetten, R. and Murphy-McMillan, L. (2008) Trauma, mental health, distrust, and stigma among HIV-Positive persons: implications for effective care, *Psychosomatic Medicine, 70*(5): 531–8.

Williams, J. (2011) Effective teamwork can improve the care of older people with diabetes, *Journal of Diabetes Nursing, 15*(3): 109–12.

Winn, K., Ozanne, E. and Sepucha, K. (2015) Measuring patient-centered care: an updated systematic review of how studies define and report concordance between patients' preferences and medical treatments, *Patient Education and Counseling, 8*(7): 811–21.

Woodall, J., Raine, G., South, J. and Warwick-Booth, L. (2010) *Empowerment and Health and Wellbeing: Evidence Review*. Centre for Health Promotion Research, Altogetherbetter. Leeds Metropolitan University. Available at: www.altogetherbetter.org.uk/our-evidence-base

World Health Organisation (2003) *Adherence to Long Term Therapies: Evidence for Action*. Available at: http://www.who.int/chp/knowledge/publications/adherence_report/en/

Yu, S., Wen, Y., Almeida, F., Estabrooks, P. and Davy, B. (2017) The effectiveness and cost of lifestyle interventions including nutrition education for diabetes prevention: a systematic review and meta-analysis, *Journal of the Academy of Nutrition and Dietetics, 117*(3): 404–22.

Yuen, E.Y.N., Knight, T., Ricciardelli, L.A., and Burney, S. (2018) Health literacy of caregivers of adult care recipients: A systematic scoping review. *Health and Social Care in the Community, 26*(2): 191–206.

CHAPTER 9

Neurological Damage

Case Studies: Richard and Steven

SARA J. WHITE AND FLEUR LOWE

CHAPTER AIMS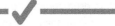

1 To explore how the history of substance misuse may delay early diagnosis and treatment.
2 To discuss the clinical decision making related to patients with spinal damage and early detection of autonomic dysreflexia.
3 To explore leadership and humanising care related to sudden catastrophic events.

INTRODUCTION

This chapter offers two case studies. The first offers a discussion regarding how the past medical history of the client hindered care and how this led to delayed treatment and dehumanised care.

The second case study explores how a patient with a spinal injury suffered a catastrophic Intracranial Haemorrhage. It explores how a HEART Choice model can be used to help humanise care for both the patient and his family at a time of critical illness. It explores how catastrophic illness impacts on patients and their families' lives.

CASE STUDY 9.1: RICHARD

This case study explores Richard's experiences after being admitted to hospital following a call to paramedics. Through marking the times at which Richard received care, the case study will indicate that a possible delay in care occurred.

(Continued)

(Continued)

Richard (aged 47) was admitted at **13:55** on a November day after his father called para-medics to his home when he found him there unresponsive. Richard had seen his GP two days before with a four-day history of flu-like symptoms, vomiting, headache, confusion and right-sided visual loss with oblique inattention. It was noted that he held his head throughout the consultation.

On arrival to hospital his neurological response fluctuated between agitation and respond-ing only to painful stimuli. Initial observations showed: Temperature 38.3°C; Blood pressure 124/76; Heart rate 82; Respiratory rate 16; O2 saturations 97% on air and an early warning score of 2. Venous blood gas analysis showed: pH 7.47; pO2 4; pCO2 4.6; Saturation 64%; Lactate 2.5. Sepsis screening occurred at **15:19** and the potential source was thought to be cerebral. Blood results were not conclusive.

Richard's records indicated that he was an ex-intravenous Drug User (ex-IVDU), opioid dependent and had depression. Previous blood results taken six months before this admis-sion were negative for Human Immunodeficiency Virus and Hepatitis C. Richard was a recov-ering drug addict and part of his rehabilitation was support from a local substance misuse service and taking Methadone.

Intravenous Ceftriaxone, aciclovir, amoxycillin and dexamethasone were prescribed; how-ever, multiple attempts at intravenous access were unsuccessful and consequently he was given intramuscular cefuroxime at **18:15**. Although an anaesthetist was contacted at **15:45** to assist with central line placement, due to other emergencies taking priority Richard was not seen until **21:30** when peripheral cannulation was achieved.

A CT scan without contrast undertaken at **18:47** indicated a possible brain abscess or tumour (see Figure 9.1, Richard's CT scan).This was discussed with the local neurological spe-cialist unit (LNSU) who requested that the CT with contrast be repeated urgently and prior to transfer. They also advised not to administer antibiotics until the second CT result was available.

Following 0.5mg of lorazepam a further CT with contrast was attempted at **01:50**, but the contrast extravasated and the procedure was abandoned. After discussion with the LNSU they agreed the patient should be transferred there immediately for drainage of a cerebral abscess. They recommended IV antibiotics, but this was not possible as Richard was too agi-tated to attempt further cannulation. Richard was moved to ITU.

During the night Richard remained agitated and confused. He accepted monitoring until **3:00 a.m.**, after which he declined monitoring. Staff recorded that he was very agitated and aggressive. He was transferred to the LNSU the next morning.

Discussion Points

- Was there a delay in treatment?
- Was the delay due to his PMH and negative reactions to drug addiction?
- Was he aggressive due to the cerebral pressure from the abscess or because he had not had his methadone or because he was being labelled and being treated inhumanely?

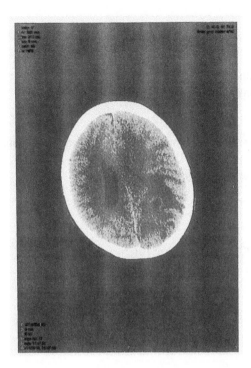

Figure 9.1 Richard's CT scan

BITE SIZE KNOWLEDGE 9.1

Brain abscess

Symptoms may develop quickly or slowly and include:

- headache, often severe, located in a single head section, not relieved with analgesia
- mental state changes such as confusion or irritability
- nerve function problems such as muscle weakness, slurred speech, paralysis
- pyrexia of = or >38C
- seizures
- nausea and vomiting
- stiff neck
- pressure on the optic nerve leading to vision blurring, greying of vision or double vision.

Causes via direct entry, blood, bacteria or fungi include:

- infection in another part of the skull or body; i.e. ear, sinusitis, dental pneumonia
- trauma; i.e. severe head injury with skull fractures
- unknown source.

(Continued)

(Continued)

Treatment includes a combination of:

- antibiotics or antifungals
- surgery: aspiration or craniotomy.

Complications include:

- reoccurring abscess (more common in people with weakened immunity or cyanotic heart disease)
- mild to moderate brain damage
- epilepsy
- meningitis.

(After: Török, et al., 2017; Estenson, 2015)

BITE SIZE KNOWLEDGE 9.2

Opiates

Historically an Opiate is a drug derived from opium. The more modern term Opioid includes natural and synthetic substances that bind to opioid receptors in the brain. Opiates act on the delta, kappa, lambda and mu subtypes of opiate receptors in the brain and mimic the actions of endorphins, which regulate pain and pleasure. The most serious drugs of addiction are cocaine, heroin, morphine and the synthetic opioids.

Opium is produced from Papaver Somniferum, a species of the poppy plant. Opium contains over 60 pharmacologically active ingredients, including codeine and morphine. For the illegal drug trade, the morphine is extracted from the opium and converted to heroin which is two to four times as potent and has a greatly reduced weight and bulk. Heroin is a Class A drug discovered by Alder Wright (British chemist) in 1847. In 1889 its potency (10 times that of morphine) was detected by Heinrich Dreser (German pharmacologist). Heroin can be sniffed or smoked or injected subcutaneously (SC) or intravenously (IV). SC or IV routes give a faster, more intense peak effect. The potency of street heroin tends to be low.

The synthetic opioid Fentanyl has a rapid onset and effects generally last less than an hour or two. Fentanyl was first made by Paul Janssen in 1960; it is similar in structure to pethidine (meperidine). It is the most widely used opioid in medicine. Side effects include nausea, constipation, sleepiness, and confusion, respiratory depression, serotonin syndrome, hypotension, or addiction. Fentanyl works in part by activating opioid receptors. It is about 75 times stronger than morphine for a given amount. Some fentanyl equivalents may be as much as 10,000 times stronger than morphine.

Recreational side effects of using Opiates: The use of non-sterile needles and syringes facilitates IV entry and dissemination into the blood of infective organisms can cause: infective endocarditis, haemorrhagic and embolic infarcts, botulism, tetanus, meningitis, cerebral abscess, septic arteritis, osteomyelitis, discitis causing extradural abscesses and cord involve-ment, HIV and AIDS, altered immune system (humoral, cell mediated, and phagocytic defects). Contaminants within the injection (talc or corn starch) may embolise in retinal arteries and/or cause infarction in the spinal cord or brain.

Effects include euphoria, drowsiness, anxiety, increased alertness, nausea, vomiting, auto-nomic effects include small pupils, difficulty passing urine, flushing, and dry mouth.

Overdose causes: coma, deep respiratory depression, bradycardia, hypotension, non-cardiogenic pulmonary oedema, aspiration, post-anoxic encephalopathy, cardiorespiratory arrest, stroke (caused by infective arteritis/mycotic aneurysm, infective endocarditis or par-adoxical embolism).

(After: Török et al, 2017; UNODC, 2017; Joint Formulary Committe, 2017; Hoffbrand and Moss 2015; BMA, 2015; Olson, 2012).

· DISCUSSION

A brain abscess is a pus-filled swelling in the brain and usually occurs when bacteria or fungi enter the brain tissue after an infection or severe head injury. The risk of developing a brain abscess is extremely low. However, because swelling caused by the abscess can disrupt the blood and oxygen supply to the brain, it is a life-threatening condition and should be treated as a medical emergency. There is also a risk of the abscess bursting (Hoffbrand and Moss, 2015). Central nervous system infections in injection drug users are often devastating in terms of excess morbidity and mortality. In injection drug users with infective endocarditis, embolisation from infected valvular vegetations may cause cerebral infarction, intracranial haemorrhage, and the formation of brain abscess. Focal intracranial infections (i.e. brain abscess and spinal epidural abscess) may occur in the absence of infective endocarditis, resulting from bacteraemia that seeds the brain or epi-dural space. Toxin-mediated diseases (especially tetanus and wound botulism) are also seen in injection drug users. Inoculation of Clostridium spp at injection sites may lead to toxin generation and disease (Török, et al., 2017; Olson, 2012). Clinicians must maintain a high level of thought for these diagnoses in injection drug users.

Substance use disorders are severely stigmatised, and more often evoke more disapproval and negative opinions than other mental illnesses. Stigmatisation of substance use disor-ders has been investigated from different perspectives such as among the general public, healthcare professionals and clients in treatment for substance abuse. For instance, the Dutch general public showed high intentions to impose far-reaching restrictions on people with an alcohol or drug addiction which minimise their participation within society (Van Boekel et al., 2013a, 2013b). Amongst others Gilchrist et al. (2011) and Van Boekel et al. (2014) found that some healthcare professionals have negative attitudes related to clients with an alcohol or drug addiction. The experiences of rejection and anticipation of discrimination were prevalent among individuals in treatment for substance use disorders; and the stigma attached to addiction affects different aspects of their life and can have major consequences (Schomerus et al., 2011; Room et al., 2001; Crisp et al., 2000, Pescosolido et al., 1999). Apart from the adverse consequences for the quality of life of individuals and their life wants or needs or opportunities (such as employment or housing) the stigma attached to addiction may also prevent individuals from seeking help for substance use problems, as fear of negative reactions is a barrier for seeking treatment (Van Der Pol et al., 2013; Alonso et al., 2009).

Discussion Point

- Could stigmatisation have affected Richard's GP when he presented at the surgery?
- Did stigmatisation contribute to a delay in any of Richard's investigations, procedures, treatment and care?

Richard was an ex-IVDU who was opioid dependent and being treated with methadone. The effects of opioids can mask symptoms of other underlying neurological pathology and deterioration (see Bite Size Knowledge 9.2: Opiates). The recognition of drug addiction should raise suspicion that the presenting neurological syndrome may have an unusual aetiology and pathogenesis, with the potential for multiple pathologies and may, therefore, be complex to manage. According to Olson (2012) certain common clinical themes are useful, partly because their recognition may act as an early warning sign for drug abuse, such as their age, very late presentation, inconsistent or unreliable history, and the tendency to abscond.

It is sometimes difficult to attribute a particular clinical syndrome to a particular drug type. Certain common features emerge which may be related directly and specifically to the drug, but other clinical features may arise in a non-specific way from complications of injection and/or coma. Addicts may use multiple drugs (wittingly or unwittingly), and the dose and the constituents of what they take, in terms of contaminants and other substitutes, can vary according to the source and consignment. The effects of the drug may vary considerably according to the method of intake, and they may be intensified by coincidental alcohol use. Whilst in many instances of drug misuse the effects of the drug wear off without incident, problems can arise directly due to the drug and its constituents and identifying these in individual cases is very difficult, causing a variable clinical picture (Garland and Howard, 2012; Howard et al., 2008; Haddad et al., 2007).

Discussion Point

- Could any of these factors have been thought out when Richard first presented at his GP?

NEUROIMAGING

There are difficulties in clinically diagnosing brain abscess and neuroimaging is essential (Love et al., 2015). In general, radiographic abnormalities depend on the particular stage of the brain abscess. Neuroimaging can estimate the age of the brain abscess. This is important as a lesion in the early or late cerebritis stage may be managed somewhat differently compared with a mature, walled-off abscess (see 'Treatment' below). CT scanning with contrast during early cerebritis may show only oedema, which may or may not enhance with contrast. If done very early in the course of infection, a contrast-enhanced CT may be normal. During later stages, there is the development of a space-occupying lesion, which is often surrounded by a large area of oedema. Although contrast-enhanced CT scanning is considered sensitive for the detection of brain abscesses, it is not specific. Brain abscesses tend to have smooth thin-walled capsules, whereas tumours tend to have more irregular capsules. There are additional characteristics of brain tumours, but some overlap exists with brain abscesses. It is important to note that brain abscesses and brain tumours may have an identical appearance on the CT scan. MR imaging is more sensitive than CT, and MRI can usually detect infection in the early cerebritis stage (Love et al., 2015).

Discussion Point

- The neurological specialist unit requested a repeat CT with contrast – explore the necessity of this and how it helped Richard's treatment.

Treatment

The optimal treatment of brain abscess is complex and requires a coordinated approach among multiple teams. There are no large, randomised, clinical trials comparing different antimicrobial regimens or different neurosurgical approaches, but several studies have demonstrated dramatic improvement in survival using a combination of antimicrobial therapy combined with surgical drainage (Helweg-Larsen et al., 2012; Muzumdar et al., 2011; Brook, 2009; Carpenter et al., 2007). In most patients, particularly those with abscesses larger than 2.5 cm, stereotactic aspiration or open brain biopsy with evacuation should be strongly considered for microbiologic diagnosis, given the wide range of possible pathogens and the prolonged course of IV antibiotics required. Neurologically stable patients with early infections in the cerebritis stage can be treated with IV antibiotics alone, with aspiration attempted when the infection later appears more encapsulated and liquefied, to maximise the yield of an aspiration procedure (Estenson, 2015). Alternatively, an area of focal cerebritis without a frank abscess may still be aspirated through a burr hole, but the volume of fluid and tissue may be small. Large abscesses (>2.5 cm) should generally be aspirated, drained, or completely excised.

For patients with multiple abscesses of varying sizes, large collections may be aspirated and/or evacuated, and smaller abscesses treated medically. Serial CT scans need to be obtained afterwards to assess the stability of the remaining abscesses, because repeat aspirations may be necessary. Patients with multiple small (<2 cm) abscesses may respond to medical therapy alone, particularly if the lesions are smaller than 1 cm, but these patients also need serial neuroimaging. Medical treatment is usually attempted when abscesses are also in deep locations, such as the brainstem. However, a medical approach carries a significant risk of selection of incorrect antibiotics. This is particularly problematic for the immunocompromised patient, in whom the spectrum of pathogens is even more unpredictable (Haddad et al., 2007).

In summary this case study has multiple questions related to delay in treatment, negative perceptions and stigmatisation of drug users amongst health professionals and as such is a good study for open frank discussion, reflection and development.

REFLECTIVE EXERCISE 9.1

- What are the common key 'red flag' features that would raise suspicion of drug misuse?
- What factors may influence adverse effects with recreational drugs?
- Drawing on Chapters 1 and 2 consider writing a humanising healthcare framework for Richard.
- Substance abuse affects all members of the family in some way. How could healthcare professionals educate and support Richard's father to cope with his feelings generated by his son's critical illness?

CASE STUDY 9.2: STEVEN

This case study is about 'Steven', an active 60-year-old married man who is a full time engineer, whose only past medical history is a myocardial infarction 13 years ago. Steven fell from a ladder in the summer which caused a fracture dislocation of C5 & C6 – which was fixed anteriorly. In September he had cardiac arrhythmia and a permanent pacemaker was inserted. He was transferred to a regional spinal unit for rehabilitation in October. In mid-November staff noticed that he was very tired and sleepy and that his chest had bilateral crepitations. Examination showed that his PO2 was reduced and 2L of nasal O2 was administered. It was noted that he was tolerating his Nasogastric feed and in the last 24 hours he had a negative fluid balance 245mls. He had not had his bowels open for two days. He remained unwell during the shift and was regularly monitored. During the 21:00 p.m. monitoring it was noted that his respiratory rate and systolic blood pressure had increased and his early warning score was now indicating 3 out of 4. (National Early Warning Score (NEWS) was launched in 2012 in the NHS and it improves the detection and response to clinical deterioration in adult patients and is a key element of patient safety and improving patient outcome: NHS England, 2017). An abdominal examination was undertaken and this questioned if cholecystitis or autonomic dysreflexia was occurring and an abdominal ultrasound was ordered. Whilst waiting for this IV fluids were administered; a chest X-ray, ECG, catheter specimen of urine (CSU), blood screen and hourly observations were requested. Over that evening and night he remained unwell but stable. To help with respiratory distress non-invasive BiPAP was commenced (see Chapter 5: Bite Size Knowledge 5.4 - re BiPAP).

At 6:30 the next morning he was reassessed and this showed that his respiratory rate had increased to 30 BPM, his blood pressure had risen to 152/90, his heart rate was 89 bpm, his BM 7, and that his blood results were within normal parameters. However, whilst being assessed Steven started 'snoring'; a jaw thrust occurred and the resuscitation team were called. Unfortunately his pupils became dilated and fixed and a catastrophic brain injury appeared to have occurred. An urgent brain scan showed an intracranial haemorrhage (see 9.1: Bite Size Knowledge: Brain abscess). Having been orally intubated and ventilated he was transferred to the ITU where upon suction thick yellow secretions were obtained (see Chapter 3: Bite Size Knowledge 3.1: Respiratory Failure and Bite Size Knowledge 3.2: Sepsis).

Meanwhile the on-call Neurologist at an Local Specialist Neurological Unit (LSNU) was contacted for advice; who having reviewed Steven's notes and scan suggested that the injury was un-survivable and no neurosurgical intervention would help. As soon as possible 'during' the event Steven's wife and daughter were contacted and at 15:30 that day they were informed that he was unlikely to survive. Meanwhile cranial diabetes insipidus occurred. His blood sodium gradually started to rise. Treatment was shortly discontinued and Steven died.

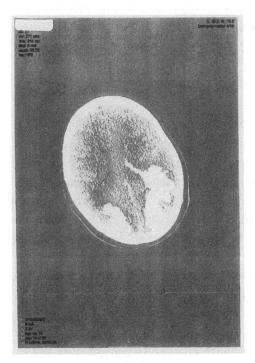

Figure 9.2 Steven's CT scan

DISCUSSION

This chapter section does not aim to explore spinal injuries but draws upon the case study to explore how staff should:

- be mindful of the need to report subtle changes in observations
- seek advice regarding reduction in post-surgical/injury/trauma complications; symptom control and care management
- understand the implications of catastrophic intracranial haemorrhage in order to assist the family.

Patients with spinal cord damage have a loss or total absence of sensory and motor functions in the lowest sacral segments and as such staff need to be aware that presentation of symptoms can be very subtle. Steven was being cared for in a specialist ward but we need to remember that most spinal patients admitted to hospital are admitted to general wards for surgery or medical care. Therefore you might like to:

- explore what your staff know about conditions outside of their own specialism

- explore how staff can obtain knowledge reasonably quickly when needed, e.g. spinal injury and Autonomic dysreflexia (AD), and how the clinical leader creates this progression
- use Steven's case study to explore what may have occurred; what the slight changes in cardiovascular readings indicated and what may have contributed to Steven's deterioration.

What is Autonomic Dysreflexia?

Autonomic dysreflexia (AD) is a syndrome whereby a sudden, massive reflex sympathetic discharge associated spinal cord injury at or above T5–T6. AD is triggered by a somatic or visceral stimulus below the spinal cord lesion, where supraspinal control of the sympathetic nervous system is disrupted causing an imbalance between sympathetic and parasympathetic nervous systems. Most commonly this can be from stimulus from the bladder or bowel (colorectal distension) where sympathetic mediated vasoconstriction occurs together with hyperactivity of the adrenal medulla with associated rises in norepinephrine and epinephrine levels. Caruso et al. (2015) also report that there may be an upregulation of alpha-1 and alpha-2 adrenoreceptors which leads to increased vascular reactivity. These lead to uncontrolled hypertension (AD) and if left untreated AD results in intracerebral haemorrhage, seizure, retinal detachment and death (Wan and Krassioukov, 2014) (see Bite Size Knowledge 9.2: Autonomic Dysreflexia – Causes, Symptoms and Treatment).

━━ BITE SIZE KNOWLEDGE 9.2 ━━━━━━━━━━━ ━━━━━━━

Autonomic Dysreflexia – causes, symptoms and treatment

Causes:

- spinal cord injury (the most common cause)
- Guillain-Barré syndrome
- severe head trauma and other brain injuries
- subarachnoid haemorrhage
- recreational drugs such as cocaine and amphetamines.

Debilitating symptoms include:

- bradycardia (30–40BPM)
- paroxysmal hypertension
- pounding headache and dizziness
- sweating
- muscle spasms
- skin colour changes: paleness, redness, blue-grey
- nausea
- blurred vision
- fever
- distended bladder or rectum.

Treatment:

- elevate head of bed
- establish cause and remove stimulus
- empty bladder and bowel
- Calcium Channel blockers/adrenergic receptor blocking agents.

(After: Caruso et al., 2015; McCance and Huether, 2014; Copstead and Banasik, 2000)

Clinical decision making in this case study involves a multifaceted interplay of elements in the situation, for example due consideration of the subtle changes in cardiovascular observations, lack of bowel action as a contributing factor to AD and early detection and management of potential complications. The nurse caring for Steven needed to demonstrate patient-centred care (see Chapter 1), working collaboratively to offer care of the highest possible quality, which was safe, effective, person-centred, timely, efficient and equitable (The Health Foundation, 2016). S/he needed to be an adaptive decision maker using a variety of strategies to make judgements and choices about the care Steven needed. Micro-decisions when caring for Steven may have involved the routine interventions, for example hygiene needs, medication administration, and probably involved continuous thinking about planning care needed and actions to be taken. But did the nurse move to the next level of clinical decision making (i.e. the meso level)? Here meso-decisions needed were related to more structural factors such as calling upon the specialist nurse or outreach to review him. It may have involved cultural considerations and ethical decision making, i.e. that of individual freedom to make choices (Thiroux and Krasemann, 2014). But did Steven have the knowledge base regarding the importance of bowel action for spinal patients and if this was considered when asking him if he wanted to have his bowel evacuated?

SO WHAT IS THE ROLE OF THE LEADER IN THIS CASE STUDY?

Gopee and Galloway's (2017) HEART Choice model (*Holism, Empowerment, Advocacy, Respect, Trust, Choice*) can be used to achieve patient-centred care in everyday practice and is applicable to the care of Steven. When applied to the situation being discussed, each central node can be understood as follows:

Holism – Due consideration of humanising care for Steven as he is 'viewed' via the eight humanising care dimensions – see Table 9.1.

Empowerment – Empower Steven by giving evidence based knowledge for the care needed.

Advocacy – The nurse caring for Steven could liaise with the specialist or outreach nurse.

Respect – The nurse–patient relationship is a mutual and helping relationship based on the nurturing of faith and hope and offering humanised health care.

Trust – The nurse needs to show confidence in care so that Steven knows that s/he was both reliable and knowledgable and acting in his best interests.

Choice – Whilst Steven needed to be given choice on the micro level of care, the time to develop his understanding at a meso level would have been limited because the nurse needed to act quickly in his best interests (NMC, 2015).

To achieve the elements of HEART Choice the clinical leader could develop staff by using the GROW model. The GROW model is a well-established and successful coaching model (Whitmore, 2009), used for goal setting and problem solving. GROW stands for Goals, Reality, Options, and Will, these steps being necessary in a problem solving processes. When applying this to establishing staff development and using Steven's case study this could consist of meeting individuals or teams to ask:

Goal: What goal do you/we want to achieve? How would you/we know that you/we had achieved it? What is your/our sphere of influence?

Reality: What is the current situation? What is not occurring? What have you/we done so far? What obstacles are in the way?

Options: What could you/we do? What else could you/we do? What do you/we want managers to do?

Will: When will you/we start? How long will it take? Who needs to help you/us?

One goal could be related to knowledge about catastrophic intracranial haemorrhage.

What is Catastrophic Intracranial Haemorrhage?

Figure 9.2 shows Steven's CT scan, post-injury. Intracranial haemorrhage (ICH) is a serious medical emergency and is a significant cause of morbidity and mortality throughout the world. ICH can be spontaneous and non-traumatic and if diagnosed early and appropriate intervention undertaken then many can survive (Steiner et al., 2013; Morgenstern et al., 2010; Runchey and McGee, 2010). Naidech (2011) high-lighted that critical care staff need to assess the possible cause, minimise the risks of further haemorrhage by controlling blood pressure, correct coagulopathy, and eradicate vascular lesions that may lead to re-bleeding. Unfortunately Steven's ICH was large and no intervention was taken.

Discussion Points

Using the GROW model consider:

- What do your staff need to know about ICH and what is your goal?
- What obstacles are in the way of them gaining that knowledge?
- What do you as the clinical leader need to do?
- What actions do you need to take to explore your staff's perceptions of their developmental needs?

This now moves us to explore how care could be humanised for Steven's wife and daughter in the last few hours of his life.

Fett (2000) writes of the benefits of science and technology and cites Bunker et al. (1994) who estimated that, over the twentieth century, life expectancy in industrialised countries increased from around 45 to 75 years. They suggest that about five years of the improvement to life expectancy is due to clinical care. One could suggest that in the previous century Steven would not have survived his fall and the effectiveness of health provision enabled him to have four months more time with his family. Whilst they could not have been aware of his impending death nor had time for making informed choices about dying (DoH, 2015) they had been coming to terms with his critical illness. Hickman and Douglas (2010) discuss how critical illness of a chronic nature, such as Steven's, exposes the patient and their family, to 'heightened levels of psychological distress' (2010: 80). Family members require a sense of trust in the critical care team and the principles of the HEART Choice model can be equally applied to care of the family, for example:

Holism – As Steven's care is considered via the eight humanising care dimensions the nurse needs to fully involve his wife (see Table 9.1).

Empowerment – The family need to be given the evidence based knowledge for the care being offered. They need to be updated on Steven's condition very regularly remembering that stress caused by an emotional trauma can lead to memory loss. Davidson et al. (2007) reviewed over 300 studies and discuss how information giving and truth telling enhances family relationships with staff and enhances coping.

Advocacy – The advantages of a multifaceted care approach to his care and the discussion of care with the specialist or outreach nurse needs to be explained; Davidson et al. (2007) discuss the need for consistency in communication. Therefore the bedside nurse needs to be present when the specialist or outreach nurse or doctors speak with the family.

Respect – The nurse–family relationship is also based on a mutual helping and trusting relationship. Leske and Jiricka (1998) noted that interventions such as problem solving communication may be effective in promoting the adaptation of families of critically injured patients.

Trust – The nurse needs to show confidence in the care being offered and demonstrate that s/he is reliable, knowledgable and acting in Steven's best interests.

Choice – Steven's family need to be given the choice to stay with Steven or be confident in the care being offered so that they can leave him. Alvarez and Kirby (2006) reviewed the literature on the perspective of the family during their loved one's critical illness and showed that they favoured not just good communication but having close proximity to the patient and flexible visiting; since then the majority of intensive care units have 'open' visiting.

Table 9.1 Humanising health care for Steven

Humanising dimensions	Bio-psychosocial triggers	Managing stressors and coping strategies	Role of expert nurse in support strategies
Insiderness/ objectification	Steven was an active electrician. Having sustained a fractured spine following a fall from a ladder he was slowly coming to terms with the ramifications and the necessary rehabilitation and dependency on the MDT. Having sustained an intracranial haemorrhage his life expectancy is deemed to be very short.	Steven is being given 1:1 care. Steven's family need to be with him in his last hours of life. Steven needs to know that he is loved and cherished.	Enable connectedness by helping staff understand that Steven requires a peaceful death and that his family need to be able to remember his death as peaceful.
Agency/passivity	Steven is not able to voice his needs so needs all care. He cannot voice if he has pain. Presently life is being sustained by invasive ventilation.	Steven needs all physical and psychological care.	Encourage staff to ensure that necessary ADL's are being met. Support staff to encourage his family to express their love and help them recognise that hearing is one of the last senses to leave a dying patient.
Uniqueness/ homogenisation	Steven is dying but he still needs to be made comfortable with his surroundings, treatment and comfort needs.	Steven needs regular review of treatments to ensure his comfort needs are being met despite not being able to voice his needs.	Facilitate staff to appreciate that a dying patient still needs to be helped with awareness of time, location and treatments.
Togetherness/ isolation	As Steven deteriorates, he wants his family near him. Constant vigilance is affecting the family as they struggle to cope with his imminent death.	His family are attentive to his needs and want to help ease any discomfort and anxiety he may feel.	Assist staff to consider the impact of Steven's illness since his fall and intracranial haemorrhage and let them voice their emotional needs at the same time as promoting a dignified and comfortable death for Steven. Encourage staff to explore their personal coping with death and who they can turn to for help when death occurs. Encourage family to tell Steven of their support.

(Continued)

Table 9.1 (Continued)

Humanising dimensions	Bio-psychosocial triggers	Managing stressors and coping strategies	Role of expert nurse in support strategies
Sense making/ loss of meaning	Steven was referred to the spinal unit for specialist rehabilitation and the immediacy of the intracranial bleed could not have been determined. However Steven still needs help to make sense of what he may be feeling even if he cannot express his concerns and anxieties.	Steven needs to be given constant reinforcement of what is occurring and that his family are with him.	Enable staff to make sense of: (a) the impact on family members when a loved one is dying (b) feelings of desperation and powerlessness in coping with the situation.
Personal journey/loss of personal journey	Steven's optimism and hope of making a meaningful recovery and living with a spinal injury is now not an option as the bleed is not survivable. His family's world was deeply troubled following the spinal injury and now their worst fears have been confirmed.	Steven needs continuous technical intervention and monitoring.	Enable humanised care by encouraging staff to get to know who Steven is as a person, what he has enjoyed during his life and what he may presently be concerned about and offer comfort strategies.
Sense of place/ dislocation	ICU is a strange and frightening environment which Steven knows nothing of.	Steven needs staff to attend to his needs who are knowledgeable, competent and confident to manage the necessary equipment whilst keeping disruption to a minimum and maintaining a peaceful environment.	Encourage staff, and family, to create an environment that reminds Steven of happy times in his life.
Embodiment/ reductionist body	Steven may not know of the intracranial bleed but may remember his spinal injury and rehabilitation.	Staff are focused on monitoring physical signs, symptoms and technical observations.	Inspire staff to view Steven as a man who has lived a full life and made meaningful contributions to the world in which he lived.

Discussion Points

Using the GROW model consider:

- What are your staff's issues/needs are when caring for a distressed family?
- What do they want to achieve?
- What is the goal?
- What obstacles are in the way?
- What do you as the clinical leader need to do to help them achieve their goal?
- What are their developmental needs?
- How can these be achieved?
- Who can be contacted for help?

This case study has shown how subtle changes in cardiovascular monitoring could lead to issues such as respiratory failure, septic shock, Autonomic Dysreflexia, intracranial haemorrhage and how, alongside the humanising framework, the HEART Choice and GROW models can be used to facilitate learning and development.

REFLECTIVE EXERCISE 9.2

1 Review Steven's case study and explore what else could have been done.
2 How can staff assist patients and families to cope with critical illness and pending death? And what learning and help do staff need to improve confidence?
3 Consider what communication strategies were needed and would staff have these when caring for patients and families of patients such as Steven?
4 Critically analyse the Humanising Dimensions offered in Table 9.1.
5 Explore the HEART Choice and GROW models to see if these could be utilised in your clinical area.

CHAPTER SUMMARY

This chapter has explored two very different neurological conditions and associated care. However both proved challenging in respect to treatment of clients by staff and caring requirements of family. We hope it challenges nurses to think about their own practice and that of others when considering areas of prejudice and limited knowledge. We hope it enables facilitation and reflection.

FURTHER READING

Dorenbeck, U., Butz, B., Schlaier, J., Bretschneider, T., Schuierer, G. and Feuerbach, S. (2003) Diffusion-weighted echo-planar MRI of the brain with calculated ADCs: a useful tool in the differential diagnosis of tumour necrosis from abscess? *Journal of Neuroimaging, 13*(4): 330–8.

Royal College of Nursing (RCN) (2010) *Specialist Nurses: Changing Lives, Saving Money*. www. rcn.org.uk/professional-development/publications/pub-003581

Sener, R.N. (2004) Diffusion MRI findings in neonatal brain abscess, *American Journal of Neuroradiology*, *31*: 69–71.

Spijkerman, I., van Ameijden, E., Mientjes, G., Coutinho, R. and van den Hoek, A. (1996) Human immunodeficiency virus infection and other risk factors for skin abscesses and endocarditis among injection drug users, *Journal of Clinical Epidemiology, 49*: 1149–54.

Sudhakar, K.V., Agrawal, S., Rashid, M., Hussain, R., Hussain, M. and Gupta, R.K. (2001) MRI demonstration of haemorrhage in the wall of a brain abscess: possible implications for diagnosis and management, *Neuroradiology, 43*: 218–22.

REFERENCES

Alonso, J., Buron, A., Rojas-Farreras, S., De Graaf, R., Haro, J.M. and De Girolamo, G. (2009) Perceived stigma among individuals with common mental disorders, *Journal of Affective Disorders, 118*(1–3): 180–6.

Alvarez, G.F. and Kirby, A.S. (2006) The perspective of families of the critically ill patient: their needs, *Current Opinion in Critical Care, 12*(6): 614–18.

British Medical Association (BMA) (2015) *New Guide to Medicines and Drugs* (9th edn). London: Penguin Random House.

Brook, I. (2009) Microbiology and antimicrobial treatment of orbital and intracranial complications of sinusitis in children and their management, *International Journal of Pediatric Otorhinolaryngology, 73*(9): 1183–6.

Carpenter, J., Stapleton, S. and Holliman, R. (2007) Retrospective analysis of 49 cases of brain abscess and review of the literature, *European Journal of Clinical Microbiology and Infectious Diseases, 26*: 1–11.

Caruso, D., Gater, D. and Harnish, C. (2015) Prevention of recurrent autonomic dysreflexia: a survey of current practice, *Clinical Autonomic Research, 25*: 293–300.

Copstead, L.E. and Banasik, J.L. (2000) *Pathophysiology: Biological and Behavioural Perspectives* (2nd ed). London: Saunders.

Crisp, A.H., Gelder, M.G., Rix, S., Meltzer, H.I. and Rowlands, O.J. (2000) Stigmatisation of people with mental illnesses, *British Journal of Psychiatry, 177*: 4–7.

Davidson, J.E., Powers, K., Hedayat, K.M., Tieszen M., Kon, A.A., Shepard, E., Spuhler, V., Todres, I.D., Levy, M., Barr, J., Ghandi, R., Hirsch, G. and Armstrong, D. (2007) Clinical practice guidelines for support of the family in the patient-centered intensive care unit: American College of Critical Care Medicine Task Force 2004–2005, *Critical Care Medicine, 35*(2): 605–22.

Department of Health (DoH) (2015) *Choice in End of Life Care*. Available at: www.gov.uk/ government/publications/choice-in-end-of-life-care

Estenson, J. (2015) *Brain Abscess: Resource and Reference Guide for Patients and Health Care Professionals*. Seattle, WA: Capitol Hill Press.

Fett, M. (2000) *Occasional Papers: Health Financing Series*. Volume 5. Commonwealth Department of Health and Aged Care. Available at: www.health.gov.au/internet/main/ publishing.nsf/Content/DA8177ED1A80D332CA257BF0001B08EE/$File/ocpahfsv5.pdf

Garland, E. and Howard, M. (2012) *Volatile Substance Misuse: Clinical Considerations, Neuropsychopharmacology and Potential Role of Pharmacotherapy in Management*. Switzerland: Springer International Publishing.

Gilchrist, G., Moskalewicz, J., Slezakova, S., Okruhlica, L., Torrens, M. and Vajd, R. (2011) Staff regard towards working with substance users: a European multi-centre study, *Addiction*, *106*(6): 1114–25.

Gopee, N. and Galloway, J. (2017) *Leadership and Management in Health Care* (3rd edn). London: Sage.

Haddad, L., Shannon, M. and Winchester, J. (2007) *Clinical Management of Poisoning and Drug Overdose* (4th edn). Philadelphia: Saunders.

Helweg-Larsen, J., Astradsson, A., Richhall, H., Erdal, J., Laursen, A. and Brennum, J. (2012) Pyogenic brain abscess, a 15 year survey, *Biomedic Enctral Infectious Diseases*, *12*: 332.

Hickman, R.L., and Douglas, S.L. (2010) Impact of chronic critical illness on the psychological outcomes of family members, *American Association of Critical – Care Nurses, Advanced Critical Care*, *21*(1): 80–91.

Hoffbrand, A.V. and Moss, P.A.H. (2015) *Hoffbrand's Essential Haematology*. Chichester: Wiley Blackwell.

Howard, M., Balster, R. and Cottler, L. (2008) Inhalant use among incarcerated adolescents in the United States: prevalence, characteristics and correlates of use, *Drug Alcohol Depend*. *93*(3): 197–209.

Joint Formulary Committee (2017) *BNF 73*. London: British Medical Association and Royal Pharmaceutical Society.

Leske, J.S., and Jiricka, M.K. (1998) Impact of family demands and family strengths and capabilities on family well-being and adaptation after critical injury, *American Journal of Critical Care*, *7*(5): 383–92.

Love, S., Perry, A., Ironside. J. and Budka, H. (2015) *Greenfield's Neuropathology* (9th edn). London: CRC Press.

McCance, K.L. and Huether, S.E. (2014) *Pathophysiology. The Biologic Basis for Disease in Adults and Children* (7th edn). Canada: Elsevier.

Morgenstern, L.B., Hemphill III, J.C., Anderson, C., Becker, K., Broderick, J.P., Connolly, E.S., Greenberg, S.M., Huang, J.N., Macdonald, R.L., Messé, S.R., Mitchell, P.H., Selim, M. and Tamargo, R.J. (2010) *Guidelines for the Management of Spontaneous Intracerebral Hemorrhage*. American Heart Association/American Stroke Association.

Muzumdar, D., Jhawar, S. and Goel, A. (2011) Brain abscess: an overview, *International Journal of Surgery*, *9*(2): 136–44.

Naidech, A.M. (2011) Intracranial Hemorrhage, *American Journal of Respiratory and Critical Care Medicine*, *184*(9): 998–1006.

NHS England (2017) National Early Warning Score (NEWS) www.england.nhs.uk/nationalearlywarningscore

Nursing and Midwifery Council (NMC) (2015) *The Code. Professional Standards of Practice and Behaviour for Nurses and Midwives*. Available at: www.nmc.org.uk/standards/code/

Olson, K.R. (ed.) (2012) *Poisoning and Drug Overdose* (6th edn). New York: McGraw-Hill.

Pescosolido, B., Monahan, J., Link, B., Stueve, A., and Kikuzawa, S. (1999) The public's view of the competence, dangerousness, and need for legal coercion of persons with mental health problems, *American Journal of Public Health*, *89*(9): 1339–45.

Room, R., Rehm, J., Trotter, R., Paglia, A.,and Üstün, T. (2001) Cross-cultural views on stigma, valuation, parity and societal values towards disability, in Üstün, T.B., Chatterji, S. and Bickenbach, J.E. (eds), *Disability and Culture: Universalism and Diversity* (pp. 247–91). Seattle, WA: Hofgrebe and Huber.

Runchey, S. and McGee, S. (2010) Does this patient have a hemorrhagic stroke? Clinical findings distinguishing hemorrhagic stroke from ischemic stroke, *Journal of the American Medical Association*, *303*(22): 2280–6.

Schomerus, G., Lucht, M., Holzinger, A., Matschinger, H., Carta, M.G. and Angermeyer, M.C. (2011) The stigma of alcohol dependence compared with other mental disorders: a review of population studies, *Alcohol and Alcoholism*, *46*(2): 105–12.

Steiner, T., Juvela, S., Unterberg, A., Jung, C., Forsting, M. and Rinke, G. (2013) European stroke organization guidelines for the management of intracranial aneurysms and subarachnoid haemorrhage, *Cerebrovascular Disease*, *35*: 93–112.

The Health Foundation (2016) *Person Centred Care Resource Centre*. Available at: http:// personcentredcare.health.org.uk/about-us-0

Thiroux, J. and Krasemann, K. (2014) *Ethics, Theory and Practice* (11th edn). Hoboken, NJ: Pearson and Prentice Hall.

Török, E., Moran, E. and Cooke, F. (2017) *Oxford Handbook of Infectious Diseases and Microbiology* (2nd edn). Oxford: Oxford University Press.

United Nations Office on Drugs and Crime (UNODC) (2017) Commission on Narcotic Drugs takes decisive step to help prevent deadly fentanyl overdoses. www.unodc.org/unodc/en/ frontpage/2017/March/commission-on-narcotic-drugs-takes-decisive-step-to-help-prevent-deadly-fentanyl-overdoses.html

Van Boekel, L.C., Brouwers, E.P.M., Van Weeghel, J. and Garretsen, H.F.L. (2013a) Public opinion on imposing restrictions to people with an alcohol- or drug addiction: a cross-sectional survey, *Social Psychiatry and Psychiatric Epidemiology*, *48*(12): 2007–16.

Van Boekel, L.C., Brouwers, E.P.M., Van Weeghel, J. and Garretsen, H.F.L. (2013b) Stigma among health professionals towards patients with substance use disorders and its consequences for healthcare delivery: systematic review, *Drug and Alcohol Dependence*, *131*(1–2): 23–35.

Van Boekel, L.C., Brouwers, E.P.M., Van Weeghel, J. and Garretsen, H.F.L. (2014) Healthcare professionals' regard towards working with patients with substance use disorders: comparison of primary care, general psychiatry and specialist addiction services, *Drug and Alcohol Dependence*, *134C*: 92–8.

Van Der Pol., P., Liebregts, N., De Graaf, R., Korf, D. J., Van Den Brink, W. and Van Laar, M. (2013) Facilitators and barriers in treatment seeking for cannabis dependence, *Drug and Alcohol Dependence*, *133*(2): 776–80.

Wan, D. and Krassioukov, A.V. (2014) Life-threatening outcomes associated with autonomic dysreflexia: a clinical review, *The Journal of Spinal Cord Medicine*, *37*(1): 2–10.

Whitmore, J. (2009) *Coaching for Performance: GROWing Human Potential and Purpose – The Principles and Practice of Coaching and Leadership* (4th edn). London: Nicholas Breayley.

CHAPTER 10

Legal and Ethical Issues in Critical Care

Case Study: Ms B

MARK GAGAN AND DESIREE TAIT

━━ CHAPTER AIMS ━━━━━━━━━━━━━━━━━━━ ━

1 To critically discuss some legal and ethical influences that affect clinical decision making in critical care environments.
2 To be able to recognise and manage personal and professional values and their limitations in the context of suffering and loss, often on a daily basis.
3 To explore how reflecting on practice can manage guilt and promote positive humanising outcomes for others.

INTRODUCTION

This chapter considers some of the key legal and ethical issues that can occur in critical care areas. The issues chosen are not exhaustive and there are many other concerns such as Deprivation of Liberty, and arguments around passive or active euthanasia that provoke debate. The information given is an attempt to explain how the law and ethical frameworks might impact on the care given; it is not an explicit statement of legal or ethical advice. It uses a case study that came to public attention in 2002, some years before the Mental Capacity Act 2005 became enshrined in statute in the United Kingdom. It could be argued that this case was instrumental in the development of the establishment of the 'advance directive' in medico-legal practice.

The discussion of ethical frameworks may appear simplistic; however, there are many journals and books regarding ethics that can be utilised should the reader wish to develop a deeper understanding of the subject.

The chapter examines and discusses concepts such as emotional labour, moral distress, and feelings of powerlessness and oppression and the effects these can have on those who deliver the care. There also is an outline of how the use of ethical, legal and professional frameworks can enhance and encourage the humanisation of care for the benefit of patients, their families and significant others and for healthcare professionals too.

Working in a critical care area is worthwhile and exciting and has many rewards, especially when a critically ill person is helped back to recovery from an initially desperate situation. However, not all cases are able to survive the experience and insult of disease or trauma and the burden of caring for these people can exact a heavy price on the patient and those who care for them (in all senses of that word) and how that care might become more humanised. First there must be an understanding of key terms such as ethics, morals and values (see Bite Size Knowledge 10.1 Ethics, values and morals).

BITE SIZE KNOWLEDGE 10.1

Ethics, values and morals

Ethics can be defined as 'the philosophical study of the moral value of human conduct and the rules and principles that ought to govern it' (Collins English Dictionary 2014), or, 'a social, religious or civil code of behaviour especially that of a particular group or profession or individual' (ibid.). The critical care environment is a multi-disciplinary team environment, with healthcare professionals who may share the same goals (the care of critically ill persons) but who have different professional standards, outlooks and regulation.

Values are explained as 'the usual principles and beliefs or accepted standards of a person or social group' (ibid.).

Morals are 'principles of behaviour in accordance with standards of right and wrong' (ibid.).

The essence of being a Registered Nurse (RN) is to demonstrate the ability to assess, plan, implement and evaluate holistic nursing care and to deliver it in a safe, knowledgeable and competent manner. As the NMC Code (2015) states at section 6 (p. 7), 'You assess need and deliver or advise on treatment, or help (including preventative or rehabilitative care) without too much delay and to the best of your abilities, on the basis of the best evidence available and best practice.' According to the Royal College of Nursing (RCN, 2014: 3), nursing is 'The use of clinical judgement in the provision of care to improve, maintain, or recover health, to cope with health problems, and to achieve the best quality of life, whatever their disease or disability, until death.' Furthermore one of the key defining characteristics is 'A particular value base: nursing is based on ethical values which respect dignity, autonomy, and uniqueness of human beings, the privileged nurse–patient relationship, and the acceptance of personal accountability for decisions and actions. These values are expressed in written codes of ethics and supported by a system of professional regulation' (ibid.). Consequently it is important to define key words such as 'ethics', 'values' and 'accountability' because they collectively inform clinical decision making and the delivery of individualised, holistic nursing care.

These are not simple definitions to understand or enact and there are many questions to be asked about whose values are taking priority. One civil society's values and conduct might be totally against another society's established beliefs and practices (for example some societies could not countenance the consumption of alcohol, yet in other cultures it is used in many social interactions) so the adoption of morals and values is not as straightforward as might be imagined.

Another question might be centred around who has the power to make one group of people accept a value system that another group does not share. This can lead to stress, strains and miscommunication or misunderstanding which if unresolved can impact on the wellbeing of the group and delivery of poor quality care for patients.

None of the definitions offered give a concrete answer as to the best way to act in an ethical and moral way. This might be why there are ethical dilemmas, situations that seem intractable (should treatment be commenced or withdrawn? Who is the most in need of care?). This is why nurses have to be assertive, articulate, knowledgeable, reflective and rational when advocating for those in their care who cannot speak for themselves, with other groups who might not share the same philosophical basis for treatment that nurses do.

DEONTOLOGICAL AND UTILITARIAN FRAMEWORKS

Two approaches to developing ethical practice in health care use 'deontological' and 'utilitarian' frameworks. Deontology is mainly concerned with duties, rights and wrongs and the following of rules to achieve the right outcome regardless of the consequences. The professional codes of conduct such as the Nursing and Midwifery Council (NMC) Code (2015) highlight what should be done and that nurses should follow this code in dealing with patients under their care. Although one could argue that to follow the code is mandatory, patients come in all shapes and sizes (metaphorically speaking) and a one-size-fits-all code of conduct may raise some ethical questions that are not easily resolved. At least one other effect a deontological approach provides is a degree of certainty and that can enable nurses to proceed with some degree of confidence that their actions or inactions, if in line with the code, will offer some protection against committing ethically and professionally incorrect behaviour.

The second pathway is the utilitarian approach. This method supports the idea that those actions which produce the greatest good for the greatest number are intrinsically morally correct. For example, most people would like the government to take less tax from their wage packets at the end of the month. However, the finances raised help support the provision of a National Health Service, which provides universal care to those entitled to receive it, free at the point of delivery. This is regarded as a moral and societal 'good' whereby those who can afford money to be taken support those who cannot contribute financially (e.g. children, the aged, the sick or unemployed persons). Universal health care provides the greatest overall good to more members of society than it disadvantages and therefore brings the greatest happiness to the greatest number.

DISCUSSION

This brief explanation of some ethical approaches will not equip the reader with the panacea for all ethical issues. However it does serve to highlight that when healthcare professionals engage with patients and each other a shared ethical framework may reduce some of the stresses and strains produced in the critical care area, particularly around who makes decisions about treatment or withdrawal of treatment and who ultimately has the power over life, quality of life or death. It is how these decisions are made and enacted that can cause the greatest dissatisfaction and distress. Caring for critically ill people not only has ethical but also professional and legal implications. At section 20.4 in the NMC Code (2015) it clearly states that the RN should 'Keep to the laws of the country in which you are practising.' A registered nurse cannot use the legal defence of ignorance, i.e. the nurse could not claim that they did not know that their actions (or omissions) were illegal or unlawful and therefore should not be liable or accountable as a result.

CASE STUDY 10.1: MS B

In the case study being used, it is interesting to consider whether any of the healthcare staff looking after Ms B were acting in an unethical, illegal or unlawful manner. Key points from the case study of Ms B (Ms B and An NHS Trust [2002] EWHC 429 (Fam)) are:

- In August 1999 Ms B was hospitalised following a haemorrhage in her spinal column. The prognosis was such that a second haemorrhage could occur which would cause severe disability. She completed an advance directive in September 1999 stating that in the event of her becoming permanently unconscious, permanently impaired mentally or suffering a life-threatening illness that treatment should be withdrawn.
- In February 2001 she was admitted to hospital with an intramedullary spinal cavernoma, an abnormal collection of blood vessels that can leak blood within the spinal cord, which caused a total paralysis from the neck down and she developed breathing problems requiring her to be attached to artificial respiratory support.
- Ms B advised the medical team in February 2001 that she had completed an advance directive but was informed by them that the terms of the advance directive were not

specific enough to withdraw the ventilator support. An operation in March 2001 followed to try to alleviate the problems the cavernoma caused but this had limited success.

- Following this Ms B requested that her ventilation support be switched off. This did not happen and in April 2001 she instructed her legal team to ask that the machine be switched off. A case conference was held to discuss the issue and it was decided that two independent psychiatrists should assess Ms B's mental capacity before any changes to treatment were made.

- The assessments took place in April 2001 and it was decided that Ms B did not have capacity and so the treatment continued supplemented by the prescription of antidepressant medication.

- Ms B's assessments continued in June and July 2001 but no firm conclusions as to the state of her mental capacity were made.

- In August 2001, another mental capacity assessment was performed and Ms B was declared to have capacity to make decisions concerning her further treatment.

- She created an advance directive on 15 August 2001 but remained on the ventilator whilst discussions were made about how best to manage her removal from the ventilator, as the clinicians were not prepared to remove the respiratory support.

- This continued until March 2002 when the case was heard in the High Court of Justice where it was found that she was mentally competent and the action of the medical staff in placing her on a ventilator was against her wishes was a trespass to her person and the judge allowed Ms B's request that the respiratory support be switched off.

- Following the judgement ventilation support was discontinued and Ms B died in her sleep several days later.

Legal and Ethical Dilemmas of the Case of Ms B

The above case highlights the complex nature of caring for critically ill persons and their family members or significant others. Not only do healthcare professionals need to be aware of the inherent psychological and environmental issues but also their legal and ethical responsibilities particularly regarding refusal of treatment and in making judgements about end of life care. The following discussion will outline some of the legal and ethical dilemmas that can occur in a case such as Ms. B and how these can affect clinical decision making as a result.

Consent is closely allied to autonomy and has legal ramifications as noted below.

In the case of Schloendorff v. Society of New York Hosp, 105 N.E. 92, 93 (N.Y. 1914) Cardozo J stated: 'Every human being of adult years and sound mind has a right to determine what shall be done with his own body; and a surgeon who performs an operation without his patient's consent, commits an assault, for which he is liable in damages.'

The language is now outdated but the sentiment remains important in that any adult, competent individual can refuse to have treatment suggested by a healthcare professional regardless of the consequences (even death) of that refusal. If a nurse were to treat a person without their consent they could face serious legal and professional repercussions including removal from the NMC register if they were found to have acted improperly.

The most recent notable case regarding consent and patient autonomy was Montgomery v Lanarkshire Health Board [2015]. Mrs Montgomery was expecting her first child. She had a small pelvis and was diabetic. These factors can combine to make the delivery of the child problematic as babies of diabetic mothers can have more body weight distributed around the shoulder area, which can make the passage through the pelvis difficult. The estimated risk of this happening was calculated as around 9–10%.

The remedy to reduce the risk is to deliver the child via a Caesarean section. The consultant did not advise Mrs Montgomery of this possibility and alternative means of delivery because she felt that a natural delivery was better and most women would opt for a Caesarean if they were told there was a chance that the baby was at risk by being delivered naturally.

During delivery, the baby became wedged in the pelvis for a 12-minute period causing oxygen deprivation. The child was born with severe disabilities as a result. The judgement went against the Health Board which were found liable and ordered to pay £5.2 million in damages.

This decision has implications for healthcare professionals regarding the amount of information they give to patients about their treatment. Any risks as a result of the treatment should be disclosed, as well as alternative treatment strategies discussed so that the person has the opportunity for informed consent before making any decision that can materially affect their life. One way of describing this is that the patient decides and the healthcare professional advises rather than the decision being made for the patient. In this way autonomy and agency can be developed leading to more effective care being delivered. It is no longer acceptable for patients to be treated in a paternalistic way by healthcare providers. 'Paternalism' is defined as 'acting for the benefit of another, or in another's best interests, without the specific consent of the person concerned (Mason and Laurie, 2006: 8). Although the intent of paternalistic behaviour might arguably be grounded on the notion of doing good (beneficence), it is also open to the charge that it removes a person's autonomy with the result that actions are done to the person rather than discussed and agreed with the person because the healthcare professional knows best.

Although the example of childbirth might have no obvious link to nurses working in critical care areas, it is important to remember that the law of the land applies to everyone in that jurisdiction (where the law is enforced) and legal precedent applies. This is where the common law (judge-made law based on legal cases) rather than statutory law (law passed by parliament) applies to seemingly different situations. Hence the Montgomery case was an issue about informed consent to treatment and its implications go across the whole spectrum of consent in healthcare cases.

The Mental Capacity Act 2005 (MCA) determines the legal regulations regarding the establishment of capacity. There are five principles underpinning the Act including that a person must be assumed to have capacity unless it is established that she or he does not have capacity (MCA, section 2) The person must not be treated as not being able to make a decision unless all practicable steps to enable them to make that decision have been implemented without success (MCA section 3).

Similarly a person cannot be treated as unable to make a decision simply because they make an eccentric or unwise decision regarding treatment (MCA, section 4).

If a person lacks capacity any decision made on their behalf must be made in the best interests of that person (MCA, section 5). The decision made and its actions must be the least restrictive option in its restriction of the person's rights (MCA, section 6).

The definition of a person lacking capacity is given in the Mental Capacity Act 2005 (section 2.1) which states: 'a person lacks capacity in relation to a matter if at the material time he is unable to make a decision for himself in relation to the matter because of an impairment of, or a disturbance in the functioning of, the mind or the brain.'

In terms of critical care, where a person's situation renders them unconscious and unable to communicate, then actions may need to be taken quickly, without consultation with the patient, family or significant others to prevent further deterioration to administer life-saving treatment, which is 'treatment which in the view of the person providing health care for the person concerned is necessary to sustain life' (Mental Capacity Act 2005, section 4.10).

Best Interests

In this type of scenario acting in the person's 'best interests' is obviously the appropriate path to follow. Best interests can be defined as 'anything done for a person who cannot make decisions for themselves must be in their best interests. This means, thinking about what is best for the person and not about what anyone else wants' (Martin et al., 2012).

In terms of types of care decisions there are different levels of intervention ranging from day-to-day care decisions which a patient's family would wish to be involved with, or medical care decisions which rely on input and implementation from medical and nursing staff including treatments and invasive procedures, which can require the permission of a personal welfare Lasting Power of Attorney (LPA) who has the legal authority to make medical or healthcare decisions on behalf of the incapacitated patient (Mental Capacity Act 2005, section 9.1).

It is necessary for all the parties concerned in the care of the incapacitated person to communicate effectively and efficiently with each other. Indeed the NMC Code (2015) encourages nurses to:

- 'Treat people as individuals and uphold their dignity (1)
- ... avoid making assumptions and recognise diversity and individual choice (1.3)
- ... respect and uphold people's human rights' (1.5).

Similarly the NMC Code (2015) continues to advise on listening to people and to respond to their preferences and concerns (section 2 of The Code (NMC 2015)).

- 'You must work in partnership with people to make sure you deliver care effectively (2.1)
- ... recognise and respect the contribution that people can make to their own health and wellbeing (2.2)
- ... respect the level to which people receiving care want to be involved in decisions about their own health, wellbeing and care (2.4)
- ... respect support and document a person's right to accept or refuse care and treatment (2.5).'

However, if the incapacitated person had previously made a valid advance directive, those instructions would form the basis of intervention and non-intervention strategies around the person's care.

Advance Directive or Decision

An advance directive or decision is where a person (over 18 years of age) and with capacity at the time of making the advance directive, specifies the type of medical and nursing treatment they do not wish to be given to them at a future date should they become incapacitated and unable to refuse that treatment (Mental Capacity Act 2005, section 24.1).

This instruction will not apply to life-saving treatment unless 'the [advance] decision is verified by a statement by P [the person making the decision] to the effect that it is to apply to that treatment even if life is at risk and:

1 ... it is in writing
2 ... it is signed by P or by another person in P's presence and by P's direction
3 ... the signature is made of/acknowledged by P in the presence of a witness, and
4 ... the witness signs it, or acknowledges his signature, in P's presence.' (Mental Capacity Act 2005, sections 5 and 6)

The advance decision, if valid and applicable to a treatment being considered has the same effect as if the person had refused the treatment as a capacious person and therefore means that the treatment should not be commenced or continued. As a protection for healthcare staff the Act also states that there is no liability for withholding or withdrawing medical treatment, provided it is reasonably believed a valid and applicable advance decision exists (section 26(3)).

Reflection

A key issue in the case of Ms B was the knowledge that if she were disconnected from the ventilator this would inevitably lead to her death, as she could not support her respiratory function without it. This being so, if the medical team allowed the ventilator to be removed was there the possibility they could be charged with murder or manslaughter following her death or be accused of assisting a suicide which is illegal under the Suicide Act 1961?

The Nursing and Midwifery Council Code (2015, section 4) states that registered nurses should: 'Act in the best interests of people at all times' (4). To achieve this, you must: 'balance the need to act in the best interests of people at all times with the requirement to respect a person's right to accept or refuse treatment' (4.1).

This issue goes to the notion of autonomy, which is defined by Gillon (1986: 60) as 'the capacity to think and decide and act (on the basis of such thought and decision) freely and independently'. Similarly Beauchamp (2010: 37) states:

> Autonomy means freedom from external constraint and the presence of actual
> mental capacities such as understanding, intending and voluntary decision
> making ...

The concept of autonomy therefore links closely into the idea in the humanising framework of 'agency' – being able to choose and make decisions unhindered by others. As Todres et al. (2009: 70) state:

> To be human is to experience oneself as making choices and being generally
> held accountable for one's actions. This constitutes a sense of agency in which
> we do not experience ourselves as merely passive or totally determined but have
> the possibility of freedom to be and act within certain limits. A sense of agency
> appears to be very closely linked to the human sense of dignity. When this is
> taken away, one's sense of personhood is diminished.

It can be argued that Ms B's sense of personhood was not supported during her time in the intensive care unit, yet this should be anathema to healthcare professionals, particularly nurses who claim to be the foremost patient advocates, as the NMC (2015) Code states at 3.4 that nurses must '...act as an advocate for the vulnerable, challenging poor practice and discriminatory attitudes and behaviour relating to their care'. Yet as Beauchamp and Childress (2012: cited Zenz, 2017) argue, autonomy alone is not the single criterion to establish an appropriately ethical action because the other three biomedical principles, beneficence, non-maleficence and justice, are also important to consider when making decisions regarding a person's care.

BIOMEDICAL PRINCIPLES OF BENEFICENCE, NON-MALEFICENCE AND JUSTICE

The term beneficence is described as 'acts of mercy, kindness and charity. It is suggestive of altruism, love, honesty and promoting the good of other persons ... it is a statement of moral obligation to act for others' benefit, helping them further legitimate interests, often by preventing or removing possible barriers' (Beauchamp (2013) in the *Stanford Encyclopaedia of Philosophy*).

Non-maleficence can be defined using the Latin term 'primum non nocere'. This means 'first of all do no harm'. In other words the care given should not harm the person receiving that care. This can be a difficult balancing act as sometimes the medication administered can have an adverse effect on the recipient, say in the case of chemotherapy where unaffected cells are also killed by the treatment and this causes unpleasant or painful side effects. There is evidence to suggest that in the drive to utilise medical technology to its limits, there are occasions where medical and nursing staff have different opinions about continuing 'futile treatment'.

Justice essentially considers the distribution of resources and benefits in a fair manner so each person is owed his or her due. However, it is not about limitless resources being made available to every person. There has to be an economic affordability or a rationing of resources when demand is greater than supply. This is sometimes known as 'distributive justice'. For example, according to the *Guardian* newspaper (2014), the cost of caring for a newborn in a neonatal intensive care unit was £1,118 per day, with an average stay of 5 days (4.9 days) leading to a total cost of £5,590 per child. Figures released for 2013 in England stated there were 80,251 neonatal admissions (South West Neonatal Network, 2013). The assumed cost of this care to the NHS in England would be £448,603,090.

In the adult intensive care unit, the costing for level 3 care was estimated at £1,932 per day (Wales.nhs.uk, 2013) with the average stay being usually 2 days in duration (Ridley and Morris, 2007). In England records show that 271,079 medical admissions to critical care areas were made in 2015–16 (NHS Digital, 2017). Given the cost of each admission, it is easy to see that there has to be an element of distributive justice simply to enable limited resources to be applied fairly. What is the best return one might expect for all the effort expended in the care of a person who is critically ill and who might not survive the disease process that caused the illness originally and the effects of the treatments given? It could be argued in that type of scenario that quality of life might be more important than duration of life and that any future treatment would be prolonging the agony for the person and their family.

The costs of maintaining universal health care in a state where people are living longer with complex co-morbidities are challenging. Robust resource management is a key element in reducing expenditure and national and local targets are set by governments anxious to keep tight fiscal control on tax receipts. In the United Kingdom, the cost of the National Health Service is expected to be £127 billion during the 2020–21 time period (NHS Confederation, 2017) or just around 8% of gross national product (GDP).

Reflection

What answer would you give to someone who asked, 'Given the length of time Ms B was in level 3 care and the cumulative cost of her care and the eventual outcome, how can this type of care be justified?'

The effect of this type of monetary control has led to some hospital managers becoming more focused on budgets rather than quality of patient care.

The Mid Staffordshire NHS Trust Public Inquiry (2013) was scathing in its findings about the working environment of the hospital:

> The culture of the Trust was not conducive to providing care for patients or providing a supportive working environment for staff; there was an atmosphere of fear of adverse repercussions. A high priority was placed on the advancement of targets. There was low morale amongst staff. There was a lack of openness; there was an acceptance of poor standards. Management thinking was dominated by financial pressures and delivering FT (Foundation Trust) status to the detriment of quality of care. (p. 6)

Oppressive Behaviour

Tinsley and France (2004) had previously discussed this type of issue in their study of nurses leaving the profession because of oppressive behaviours caused by the acuity of the workload, the attitude of other nurses and doctors and pressures from administrators who controlled their workplace environment. Cox (1991, cited Tinsley and France 2004), argued that nurses feel oppressed because 'they are controlled by external forces that have greater prestige, power and status' (p. 32) Similarly, Young (1990, cited Dubrosky, 2013: 205) discussed the 'Five Faces of Oppression' where she defined oppression as 'The disadvantage and injustice some people suffer not because a tyrannical power coerces them but because of the everyday practices of a well intentioned liberal society' and furthermore that:

> oppression is structural because it is embedded in the unquestioned norms, habits and symbols, in the assumptions underlying institutional rules and the collective consequences of following those rules. (ibid.)

Cultural Imperialism

This powerlessness and distress is further exacerbated by what Young (1990, cited Dubrosky 2013, p207) referred to as 'Cultural Imperialism' where 'the dominant group continues to reinforce its position by bringing other groups under the control of the dominant group's domain'. Matheson and Bobay (2008, cited Dubrosky 2013, p207) claim:

> Nursing has struggled with medicine's power as the normalizing standard of health care for many years ... and has been [so much] under the domination of medicine that it has forgotten its origin.

Reflection

Given that nurses aspire to be the patient's advocate, and considering Ms B's situation regarding her advance directive, why do you think it took so long for her wishes to be complied with? What role would you have expected (and why?) the nurses involved in her care would play in making her request to discontinue treatment known?

Moral Distress

Over 20 years on from Cox's work, and as exemplified by the findings of the Francis Report (2013), nurses were still feeling they could not make holistic, clinical care decisions that would not only have a positive impact on patient and family care but would also improve the wellbeing of the nurses themselves because they felt powerless. This causes tensions between doctors and nurses in particular (though not exclusively so) and can lead to a situation known as 'moral distress' (Jameton, 1984; Corley, 1995; Hamric and Blackhall, 2007; Epstein and Delgado, 2010; Kentish-Barnes and Azoulay, 2016).

Moral distress is defined as 'a challenge that arises when one has an ethical or moral judgement about care that differs from that of others in charge' (Jameton, 2013). Nurses' moral distress, according to Corley (2002: 369) 'results from harm and distress caused to patients by pain and suffering, the treatment of patients as objects, and the medical prolongation of dying without letting the patient or family know about choices concerning care'.

There are different ideologies regarding how to care for the sick patient. Doctors are trained in the rational, scientific method allegedly leading to a more detached view of the situation whereas nurses, whilst also following a rational, evidence based approach, tend to deliver care using a humanised approach which is more inclusive and holistic in its outlook. Nurses often report that the biomedical and technical approach to care where patients are supported with technology that prolongs life (often at the expense of quality of life) is dehumanising care and is maintained because the medical staff implement treatment because it is available and is possible to do rather than withholding or with-drawing treatment for fear of upsetting the family or facing a legal challenge for 'writing the patient off too early'.

The notion of 'futile treatment' was discussed by Solomon (1993) who described such treatment as 'physiologically' ineffective'. He went on to write that it is futile 'if it merely preserves patient unconsciousness or cannot end dependence on intensive medical care' (p. 231). Benner et al. (1999: 366) discuss how it is an 'ethical breach to provide futile care or not offer patients the best standard of practice that will allow recovery'. They state that no one really knows when the tipping point between recovery and futility is likely to occur and this may lead to the 'slow dying trajectory' described by Glaser and Strauss (1965 cited ibid.) with its attendant distress and uncertainty.

These situations cause nurses 'moral distress' because the uncertainties mean nurses feel they cannot deliver the care they feel is humanising and dignifying and as a result they feel impotent, powerless and unable to meet their professional expectations of high qual-ity care. Jameton (2013: 299) describes the effects of this type of situation on nurses.

> In their position at the bedside, when patients were over treated and suffered for
> it, nurses were often hit hard with distress. Sometimes, they witnessed suffering
> they could not justify and were hands on in causing that suffering with suctioning,
> shots (giving injections), adjusting ventilator settings and so on. To nurses, up close
> physically and emotionally to suffering, unnecessary pain felt like abuse of patients
> and being complicit in and witnesses to abuse, they themselves experienced abuse.
> Meanwhile they resentfully saw physicians enter the patient's room and write orders,
> only to depart quickly and leave the management of suffering to nurses.

Dodek et al. (2016: 178) believe that 'Moral distress is higher in ICU nurses and other non-physician professionals than in physicians, is lower with older age in non-physician professionals but greater with more years of experience in nurses and is associated with a tendency to leave the job'. Moreover, 'Nurses experience high levels of moral distress which is linked to poor collaboration with physicians, burn out and attrition. Distress is associated with violations in medication practice (drug errors) and burnout is associated with failure to report errors and adverse events. It may also jeopardise the quality of clinical decision-making and care for seriously ill patients and their family members' (ibid.: 179). Musto et al. (2015) suggest that it is not only the hierarchical power and gender differences between nurses (traditionally female) and doctors (traditionally male) that lead to inequality and distress with the tensions between feminine and masculine approaches to life in general but also how nurses and doctors view the outcomes for critically ill patients. When medical intervention is ongoing, aggressive and prolonging life rather than improving quality of life (or even death) and this becomes a repeated pattern, nurses can find they begin to dwell on those situations where they feel they should have intervened with colleagues to question the direction the care was heading but failed to do so. To survive the situation a nurse might settle for a compromise that assuages their feelings at that moment in time but it comes back to haunt them later when a similar scenario occurs where they feel they have traduced their values and their standards of care again.

Emotional Labour

Hochschild (1983 cited Theodosius, 2008: 20) described the above phenomenon as 'emotional labour' which is:

> Labour that requires one to induce or suppress feelings in order to sustain the outward countenance that produces the proper state of mind in others, the sense of being cared for in a convivial and safe place. This kind of labour calls for a coordination of mind and feeling, and it sometimes draws on a sense of self that we honour as deep and integral to our individuality.

This can lead to feelings of shame, powerlessness and a failure to do the job they want to do – care for people effectively. As time goes on and these situations begin to repeat in frequency (called the 'crescendo effect' by Epstein and Hamric, 2009: 3), each episode where the nurse does not advocate (as they see it) for their patient leaves a mark on the nurse's sense of duty which is a feeling of not doing the right thing ethically or morally. This is described by Webster and Bayliss (2000, cited Epstein and Hamric, 2009) as 'moral residue' and is defined as 'That which each of us carries with us from those times in our lives when in the face of moral distress we have seriously compromised ourselves or allowed ourselves to be compromised.'

Reflection

Consider if you have ever been in this situation. How did you deal with it?

Do you have strategies to enable a disclosure of these feelings or are they simply put aside in an emotional drawer that does not get opened once it has been closed (except for the next addition to the drawer)? What can nurses do individually and collectively to reduce the emotional labour of caring for others?

Positive Aspects of Moral Distress

There are some positive aspects to consider when examining moral distress. Rodney (2017: 58) states that 'The concept of moral distress provides nurses, other healthcare providers and managers with an important lens through which to observe ethically challenging situations and initiate positive changes in practice.' He continues by saying: 'it can also be perceived as a path to positive growth prompting nurses and other health-care providers to engage in self-reflection and to be effective advocates for their patients and their patients' families' (ibid.).

This refocusing from the hopelessness of moral distress to overcoming the trauma and moving towards a positive response is termed 'moral resilience' which Rushton (2016: 112) defines as 'the capacity of an individual to sustain or restore their integrity in response to moral complexity, confusion, distress or setbacks ... In other words, choosing how one will respond to ethical challenges, dilemmas and uncertainty in ways that pre-serve integrity minimise one's own suffering and allow one to serve with highest purpose'.

It is by reflecting on experiences that strategies can be developed to allow the nurse to become empowered to overcome these challenging situations. This will require moral courage, which, according to Numminen et al. (2017: 878) is 'a highly valued element of human morality and ... an acknowledged virtue in nursing care'; they go on to define it as 'facing the pains and dangers of social disapproval in the performance of what one believed to be duty' (p. 880).

It is the ability to put oneself literally in harm's way, by speaking out or challenging oppressive environments and it is not an innate talent. It requires a professional attitude, the demonstration of a firm values base, a good knowledge of the situation that is the cause of the distress, the willingness to advocate for the patient, to be able to show personal and professional integrity by demonstrating nursing presence with the courage to challenge others (both medical staff and sometimes families) ele-gantly and the ability to listen to and deconstruct arguments in a critically reflective manner.

Challenging Elegantly

Challenging elegantly, according to Thompson (2011: 179), is 'the type of challenging that succeeds in getting the point across without alienating or antagonising the person being challenged (based on the premise that antagonism and alienation will not produce positive change)'. Communication within the critical care setting, according to Kentish-Barnes and Azoulay (2016: 1653), is perceived to be 'inconsistent, unsatisfactory or uncomforting' and it is 'physicians' and nurses' attitudes and the ability to express empa-thy, comfort and reassurance that significantly affect relatives' experience'.

It is a cry for a humanising culture to be adopted in a technological world where science and mechanisation can seem to push the patient further away from their familiar social experience and environmental support. Kentish-Barnes and Azoulay (2016: 1653) also state that:

To improve care in the ICU (Intensive Care Unit), the experience of all participants must be taken into account: when possible the patient's but also the relatives' and the care givers' experience. A holistic approach takes account of all aspects and concentrates on the interactions between its different elements. The experience is shaped by the patient's, his physician's, his nurse's experience as well as the organizational culture of the ICU.

The examination and synthesis of these experiences may provide positive ways of reducing moral distress and reinforcing moral resilience because 'Comparing experiences and respective burdens will permit one to put forward strategies to improve all participants' experiences: the patients', the relatives' and the caregivers' – all now considered active partners in decision making and care' (Kentish-Barnes and Azoulay, 2016). It seems in order to humanise the care of patients, relatives and of the staff in critical care areas, there has to be a wide ranging and deep reflection on the way the environment is shaped and the way that care is delivered.

Reflection

Given the relationships and structures in the multi-disciplinary team caring for the critically ill patient, who do you feel is the most appropriate team member to advocate for them (and why)?

Nurses in particular, are in theory, well positioned to take a pivotal role in identifying and managing solutions to the issues raised in the delivery, maintenance and cessation of critical care. Nurses are the key links in the multi-disciplinary team between fellow healthcare workers on one hand and the patients and their families on the other. Nurses spend more time with patients and families than any other members of the healthcare team and it is this continuity of care that gives nurses the insight into the condition and feelings of the patient and their relatives that others do not experience. Similarly nurses' take, by virtue of their Code of Conduct (NMC, 2015), a holistic approach, which is not required by any other caring profession's regulatory authority's code as explicitly as in their code. The deontological nature of this approach ensures an ethical basis to the care given. The NMC Code (2015) requires nurses to speak out where care might be compromised (sections 16, 19 and 25). It also encompasses a utilitarian aspect in that it requires all persons to be treated without fear of discrimination (section 1).

Allied to this is the expectation that nursing care will be informed by best evidenced practice (NMC, 2015, section 6) and reinforced by the use of the 6Cs (Cummings and Bennett, 2012) particularly in the use of communication, compassion and courage to speak with peers, colleagues and administrators about the effects of professional, managerial or governmental polices that adversely impact upon the delivery of humane care.

These attributes are those that require a personal commitment to the values each individual nurse aspires to, because they believe they are worthy values to hold, and importantly they are what society expects nurses to demonstrate when delivering care. Nurses are advocates for those in their care who cannot or do not speak for themselves and this should include fellow nurses and other healthcare professionals. It is no use trying to care for vulnerable people if those providing the care do not support each other or speak out when moral distress is being subsumed individually and tolerated collectively.

Reflection

The expectation that we can be immersed in suffering and loss daily and not be touched by it is as realistic as being able to walk through water without getting wet (Remen, 1996)

How can nurses influence this situation? How might they create the opportunities and strategies to influence change for the good of all?

━━━ REFLECTIVE EXERCISE 10.1 ━━━━━━━━━━ ━━━━━

Throughout this chapter there have been many reflection questions that the senior nurse can use to facilitate discussion with her/his team; for example ask your staff:

- How do they feel about the case of Ms B ?
- What are their perceptions of best interests?
- Discuss the cost of care and how it is justified.
- What do your staff understand by emotional labour and how do they manage it?
- Who do they feel is the most appropriate team member to advocate for patients?
- What opportunities and strategies can they offer to influence change?

CHAPTER SUMMARY

The 'solution' to many ethical issues is not held by one group, rather it is by co-operating and communicating with nurses, administrators and medical staff in creating a suitable environment to manage care effectively, then working in partnership with patients and their families in an honest and empathetic manner to foster a caring relationship. There needs to be a shared education programme about the use of ethical frameworks for the professions particularly on being open and humanised in care delivery. These frameworks should be integrated from the start of training programmes in order to familiarise healthcare personnel with the types of decisions they will have to learn to make in future and how to do this co-operatively.

A democratisation of the decision making process around the commencement, mainte-nance and withdrawal of care should be encouraged and practised, with all members of the healthcare professions involved in the immediate and ongoing care of the patient being able to express an opinion and to have it considered by other members of the team. The patient and their family should be involved in this wherever possible not only to meet ethical, legal and professional requirements but also to foster an empathetic and therapeutic relationship with those receiving the care.

The development of deep, reflective skills by healthcare professionals is vital to the suc-cess of strategies to humanise care for it is only having the ability to critically reflect on these scenarios and evaluate the strengths and weaknesses of the outcomes of the care delivery that safe, knowledgeable, competent care can be given. The audit of these out-comes gives a rational indication of how care needs can be planned for future events and how care might be expected to improve.

The acceptance that caring for the critically ill is not simply about 'doing something' to patients, it is about 'being with' people and their families. It is about understanding that professional, legal, ethical and individual factors all impact on all the actors in the situa-tion and no one is immune from the 'emotional labour' of being with and seeing other human beings (including staff) in distress. The origin of the answer to these problems lies, as does the provision of good care, with individual, holistic needs being recognised and respected.

In essence, nurses need to practise that which they preach, and share the message with all who are cared for by them. The task might seem onerous but it is by engaging and role modelling humanising care to patients, their families and peers and colleagues that changes can be made which will enhance the quality of life for all.

REFERENCES

Beauchamp, T.L. (2010) *Standing on Principles: Collected Essays*. New York: Oxford University Press.

Beauchamp, T. (2013) The principle of beneficence in applied ethics. Available at: https://plato. stanford.edu/entries/principle-beneficence

Benner, P., Hooper-Kyriakidis, P. and Stannard, D. (1999) Critical wisdom and interventions, in *Critical Care: A Thinking-in-Action Approach*. Philadelphia: W. B. Saunders Company.

Collins English Dictionary on line (2014) www.collinsdictionary.com [accessed 5 March 2018].

Corley, M.C. (1995) Moral distress of critical care nurses, *American Journal of Critical Care*, 4(4): 280–5.

Corley, M.C. (2002) Nurse moral distress: A proposed theory and research agenda, *Nursing Ethics*, 9(6): 636–50.

Cummings, J. and Bennett, V. (2012) Compassion in practice, *Nursing, Midwifery and Care Staff: Our Vision and Strategy*. London: NHS Commissioning Board.

Dodek, P.M., Wong, H., Norena, M., Ayas, N., Reynolds, S.C., Keenan, S.P., Hamric, A., Rodney, P., Stewart, M. and Alden, L. (2016) *Journal of Critical Care*, *31*(1): 178–82.

Dubrosky, R. (2013) Iris Young's Five Faces of Oppression applied to nursing, *Nursing Forum*, *48*: 3 (July–September).

Epstein, E.G. and Hamric. A.B. (2009) Moral distress, moral residue, and the crescendo effect, *Journal of Clinical Ethics*, *20*(4): 330–42.

Epstein, E.G. and Delgado, S. (2010) Understanding and addressing moral distress, *Online Journal of Issues in Nursing*, *15*(03).

Frances, R. (2013) *Report of the Mid Staffordshire NHS Foundation Trust Public Inquiry*. Available at: https://www.gov.uk/government/publications/report-of-the-mid-staffordshire-nhs-foundation-trust-public-inquiry

Gillon, R. (1986) *Philosophical Medical Ethics*. Chichester: Wiley.

The Guardian (2014) *Parents 'spend hundreds of pounds a week' to visit babies in neonatal care*. Available at: https://www.theguardian.com/society/2014/feb/27/parents-visit-babies-neonatal-care-cost

Hamric, A.B. and Blackhall, L.J. (2007) Nurse-physician perspectives on the care of dying patients in intensive care units: collaboration, moral distress and moral climate, *Critical Care Medicine*, *35*(2): 422–9.

Jameton, A. (1984) *Nursing Practice: The Ethical Issues*. Englewood Cliffs, NJ: Prentice Hall.

Jameton, A. (2013) A reflection on moral distress in nursing together with a current application of the concept, *Journal of Bioethical Inquiry*, *10*: 297–308.

Kentish-Barnes, N. and Azoulay, E. (2016) End-of-life care in the ICU: semper ad meliora (always strive for improvement), *Intensive Care Medicine*, *42*: 1653–4.

Martin, W., Freyenhargen, F., Hall, E., O'Shea, T., Szerletics, A. and Ashley, V. (2012) An unblinkered view of best interests, *British Medical Journal*, *345*: 22–4.

Mason, J.K. and Laurie, G.T. (2006) *Mason and McCall Smith's Law and Ethics* (7th edn). Oxford: Oxford University Press.

Musto, L., Rodney, P.A. and Vaderheide, R. (2015) Moving towards interventions to address moral distress, *Nursing Ethics*, *22*(1): 91–102.

NHS Confederation (2017) *NHS statistics, facts and figures* [online] Available from: www.nhsconfed.org/resources/key-statistics-on-the-nhs [accessed 9 April 2018].

NHS Digital (2017) *Hospital Adult Critical Care Activity 2015–16* [online] Available at: https://digital.nhs.uk/data-and-information/publications/statistical/hospital-adult-critical-care-activity/2015-16 [accessed 6 April 2018].

Numminen, O., Repo, H. and Leino-Kilpi, H. (2017) Moral courage in nursing: A concept analysis, *Nursing Ethics*, *24*(8): 878–91.

Nursing and Midwifery Council (NMC) (2015) *The Code: Professional Standards of Practice and Behaviour for Nurses and Midwives*. London: NMC publishing.

Remen. R.N. (1996). *Kitchen Table Wisdom: Stories that Heal*. New York: Penguin.

Ridley, S. and Morris, S. (2007) Cost effectiveness of adult intensive care in the UK, *Anaesthesia. 62*: 547–54.

Rodney, P.A. (2017)What we know about moral distress: looking over three decades of research and exploring ways to move the concept forward, *American Journal of Nursing, 117*(2): S7–S10.

Royal College of Nursing (RCN)(2014) *Defining Nursing*. London: RCN publishing.

Rushton, C.H. (2016) Moral resilience: a capacity for navigating moral distress in critical care, *Advanced Critical Care (AACN), 27*(1): 111–19.

Solomon, M.Z. (1993) How physicians talk about futility: making words mean too many things, *The Journal of Law, Medicine and Ethics, 21*(2): 231–7.

South West Neonatal Network (2013) *South West Report on Term Admissions to Neonatal Units*. [online]. London: Royal College of Paediatrics and Child Health.

The Mid Staffordshire NHS Foundation Trust Public Inquiry (2013). *Report of the Mid Staffordshire NHS Foundation Trust Public Inquiry. Executive summary HC 947*. London: The Stationery Office.

Theodosius, C. (2008) *Emotional Labour in Health Care: The Unmanaged Heart of Nursing*. Abingdon: Routledge.

Thompson, N. (2011) *Promoting Equality: Working with Diversity and Difference*. (3rd edn). Basingstoke: Palgrave Macmillan.

Tinsley, C. and France. N. (2004) The trajectory of the registered nurse's exodus from the profession: a phenomenological study of the lived experience of oppression, *International Journal of Human Caring* [online] 8: 8–12. Available from: www.researchgate.net/publication/292260102_The_Trajectory_of_the_Registered_Nurse's_Exodus_from_the_Profession_A_Phenomenological_Study_of_the_Lived_Experience_of_Oppression [accessed 4 April 2018].

Todres, L., Galvin, K.T. and Holloway, I. (2009) The humanization of healthcare: a value framework for qualitative research, *International Journal of Qualitative Studies on Health and Wellbeing*, 4(2): 68–77.

Wales NHS (2013) *Together for Health – a delivery plan for the critically ill: 2013–2016*. [online] Available from: www.wales.nhs.uk/sitesplus/documents/866/2.8%20Critical%20Illness%20Delivery%20Plan%202013-16%20ABuHB%20Final.pdf.

Zenz, J. (2017) Response to LiPuma and DeMarco's Article on 'Hastening Death'. *Health Service Insights* [online] 10: 1–2.

Legal cases

Ms B and An NHS Trust [2002] EWHC 429 (Fam).

Montgomery (Appellant) v Lanarkshire Health Board (Respondent) (Scotland) [2015] UKSC 11.

Schloendorff v. Society of New York Hospital, 105 N.E. 92, 93 (N.Y. 1914).

Legislation

Mental Capacity Act 2005, www.legislation.gov.uk/ukpga/2005/9/notes

CHAPTER 11

The Impact of Critical Illness on Recovery and Rehabilitation

Case Study: Fred

DESIREE TAIT AND SARA J. WHITE

1 To understand the complexity of Delirium and how this can lead to Post-Traumatic Stress disorder.
2 To discuss the factors that can lead to critical illness neuromyopathy and the impact this can have on patient progress and outcome.
3 To explore the role of the senior nurse in relation to humanising the care of Fred in a complex situation and associated leadership and management of staff.

INTRODUCTION

As we have seen in Chapter 2, there are often complex and multifaceted factors that can trigger critical illness that can also impact the severity and duration of people's experience of their condition. This chapter explores the case study of Fred, a 74-year-old man who was admitted to ITU following a Road Traffic Collision (RTC).

═══ CASE STUDY 11.1: FRED ═══════════════ ═══

Fred is married to Mary who is also 74 and they have been together as husband and wife for 50 years, celebrating their Golden Wedding Anniversary two months ago. Fred's career was in the army and he is a well-groomed man, liking his moustache kept trim and his hair clean and washed. He has a slim build and is 5ft 11 inches (1.8 m) tall with an average weight of

(Continued)

(Continued)

11 stone (70Kg). He does not like TV, preferring to listen to Radio 4. Mary and Fred have one son who lives in Australia and they have not seen or visited him for 15 years. They both enjoy walking and Fred makes model aircraft. Fred has no previous history of any medical conditions and had not visited his GP for 24 years, since leaving the army at the age of 50.

One clear and fine June evening, while travelling home from an evening out with friends, and only 3 miles away from his home, Fred swerved and drove head on into a stone wall which caused the air bag to inflate. No other vehicles were involved and there was no evidence of mechanical failure. Fred's friends told how he had only had a pint of stout beer shandy (50% stout beer and 50% lemonade) and a packet of cheese and onion flavoured crisps. In the absence of any other vehicle involvement two possible causes of the accident included the avoidance of a wild animal in the road or a possible transient loss of consciousness.

- On admission to emergency care Fred was breathing on his own with the support of 60% high flow oxygen. His respiratory rate was 30 and his respirations shallow, there was reduced air entry to the right apex of the lung and air entry to both bases was quiet. There was evidence of early bruising and contusion to his right shoulder and left lower area of his chest consistent with a seatbelt injury and release of the driver's airbag. Chest X-rays revealed fractures to Fred's left ribs from 4–7 and a high left rib fracture together with evidence of a left pneumothorax. Fred's oxygen saturations were 84% on 60% oxygen and arterial gases revealed evidence of hypoxia and type one respiratory failure. Other injuries identified a Right fractured shaft of femur, Right tibia and fibula and a Left open compound fracture of his tibia and fibula. Fred had a Right apical chest drain inserted and with evidence of continued respiratory distress, he was sedated and intubated with an oral size 9 endotracheal tube and his respiratory rate supported by mechanical ventilation.
- Fred was cardiovascularly compromised with a pulse of 130/minute and blood pressure of 90/60 mmHg (Mean arterial pressure of 70), with a capillary refill time of 3 seconds. Fred had an internal jugular line inserted for fluid resuscitation and both a peripheral and arterial line for haemodynamic assessment and fluid management. A urinary catheter was inserted and 100 mls of clear urine drained which tested positive to glucose. A blood glucose confirmed a hyperglycaemia of 40 mmol. Pain relief was managed by intravenous opioid and an antiemetic.
- On admission prior to sedation Fred's Glasgow Coma Scale was 13–14, his eyes were open spontaneously but he was confused and unable to respond to questions, he was making purposeful movement to painful stimuli and shouting out in pain due to his fractures.

- On examination Fred presented with a fractured right femur, fractured right tibia and fibula and a compound, comminuted fracture of his left tibia and fibula just above the ankle.

Once haemodynamically stable Fred was taken to theatre for internal fixation of his right leg fractures and external fixation of his left leg fractures before being transferred to intensive care. Whilst in ICU Fred's pain was difficult to manage and his care became more complex following a diagnosis of pneumonia and sepsis. Fred was treated actively during this time until he began to show signs of respiratory and haemodynamic improvement. After a period of 8 days Fred's respiratory support was reduced with the aim of weaning him off assisted ventilation. Unfortunately each time Fred's support and sedation was reduced he showed signs of deterioration in his respiratory function and after a further 48 hours following communication with Fred's family it was agreed that he would have a tracheostomy tube in order to provide more effective management of his respiratory function. During his time in intensive care Fred's blood sugar continued to be high and together with an admission sample of his HbA1c of >200 mmol/mol a diagnosis of Type 2 diabetes was confirmed for which he was treated with insulin. Once Fred was haemodynamically stable the physiotherapy team in collaboration with the nursing staff facilitated initially passive, but later active, exercises to support maintaining his range of movement and muscle strength. Unfortunately Fred struggled with finding the strength to maintain self-ventilation and sustain coordinated movement and after a protracted period of weaning from respiratory support, he was eventually discharged from ICU 4 weeks after his admission. Neuromuscular complications of critical illness have been recognised since the 1980s and with the increase in survival rates following admission to intensive care there has been growing evidence of post-ICU morbidity, as opposed to mortality, and a need to examine triggers and management strategies in order to reduce the impact of critical illness on a person's quality of life (Zambon and Vincent, 2008; Martin et al., 2003). Bite Size Knowledge 11.1 offers a definition of critical illness myopathy and neuropathy.

━━━ BITE SIZE KNOWLEDGE 11.1 ━━━━━━━━━━ ━━━━━

Defining critical illness myopathy (CIM), critical illness polyneuropathy (CIP) and critical illness polyneuromyopathy (CIPNM)

- Critical illness myopathy (CIM): describes a range of ICU-acquired muscle pathology associated with a reduction on oxygen and nutrients to muscles and the catabolic impact of pro-inflammatory cytokines on the production of reactive oxygen species (ROS) and mitochondrial failure that leads to cellular damage. The syndrome presents with proximal

(Continued)

(Continued)

    rather than distal weakness and muscle atrophy leading to weakness of the intercostal muscles and a patient's failure to wean from ventilatory support (Shepherd et al., 2017).

- Critical illness polyneuropathy (CIP) was first described in 1984 in association with sepsis (Bolton et al., 1984) and is characterised by distal rather than proximal weakness, sensory changes and limited atrophy (Shepherd et al., 2017).
- Critical illness polyneuromyopathy (CIPNM) describes the combination of both syndromes leading to a combination of proximal and distal weakness and variable rates of muscle atrophy (Shepherd et al., 2017).

Fred's Difficulty with Weaning from Respiratory Support and Related Muscle Weakness: the Impact of Critical Illness Neuromyopathy

While Fred met some of the diagnostic criteria for CIPNM, in his case the electrophysiological evidence for this was not explored, as illustrated in Table 11.1. Shepherd et al. (2017) argue that there are a number of technical challenges to completing the nerve conduction and electromyography studies to confirm the diagnosis of CIPNM in an intensive care environment and these include:

- artefact and interference from other electronic devices
- temperature fluctuations such as hypothermia
- generalised interstitial oedema
- evidence of delirium and/or inability to co-operate while the test are being completed.

In Fred's case, he was receiving technical support from a number of essential electronic devices, he was withdrawn and confused and seemed unable to acknowledge or comprehend his close family. According to Shepherd et al. (2017) and Fan (2012) there are a number of risk factors for critical illness neuromyopathy and these include increasing age, being female, severity of illness, particularly sepsis and organ failure, and hyperglycaemia. While Fred met a number of these risk factors, he had no pre-morbid weakness due to chronic disease apart from a new diagnosis of diabetes, and he had previously been fit and well.

The impact of critical illness neuromyopathy for Fred was that he experienced a prolonged length of stay and a high number of ventilator-dependent days in ICU. This finding is supported by Visser (2006) who in a review of the literature concluded that critically ill patients with neuromuscular weakness have increased length of stay and more ventilator dependent days than those without.

Table 11.1 Diagnostic criteria for critical illness polyneuropathy and critical illness myopathy according to Latronico (2011), as they compare to Fred's signs and symptoms

Critical illness polyneuropathy	Critical illness myopathy	Fred's signs and symptoms
1 Evidence of critical illness	1 Evidence of critical illness	1 Evidence of multiple trauma associated with critical illness, pneumonia and sepsis
2 Limb weakness and/or difficulty with weaning from respiratory support after other possible causes have been considered	2 Limb weakness and/or difficulty with weaning from respiratory support after other possible causes have been considered	2 Evidence of both difficulty to wean and limb weakness when other factors had been considered
3 Electrophysiological evidence of axonal motor and sensory polyneuropathy	3 Compound muscle action potential (CMAP) amplitudes are less than 80% of the lower limit of normal in 2 or more nerves	3 Not assessed
4 Absence of decremental response on repetitive nerve stimulation	4 Sensory nerve action potentials are more than 80% of the lower limit of normal	4 Not assessed
	5 Needle electromyography detected: increased CMAP duration or reduced muscle membrane excitability on direct muscle stimulation in non-co-operative patients	5 Not assessed
	6 Absent or decreasing response to repetitive nerve stimulation	6 Not assessed
	7 Muscle histopathological findings of primary myopathy	7 Not assessed
		NB: diagnostic criteria not confirmed

Critical Illness Neuromyopathy: What is the Evidence to Support Preventative Interventions?

Hermans et al. (2014) in a systematic review of interventions for preventing neuromyopathy concluded that there is moderate quality evidence that intensive insulin therapy reduces the risk of CIPNM and high quality evidence that it reduces the duration of mechanical respiratory support. In Fred's case, he was a newly diagnosed diabetic and experienced fluctuations in his glycaemic control thus limiting the potential for preventative management. The review also identified moderate quality evidence to support the use of early rehabilitation and this is supported by NICE (2017) who argue that patients admitted to intensive care should have a rehabilitation plan in place within 4 days or prior to discharge. There is a growing body of evidence that the impact of ICU on patient morbidity is multifactorial with neuromyopathy identified as one of several ICU survivors' symptoms. These include psychological stress, pain, pulmonary insufficiency, sleep disturbances, post-traumatic stress symptoms and fatigue (Langerud et al., 2017; Guarneri et al., 2008).

CASE STUDY 11.1: FRED (CONTINUED)

During his stay of 4 weeks in ICU, Fred's wife remained with him as much as she could and she tried with the staff to orientate him to time, place and treatments, keeping a diary of what was happening. Mary talked about the things he liked and of key trigger points such as the Summer Solstice. Their son flew over from Australia to be with them and planned to stay for six weeks. However Fred did not acknowledge his wife or son; he had no eye contact with anyone, he was withdrawn and disengaged and began to show evidence of fear by backing away and shaking his head if stimulated. Fred's problems with weakness and loss of skeletal muscle further hampered movement and it was difficult for his family to see him being well enough to leave ICU.

DISCUSSION

The discussion will focus on Fred's sudden loss of consciousness which resulted in the RTC. It will then explore the possible reasons for a diagnosis of Hypoactive Delirium and potential reasons for this, concluding with an exploration of how humanising care might have helped Fred overcome his delirium.

Loss of Consciousness

There are many causes for sudden confusion and loss of consciousness which may have contributed to Fred's loss of control of his car and these include: diabetes (hypo or hyper glycaemia), poisoning such as carbon monoxide, hypoxia, infection and sepsis, stroke, TIA, Cardiac issues (i.e. MI, cardiac syncope, arrhythmia), drugs (therapeutic or recreational), cerebral issues (encephalitis, meningitis, tumour), severe electrolyte imbalance, underactive thyroid gland, psychological distress (i.e. severe state of anxiety), and NICE (2014) warns that serious causes behind transient loss of consciousness are often under-recognised. However a thorough investigation into Fred's transient loss of consciousness only revealed previously undiagnosed Type 2 diabetes and that nothing had manifested before the RTC. There appeared to be nothing specific that identified why Fred presented as being withdrawn since the sedation and pain relief were reduced and a diagnosis of Hypoactive Delirium was confirmed. However one needs to be mindful that there could have been a number of reasons for this withdrawn state and these will now be explored.

Reflection

Consider what physical, psychological and social reasons could have led to Fred being like this. Revisit:

- Chapter 2: What Triggers Critical Illness
- Chapter 3: Respiratory Failure
  - o Bite Size Knowledge 3.1: Type I & Type II Respiratory Failure
  - o Bite Size Knowledge 3.2: Sepsis
  - o Bite Size Knowledge 3.3: Acute Delirium
  - o Bite Size Knowledge 3.6: Isolation.

Delirium

As discussed briefly in Chapter 3, delirium is a complex, serious neuropsychiatric syndrome in which cerebral function is disturbed, and during and after weaning from the ventilator Fred was showing signs of delirium, manifesting in acute changes in consciousness and cognition with inattention and inability to receive, process, recall or store information.

The three forms of delirium subtypes are offered in: Bite Size Knowledge 11.2: The 3 forms of delirium subtype. Haggstrom et al. (2017), who undertook a systematic review of the literature, identified that the pathophysiology of delirium is poorly understood but that there is good evidence to show that there are abnormalities with neurotransmissions, inflammation, stress responses and cerebral blood flow. Risk factors for delirium are both iatrogenic (hypoxia, acute infection, electrolyte imbalance, metabolic disturbance, intracranial events, medication, dehydration) and environmental (sleep deprivation, immobilisation, sensory overload, visual and hearing impairment, disorientation, isolation) (Harrington and Vardi, 2014). Indeed delirium is associated with an increased mortality (Chan et al., 2017); longer stay in hospitals (Gleason et al., 2015); risk of persistent cognitive deficits (Wolters et al., 2017) and an increased possibility of the need for a higher level of care post discharge and a decreased quality of life (Pandharipande et al., 2013; Oh et al., 2017) as well as an increase in complications such as cardiac, respiratory (Zenilman, 2017) or Acute Kidney (Siew et al., 2016) and post-operative complications

(Numan et al., 2017), and recognition that pre-operative malnutrition is a precursor to higher incidence of post-operative delirium (Mazzola et al., 2017).

Conditions that mimic delirium include depression, psychosis, drug intoxication, alcohol withdrawal, hepatic or uremic encephalopathy and dementia (Oh et al., 2017), although often delirium and dementia commonly coexist (Richardson et al., 2017).

BITE SIZE KNOWLEDGE 11.2

The 3 forms of delirium subtype

1 Hyperactive delirium - occurs in older clients such as those in ICU and is also known as ICU Psychosis, ICU syndrome and Delirium - individuals are restless, have hallucinations or delusions, pull at invasive lines or catheters, have sleep disturbance, date/ time/ place confusion, are at risk of self-harm - often associated with drug intoxication.
2 Hypoactive delirium - clients are withdrawn, apathetic, inattentive, lethargic, decreased responsiveness, and have sleep disturbance, date/ time/ place confusion.
3 Mix of Hyperactive and Hypoactive delirium with an inconsistent pattern.

(Hickin et al., 2017; Williams, 2017)

So when we reflect back on Fred's case study we can see that he was quiet and withdrawn and did not have eye contact and his wife and staff felt he also showed fear; we can therefore surmise that he has Hypoactive Delirium. So let us now consider how staff could have/did humanise his care.

Humanising the treatment of patients with delirium includes early detection (Voyer et al., 2017) and management of stressors such as pain, dyspnoea and hyperactivity (Pandharipande, 2017) as well as multicomponent interventions (see Bite Size Knowledge 11.3: Multi-component targeted interventions in delirium prevention). Siddiqi et al. (2016, p1) in a comprehensive review showed that 'there is no clear evidence that cholinesterase inhibitors, antipsychotic medication or melatonin or melatonin agonists reduce the incidence of delirium'; but that there is strong evidence supporting multicomponent interventions to prevent delirium in hospitalised patients. Loftus and Wiesenfeld (2017) highlight that delirium assessment improves the quality of care when the assessment includes use of tools such as Confusion Assessment Method (CAM) and CAM-ICU (van Eijk et al., 2011). In addition, Oh et al. (2017) and Trogrlic et al. (2015) give a good overview of tools such as 3-minute Diagnostic assessment and 4 A's test and Family Confusion Assessment Method. Voyer et al. (2017) tested RADER (Rapid Detection tools for signs of delirium), which was supported by the National Institute for Health and Care Excellence (NICE 2010) which emphasised the need for a screening tool for rapid delirium screening that can be administered by a range of professionals in a busy clinical environment, and one that can be used with patients who have sensory or functional impairments and also need a general cognitive assessment.

━━━ BITE SIZE KNOWLEDGE 11.3 ━━━━━━━

Multi-component targeted interventions in delirium prevention

- prevention of sleep disturbance and therapeutic sleep enhancement strategies
- orientation to time and place
- environmental improvements – i.e. daylight
- exercise and mobilisation
- visual and hearing aids
- oral hydration.

The cost-benefits of delirium assessment and prevention are clear (Akunne et al., 2012; Lee and Kim, 2014). However delirium appears to still be under-recognised in ICU (Selim and Ely, 2017; Hickin et al., 2017). Whitehorne et al. (2015) describe the lived experiences of patients who experienced delirium in ICU and stress the fear and anxiety of patients as they try to comprehend what is occurring to them. Here, like others, they stress the importance of assessment and early detection if effective treatment and management are to be put in place.

Reflection

What strategies do you have in your department for delirium assessment and prevention? Do you have evidence that they are effective?

POST-TRAUMATIC STRESS DISORDER POST ICU (PTSD)

Aforementioned evidence suggests that lack of knowledge and awareness of delirium and its adverse effect on patients can lead to post ICU traumatic stress (PTSD). Could Fred have had PTSD? For at least the last decade PTSD post ICU has been researched (i.e. Svenningsen et al., 2015; Griffiths et al., 2007; Kapfhammer et al., 1999) revealing that PTSD post ICU has shown that depressive symptoms, such as increase in traumatic memories, nightmares and sleep disturbances, disabilities in basic activities of daily living, intense fear, panic and helplessness are common and last for a variety of months (3–9 or more) post discharge. A variety of follow-up strategies, such as

Table 11.2 Humanising health care for Fred

Humanising dimensions	Critical illness triggers	Managing stressors and coping strategies	Role of expert nurse in support strategies
Insiderness/objectification	Fred has retired from the army. He enjoys life and the company of his wife and friends. Possible triggers include: • Psychological stress – elevated blood glucose, increases risk of mitochondrial damage and type 2 diabetes • Delayed cellular recovery.	Fred may be concerned that the peaceful retirement he has may now be stressful, and diabetic health check and living may impact on his quality of life.	Enable connectedness by helping staff understand that they need to take time to enable Fred to open up to them and express his feelings and fears. Listen to Mary's fears and anxieties.
Agency/passivity	Fred is out of his comfort zone as he is not in control and he does not understand the routine and why it is important. This increases hyperglycaemia.	Fred needs a full understanding of – ward routine – roles of staff such as physio – the type of exercise needed – healthy diet – medication – return to his normality.	Ensure staff give Mary, who will in turn help Fred, a sound evidence based rationale re why it is important to focus on the present care. Discuss recovery time, and return to normal way of living.
Uniqueness/homogenisation	Fred and Mary may fear that the life they have may be lost. They may be experiencing a sense of grief and loss of role and responsibilities.	The world in which Fred lives and his fears of what may change in that world due to the illness and diabetic diagnosis, however small, are important if Fred has a unique view of that world and this must be recognised if staff are to help him overcome his fears.	Ensure staff are not judgemental about Fred's lifestyle. Challenge assumptions and examples of modern prejudice being displayed. Enable staff to reflect and learn from any stereotypical behaviour they may show.

Humanising dimensions	Critical illness triggers	Managing stressors and coping strategies	Role of expert nurse in support strategies
Togetherness/isolation	Fred will not fully understand the RTC and diagnosis and why they occurred.	Fred loves his wife very much and may feel that he may become a burden to her, and this he may fear.	Involve Mary in exploring trigger factors of diabetes and help her to help him adjust to new lifestyle choices together.
Sense making/loss of meaning	Fred has not been in ICU before and may not understand why he is connected to the monitors or why he has a urethral catheter or cannot hear his voice (prior to Tracheostomy removal) and why staff are concerned about his health and lack of engagement with others.	Staff need to provide Fred with adequate but constant and consistent knowledge of the world he is in at present so he can make sense of the care.	Enable staff to recognise that what is 'normal' to them is fear making for Fred and Mary and their son. Help them form questions and answers that are not condescending to Fred and his family, recognising that every situation is potentially new to them.
Personal journey/loss of personal journey	Fred has pain in his legs and chest. He may feel weak and helpless.	Fred needs constant reassurance that what he feels is normal and if he expresses his pain the staff can help him overcome it with positioning, distraction therapy and medication.	Enable staff to ensure Fred has a working knowledge of the care and treatment implications.
Sense of place/ dislocation	Fred may be frightened that he may die and leave his wife alone. Age and cultural and structural factors may influence his trust in healthcare systems and care offered.	Encourage Fred to talk through his fears with members of the healthcare team and explore with Mary if Fred may like a counsellor or chaplain.	Ensure staff have a sound evidence base regarding what fears post RTC and diabetes may bring and can offer coping strategies.
Embodiment/ reductionist body	Fred may be concerned because he knows he is not his normal self but because of his army life he may not wish to tell nurses of his fears in case he is thought to be weak and unmanly.	Fred may like to talk to a male nurse or to someone who he deems as being senior to him; Mary may help determine who this person might be.	Ensure staff are enabling Fred to make some choices, however small. Ensure they have a good working knowledge of support structures that can be accessed and discuss these with Mary.

counselling post discharge have been recommended. Jones et al. (2010) identified that the provision of an ICU diary written for patients while in ICU by healthcare staff and family is an effective way of aiding psychological recovery and reducing the incidence of new PTSD, and Mary and the ICU staff were proactive in keeping a diary for Fred. However, we also need to remember that family members themselves can suffer from PTSD (Jones et al., 2008; NICE 2005; Jones et al., 2004) and an ICU diary may benefit them too as they clarify the patient journey and story. We have no data that followed Fred post discharge so we cannot surmise whether or not he had PTSD or whether his wife suffered too or indeed how his son felt having not seen his parents for over 15 years and returning to the UK for such a concerning family event. We also have no data that recorded if indeed Fred and Mary got on with their son or if the relationship was strained; if it was, this might in itself not have helped Fred's recovery. However we have considered the humanising framework and how these may have been addressed or could have been addressed – see Table 11.2: Humanising care for Fred. As you can see we have focused on possible triggers for his ill health once in ICU and the psychological stress causing elevated blood glucose, increases risk of mitochondrial damage and Type 2 diabetes and delayed cellular recovery. Fred's army background and good health will no doubt have had an impact as his lack of knowledge about the complexity of the environment of ICU and the management of his sudden illness will all have affected him. This sudden change in his way of living and his hypoactive delirium no doubt caused Mary to experience considerable stress and anxiety; however, she was very proactive in helping to 'get Fred back'. Family involvement in the care of clients in ICU as they cope with a serious illness of a loved one, while also having to adapt to the unfamiliar and intimidating ICU environment and uncertainty about the outcome of their loved one no doubt causes considerable distress to the relatives. Staff need to be aware of the simple fact that they cannot just care for the patient but the family too. Shared decision making may help relatives in many situations, and Azoulay et al. (2014) give a good account of the research exploring this. In Chapter 5 we explored motivational and management theories and leadership styles (see Bite Size Knowledge 5.5: Motivational theories, management theories and leadership styles) and you may like to revisit this and work with your staff to explore ways of working and family involvement in decision making.

▬▬▬ REFLECTIVE EXERCISE 11.1 ▬▬▬▬▬▬▬▬▬▬▬▬▬ ▬▬▬

- Is there any staff education needed regarding knowledge about Delirium in your department and if so who could you call upon to help?
- What do your staff know about post-traumatic stress disorder post ICU and how they can help minimise this during patient stay in ICU?
- If your ICU admits children, explore delirium assessment in critically ill children.

- What future strategies could be employed in your department to enable staff to keep up to date with the multitude of research being undertaken relating to post ICU syndromes such as PTSD?
- Ensure your staff have read the NICE guidelines on: (1) Transient loss of consciousness ('blackouts') in over 16s; (2) Delirium: prevention, diagnosis and management; (3) Post-traumatic stress disorder management (NICE, 2014, 2010, 2005).

CHAPTER SUMMARY

This chapter has reviewed the case study of Fred who, previously fit and healthy, suffered multiple injuries following an RTC and this event had a major impact on him and his family; this in turn may have led to long-term health issues such as PTSD, for both Fred and his wife and son. Whilst both causes of delirium and PTSD have been researched for many years there is still a vast amount of research to be undertaken and disseminated to enable staff to retain being evidence based in their knowledge. Equally the growing body of knowledge on ICU neuromyopathy adds to the complexity of needs and support required for both Fred and his family as Fred continues with his rehabilitation. Shared decision making with relatives to help them work together with staff on decisions that will best enable their loved one to either return to their normal way of life, or adjust to the new way of living, can be very demanding and stressful for staff as they too may battle with their feelings and knowledge base, and it is our belief that senior nurses are in a good position to help them develop in this area of practice and be reflective in their development.

FURTHER READING

Richardson, S.J., Davis, D.H.J., Stephan, B., Robinson, L., Brayne, C., Barnes, L., Parker, S. and Allan, L.M. (2017) Protocol for the Delirium and Cognitive Impact in Dementia (DECIDE) study: a nested prospective longitudinal cohort study, *BMC Geriatrics, 17*(98): 1–7.

REFERENCES

Akunne, A., Murthy, L. and Young, J. (2012) Cost-effectiveness of multi-component interventions to prevent delirium in older people admitted to medical wards, *Age and Ageing, 41*(3): 285–91.

Azoulay, E., Chaize, M. and Kentish-Barnes, N. (2014) Involvement of ICU families in decisions: fine-tuning the partnership, *Ann. Intensive Care*, 4: 37.

Bolton, C., Gilbert, J., Hahn, A. and Sibbald, W.J. (1984) Polyneuropathy in critically ill patients, *Journal of Neurology Neurosurgery Psychiatry, 47*(11): 1223–31.

Chan, K., Cheng, L.S.L., Mak, I.W.C., Ng, S., Yiu, M.G.C. and Chu, C. (2017) Delirium is a strong predictor of mortality in patients receiving Non-invasive Positive Pressure Ventilation, *Lung, 195*: 115–25.

Fan, E. (2012) Critical illness neuromyopathy and the role of physical therapy and rehabilitation in critically ill patients, *Respiratory Care, 57*(6): 933–44.

Gleason, L.J., Schmitt, E.M., Kosar, C.C.M., Tabloski, P., Saczynski, J.S., Robinson, T., Cooper, Z., Rogers, S.O., Jones, R., Marcantonio, E.R., and Inouye, S.K. (2015) Effects of delirium and other major complications on outcomes after elective surgery in older adults., *Journal of American Medical Association, 150*(12): 1134–40.

Griffiths, J., Fortune, G., Barber, V. and Young. J.D. (2007) The prevalence of post-traumatic stress disorder in survivors of ICU treatment: a systematic review, *Intensive Care Medicine, 33*(9): 1506–18.

Guarneri, B., Bertolini, G. and Latronico, N. (2008) Long-term outcome in patients with critical illness myopathy or neuropathy: the Italian multicentre CRIMYNE study, *Journal of Neurology Neurosurgery Psychiatry, 79*(7): 838–41.

Haggstrom, L., Welschinger, R. and Caplan, G.A. (2017) Functional neuroimaging offers insights into delirium pathophysiology: a systematic review, *Australian Journal of Aging, 36*(3): 186–92.

Harrington, C.J. and Vardi, K. (2014) Delirium: presentation, epidemiology and diagnosis evaluation, *Rhode Island Medical Journal, 97*: 18–23.

Hermans, G., De Jonghe, B., Bruyninckx, F. and Van den Berghe, G. (2014) *Interventions for Preventing Critical Illness Polyneuropathy and Critical Illness Myopathy (review).* Cochrane Library, Wiley.

Hickin, S.L., White, S. and Knopp-Sihota, J. (2017) Delirium in the intensive care unit – a nursing refresher, *Canadian Journal of Critical Care Nursing, 28*(2): 19–23.

Jones, C., Bäckman, C., Capuzzo, M., Hans Flaatten, E.I., Granja, C., Rylander, C. and Griffiths, R.D. (2010) Intensive care diaries reduce new onset post-traumatic stress disorder following critical illness: a randomised, controlled trial, *Critical Care, 14*: R168.

Jones, C., Capuzzo, M., Flaatten, H., Backman, C., Rylander, C. and Griffiths, R.D. (2008) ICU diaries may reduce symptoms of posttraumatic stress disorder, *Intensive Care Medicine, 32*: S144.

Jones, C., Skirrow, P., Griffiths, R.D., Humphris, G.H., Ingleby, S., Eddleston, J., Waldmann, C. and Gager, M. (2004) Post-traumatic stress disorder-related symptoms in relatives of patients following intensive care, *Intensive Care Medicine, 30*(3): 456–460.

Kapfhammer, H.P., Rothenhäusler, H.B., Haller, M., Briegel, J., Schmidt, M., Krauseneck, T., Durst, K. and Schelling, G. (1999) Sensitivity and specificity of a screening test to document traumatic experiences and to diagnose post-traumatic stress disorder in ARDS patients after intensive care treatment, *Intensive Care Medicine, 25*: 697– 704.

Langerud, A., Rustoen, T., Smastuen, M., Kongsgaard, U. and Stubhaug, A. (2017) Intensive care survivor-reported symptoms: a longitudinal study of survivors' symptoms, *Nursing in Critical Care, 23*(1): 48–54.

Latronico, N. and Bolton, C. (2011) Critical illness polyneuropathy and myopathy: a major cause of muscle weakness and paralysis, *Lancet Neurology, 10*(10): 931–41.

Lee, E. and Kim, J. (2014) Cost-benefit analysis of a delirium prevention strategy in the intensive care unit, *British Association of Critical Care Nurses*, *21*(6): 367–73.

Loftus, C.A. and Wiesenfeld, L.A. (2017) Geriatric delirium care: using chart audits to target improvement strategies, *Canadian Geriatric Journal*, *20*(4): 246–52.

Mazzola, P., Ward, L., Zazzetta, S., Broggini, V., Anzuini, A., Valcarcel, B., Brathwaite, J.S., Pasinetti, G M., Bellelli, G. and Annoni, G. (2017) Association between preoperative malnutrition and postoperative delirium after hip fracture surgery in older adults, *The American Geriatrics Society*, *65*: 1222–8.

Martin, G., Mannino, D., Eaton, S. and Moss, M. (2003) The epidemiology of sepsis in the United States from 1979 through 2000, *New England Journal of Medicine*, *348*(16): 1546–54.

National Institute for Health and Care Excellence (NICE) (2005) *Post-traumatic Stress Disorder: Management.* www.nice.org.uk/CG26

National Institute for Health and Care Excellence (NICE) (2010) *Delirium: Prevention, Diagnosis and Management. Clinical Guideline [CG103].* www.nice.org.uk/guidance/cg103

National Institute for Health and Care Excellence (NICE) (2014) *Transient Loss of Consciousness ('blackouts') in over 16s*, Clinical guideline [CG109]. www.nice.org.uk/guidance/CG109

National Institute for Health and Care Excellence (NICE) (2017) *Rehabilitation after Critical Illness in Adults. Quality Standard 158.* www.nice.org.uk/guidance/qs158 [accessed 26 April 2018].

Numan, T., van den Boogaard, M., Kamper, A.M., Rood, P.J.T., Peelen, L.M. and Slooter, A.J.C. (2017) Recognition of delirium in postoperative elderly patients: a multicentre study, *The American Geriatrics Society*, *65*: 1932–8.

Oh, E.S., Fong, T.G., Hshieh, T.T. and Inouye, S.K. (2017) Delirium in older persons: advances in diagnosis and treatment, *Journal of American Medical Association*, *318*(12): 1161–74.

Pandharipande, P.P. (2017) Humanizing the treatment of hyperactive delirium in the last days of life, *Journal of American Medical Association*, *318*(11): 1014–15.

Pandharipande, P.P., Girard, T.D., Jackson, J.C., Morandi, A., Thompson, J.L., Pun, B.T., Brummel, N.E., Hughes, C.G., Vasilevskis, E.E. and Shintani, A.K. (2013) BRAIN – ICU study investigators. Long-term cognitive impairments after critical illness, *New England Journal of Medicine*, *369*: 1306–16.

Richardson, S.J., Davis, D.H.J., Stephan, B., Robinson, L., Brayne, C., Barnes, L., Parker, S. and Allan, L.M. (2017) Protocol for the Delirium and Cognitive Impact in Dementia (DECIDE) study: a nested prospective longitudinal cohort study, *BMC Geriatrics*, *17*(98): 1–7.

Selim, A.A. and Ely, W.E (2017) Delirium the under-recognised syndrome: survey of healthcare professionals' awareness and practice in the intensive care units. *Journal of Clinical Nursing*, *26*(5-6): 813–24.

Shepherd, S., Batra, A. and Lerner, D. (2017) Review of critical illness myopathy and neuropathy, *The Neurohospitalist*, *7*(1): 41–8.

Siddiqi, N., Harrison, J.K., Clegg, A., Teale, E.A., Young, J., Taylor, J. and Simpkins, S.A. (2016) Interventions to prevent delirium in hospitalised patients, not including those on intensive care units, *Cochrane Database of Systematic Reviews*, Issue 3. Art. No.: CD005563. DOI: 10.1002/14651858.CD005563.pub3.

Siew, E.D., Fissell, W., Tripp, C.M., Blume, J.D., Wilson, M.D., Clark, A.J., Vicz, A.J., Ely, E.W., Pandharipande, P.P. and Girard, T.D. (2016) Acute kidney injury as a risk factor for delirium and coma during critical illness, *American Journal of Respiratory Critical Care Medicine, 195*(12): 1597–607.

Svenningsen, H., Egerod, I., Christensen, D., Tonnesen, E.K., Frydenberg, M. and Videbech, P. (2015) Symptoms of posttraumatic stress after intensive care delirium, *Biomedical Research International*, ID *876947*, 9.

Trogrlic, Z., van der Jagt, M., Bakker, J., Balas, M.C., Ely, E.W., van der Voot, P.H.J. and Ista, E. (2015) A systematic review of implementation strategies for assessment, prevention and management of ICU delirium and their effect on clinical outcomes, *Critical Care 19*(157): 1–17.

van Eijk., M.M., van den Boogaard, M., van Marum, R.J., Benner, P., Eikelenboom, P., Honing, M.L., van der Hoven, B., Horn, J., Izaks, G. J., Kalf, A. and Karakus, A. (2011) Routine use of the confusion assessment method for the intensive care unit, *American Journal of Respiratory and Critical Care Medicine, 184*: 3.

Visser, L. (2006) Critical illness polyneuropathy and myopathy clinical features, risk factors and prognosis, *European Journal of Neurology, 13*(11): 1203–12.

Voyer, P., Emond, M., Boucherm, V., Carmichaels, P., Juneau, L., Richard, H., Vu, T. and Bouchard, G. (2017) RADAR: a rapid detection tool for signs of delirium (6th vital sign) in emergency departments, *Canadian Journal of Emergency Nursing, 40*(2): 37–43.

Whitehorne, K., Gaudine, A., Meadus, R. and Solberg, S. (2015) Lived experience of the intensive care unit for patients who experienced delirium, *American Journal of Critical Care, 24*(6): 474–9.

Williams, L. (2017) Delirium assessment in critically ill children, *AACN Advanced Critical Care, 28*(1): 23–26.

Wolters, A.E., Peelen, L.M., Veldhuijzen, D.S., Zaal, I.J., de Lange, D.W., Passma, W., van Dijk, D., Cremer, O.L. and Slooter, A.J. (2017) Long-term self-reported cognitive problems after delirium in the intensive care unit and the effects of systemic inflammation, *The American Geriatrics Society, 65*: 786–91.

Zambon, M. and Vincent, J. (2008) Mortality rates for patients with acute lung injury/ARDS have decreased over time, *Chest, 133*(5): 1120–7.

Zenilman, M.E. (2017) Delirium. An important post-operative complication, *Journal of American Medical Association, 317*(1): 77–8.

Conclusion: The Way Forward

SARA J. WHITE AND DESIREE TAIT

In this book, we have used real-life case histories to explore how senior staff can facilitate and enable peers to ensure they offer a personalised humanised approach to the care they offer to patients, their family and members of the healthcare team. As experienced healthcare practitioners we appreciate the complexity of the critical care world; the changing demands on healthcare practitioners; the complex health and co-morbidity needs of patients in critical care; the extensive knowledge needed to be able to care for these individuals. Indeed, we fully understand that to do this effectively needs constant knowledge development and enhancement.

Undeniably, the role of the senior nurse is also multifaceted and complex and only a small part of this is to enable their staff in their knowledge development and enhancement of these skills. Consequently, to help this we have given bite size knowledge segments, reflection points and exercises, as well as further reading to help in this quest. To set the scene the first two chapters explored the philosophical, theoretical and evidence base factors that inform critical care nursing and clinical decision making. We also explored the bio-psychosocial factors that influence critical illness and the concept of lifeworld and the humanising framework, used throughout the book. The following nine chapters took a variety of patient stories and explored them from a variety of perspectives to enable the reader to see the humanising framework in action and make it real. Consequently, we have looked at critical illness from the perspective of a young previously fit person, a middle-aged woman with co-morbidity and a middle-aged man who is a non-British national. We have considered the viewpoint from the perspective of the patient and their family as the patient faces their critical illness, its outcome, and feelings of isolation, anxiety, fear and periods of low mood during and after discharge from ICU. We have also looked at matters relating to culture, cultural reasoning, autonomy and advocacy, legal and ethical issues, emotional labour, moral distress, and feelings of powerlessness and oppression.

Throughout the book, we have also reflected on issues from the standpoint of staff in the ICU and CCU, members of CCOT and specialist nurses and matters related to capability, competency and leadership. Whilst there are many barriers to effective patient-centred care (see Jakimowicz et al., 2017, who note staff stress, ethical dilemmas, frustration, communication issues, relationships with other staff and relatives, and ICU ideology related to cost and 'false' hope'), it is important for senior nurses to understand the hurdles from an individual perspective. Throughout the book we have considered possible ways to move forward and some useful tools and resources that senior nurses may draw upon to help encourage and facilitate staff development using the humanising framework. We suggest that the first starting point is to explore the human dimensions of care as identified by Todres et al. (2009) and how these may be being compromised by staff, thus leading to dehumanised care. As a reminder, the dimensions of humanised care as applied to ICU are:

Insiderness: Care that takes account of the feelings of the patient and family and how they may be feeling uncertain or scared.

Agency: Care that enables the patient and family to have a say and make choices about their care and have a sense of control and ability to make knowledgeable decisions about their care and treatments.

Uniqueness: Care that treats every patient and family as an individual who has their own likes and preferences and priorities.

Togetherness: Care that enables the patient and family to feel a sense of belonging and community.

Sense Making: Care that helps the patient and family understand what is happening to them and the associated treatments and recovery.

Personal Journey: Care that helps the patient and family find continuity whilst connecting their past with the now and future.

Sense of Place: Care that helps the patient and family feel familiar with the environment and culture of the hospital to enable a sense of ease.

Embodiment: Care that recognises and helps the patient and family to understand their body, mind, mood and makes connections with the world.

We recognise that these constructs merge and are ultimately complex entities, but throughout the book we have kept them separate as it enabled analysis of the humanising framework. Indeed the *Humanising Care Toolkit: Sharing Experiences and Learning* (Pound et al., 2016) funded by the Burdett Trust for Nursing, is an excellent resource to use when exploring Todres et al.'s (2009) framework.

During our time as senior nurses, we have been thrilled to see how many organisations integrate the concepts of respect, choice, empowerment, patient-centred health care, patient access to support and organisational information as well as patient involvement in health policy and changes. Nonetheless as organisations evolve and embrace humanised care we should not be complacent, and consequently we suggest that clinical leaders explore enablers that do not compromise on quality and standards. As well as the humanising framework other enablers senior nurses might like to draw upon, some of which are mentioned in this book, are:

- Conditions necessary for nurses' clinical decision making (Chapters 1 and 6).
- Thompson's PCS model (Thompson (2006) – Chapter 2).
- *The Communication Quiz* (Mindtools – Chapter 3).
- Management theories (Bite Size Knowledge 5.5: Motivational theories, management theories and leadership styles – Chapter 5).
- GROW model (Whitmore (2009) – Chapter 9).
- RADER (Rapid detection tools for signs of delirium) (Voyer et al. (2017) – Chapter 11).
- Developing caring conversations (Dewar et al., 2010; Dewar and MacBride, 2017).
- Developing the 7 Cs needed for caring conversations (Roddy and Dewar, 2016).
- Exploring the enablers to enhance compassion awareness and training in the NHS (Curtis et al., 2017).
- Developing person-centred care in nursing (McCormack and McCance, 2016).
- Enhancing active listening and active responding techniques for educators (Rogers and Farson, 2015; Topornycky and Golparian, 2016).
- Developing communication skills to enable reflection, self-recognition and self-disclosure (Bulus et al., 2017).
- Developing intuition as a way of knowing (Holm and Severinsson, 2016).
- Improving Humanisation in Intensive Care Units (Heras La Calle et al., 2017).

We wish you well with exploring, questioning and applying these concepts and theories to both critical care and other area of healthcare practice.

REFERENCES

Bulus, M., Atan, A. and Sarikaya, H.E. (2017) Effective communication skills: a new conceptual framework and scale development study, *International Online Journal of Educational Sciences*, *9*(2): 575–90.

Curtis, K., Gallagher, A., Ramage, C., Montgomery, J., Martin, C., Leng, J., Theodosius, C., Glynn, A., Anderson, J. and Wrigley, M. (2017) Using appreciative inquiry to develop, implement and evaluate a multi-organisation 'Cultivating Compassion' programme for health professionals and support staff, *Journal of Research in Nursing*, *22*(1–2): 150–65.

Dewar, B. and MacBride, T. (2017) Developing caring conversation in care homes: an appreciative inquiry, *Health and Social Care in the Community*, *25*(4): 1375–86.

Dewar, B., Mackay, R., Smith, S., Pullin, S. and Tocher, R. (2010) Use of emotional touchpoints as a method of tapping into the experiences of receiving compassionate care in a hospital setting, *Journal of Research in Nursing*, *15*(1): 29–41.

Heras La Calle, G., Alonso Ovies, A. and Gomez Tello, V. (2017) A plan for improving the humanisation of intensive care units, *Intensive Care Medicine*, *43*: 547–9.

Holm, A.L and Severinsson, E. (2016) A systematic review of intuition – a way of knowing in clinical nursing, *Open Journal of Nursing*, *6*: 412–25.

Jakimowicz, S., Perry, L. and Lewis, J. (2017) An integrative review of supports, facilitators and barriers to patient-centred nursing in the intensive care unit, *Journal of Clinical Nursing*, 26: 4153–71.

McCormack, B. and McCance, T. (eds) (2016) *Person-centred Practice in Nursing and Healthcare*. Chichester: Wiley-Blackwell.

Mindtools: *The Communication Quiz*. Available at: www.mindtools.com/pages/article/newCS_99.htm

Pound, C., Sloan, C., Ellis-Hill, C., Cowdell, F., Todres, L. and Galvin, K. (2016) *The Humanising Care Toolkit: Sharing Experiences and Learning*. Available at: www.btfn.org.uk/library/directory_listings/337/Humanising%20Care%20Toolkit.pdf

Roddy, E. and Dewar, B. (2016) A reflective account on becoming reflexive: the 7Cs of caring conversations as a framework for reflexive questioning, *International Practice Development Journal*, 6(1): 1–8.

Rogers, C. and Farson, R. (2015) *Active Listening*. Eastwood, CT: Martino Publishing.

Thompson, N. (2006) *Anti-Discriminatory Practice*. London: Palgrave Macmillan.

Todres, L., Galvin, K. and Holloway, I. (2009) The humanisation of healthcare: a value framework for qualitative research, *International Journal of Qualitative Studies on Health and Wellbeing*, 4(2): 68–77.

Topornycky, J. and Golparian, S. (2016) Balancing openness and interpretation in active listening, *Collected Essays on Learning and Teaching*, IXL: 175–85.

Voyer, P., Emond, M., Boucherm, V., Carmichaels, P., Juneau, L., Richard, H., Vu, T and Bouchard, G. (2017) RADAR: a rapid detection tool for signs of delirium (6th vital sign) in emergency departments, *Canadian Journal of Emergency Nursing*, 40(2): 37–43.

Whitmore, J. (2009) *Coaching for Performance: GROWing Human Potential and Purpose – The Principles and Practice of Coaching and Leadership* (4th edn). London: Nicholas Brealey.

Index

Page numbers in *italics* refer to information in boxes, figures and tables.

Printed in October 2021
by Rotomail Italia S.p.A., Vignate (MI) - Italy